Critical Care Nursing Certification

Second Edition

Joseph T. Catalano, RN, PhD, CCRN

Springhouse Corporation
Springhouse, Pennsylvania

Staff

Senior Publisher
Matthew Cahill

Clinical Director
Judith A. Schilling McCann, RN, MSN

Editorial Director
Donna O. Carpenter

Art Director
John Hubbard

Managing Editor
David Moreau

Acquisitions Editors
Patricia Kardish Fischer, RN, BSN;
Louise Quinn

Senior Editor
Karen Diamond

Clinical Consultants
Collette Bishop Hendler, RN, CCRN; Lori
Musolf Neri, RN, MSN

Copy Editors
Cynthia C. Breuninger (manager),
Karen Comerford, Barbara Hodgson,
Brenna Mayer

Designers
Arlene Putterman (associate art
director), Cindy Marczuk

Production Coordinator
Stephen Hungerford, Jr.

Editorial Assistants
Beverly Lane, Mary Madden

Manufacturing
Deborah Meiris (director), Pat
Dorshaw (manager), Otto Mezei

Printed in the United States of America.

A member of the Reed Elsevier plc group

CCRN2-010298

Library of Congress Cataloging-in-Publication Data

Contents

Contributors

EXECUTIVE CLINICAL EDITOR

Joseph T. Catalano, RN, PhD, CCRN
Professor of Nursing
East Central University
Ada, Okla.

CONTRIBUTORS

Janice H. Bruce, RN, MSN, ACLS, CCRN
Staff Nurse, Clinical Instructor
Valley View Regional Hospital
East Central University
Ada, Okla.

Linda J. Duval, RN, BSN, CCRN
Quality Assurance Assistant for Medical Case Review
ESRD Network 13
Oklahoma City, Okla.

Terry Ferguson-Dries, RN, BSN
Staff Nurse
Department of Veterans' Affairs Medical Center
Oklahoma City, Okla.

Trudi L. Freeland, RN,C, MS, CNS, CCRN
Instructor of Nursing
East Central University
Ada, Okla.

Cynthia Linzy Gaston, RN,CS, MS, CNS, CCRN
Critical Care Clinical Nurse Specialist
Muskogee (Okla.) Regional Medical Center

A. Renee Leasure, RN, PhD, CCRN
Assistant Professor
College of Nursing
University of Oklahoma
Oklahoma City

Teresa E. Newsom, RN, MSN, CCRN
Head Nurse, Cardiovascular Intensive Care Unit
Department of Veterans' Affairs Medical Center
Oklahoma City, Okla.

Susan M. Park, RN, MEd, CCRN
Critical Care Instructor
Department of Veterans' Affairs Medical Center
Oklahoma City, Okla.

Toni Pratt-Reid, RN, BSN
Assistant Head Nurse, Education Coordinator
Critical Care Unit
Deaconess Hospital
Oklahoma City, Okla.

BOOK DEVELOPMENT

F. William Balkie, RN, CRNA, MBA
President
American Nursing Review

Jenkin V. Williams
Executive Vice President
American Nursing Review

Preface

Rapid and continual advances in technology make critical care nursing one of the most demanding areas of practice for professional nurses. To keep pace with the changes that occur constantly in this area of health care, critical care nurses must continually update their knowledge and skills. Passing the critical care certification examination is one method by which you can demonstrate that you have put forth time and effort in gaining this advanced knowledge.

American Nursing Review for Critical Care Nursing Certification, Second Edition, has been written to help the experienced critical care nurse pass the Critical Care Certification Examination for Registered Nurses (CCRN examination). The general framework of the book is based on the outline of the CCRN examination as published by the American Association of Critical Care Nurses (AACN), the organization that administers the CCRN examination. Within individual chapters, specific content areas are based on material found in the Core Curriculum, also published by the AACN.

Chapter 1 serves as an introduction to the CCRN examination, providing eligibility requirements, application information, valuable insight on the certification test plan, helpful study tips, and proven test-taking strategies. The text acquaints you with the types of questions most likely to appear on the examination and suggests effective ways to minimize anxiety and improve your test performance.

Chapters 2 through 9 are organized by body system for convenient study. Each chapter begins with a review of anatomy and physiology and then outlines the major disorders of the body system under discussion, including pertinent signs and symptoms, key laboratory values, diagnostic tests, and medical and nursing management (with rationales).

Chapter 2 reviews cardiovascular problems, including arrhythmias; acute myocardial infarction; heart failure; peripheral vascular insufficiency; angina; atrioventricular blocks; aortic aneurysm, dissection, regurgitation, and stenosis; cardiac trauma; cardiogenic and hypovolemic shock; cardiomyopathies; endocarditis; mitral stenosis and insufficiency; myocarditis; pericarditis; and pulmonary edema.

Chapter 3 presents pulmonary disorders, such as acute pulmonary embolism, acute respiratory failure, respiratory tract infection, adult respiratory distress syndrome, flail chest, hemothorax, pneumothorax, pulmonary contusion, rib fracture, and status asthmaticus.

Chapter 4 looks at endocrine disorders, including acute hypoglycemia, diabetes insipidus, hyperosmolar hyperglycemic nonketotic syndrome, diabetic ketoacidosis, and syndrome of inappropriate secretion of antidiuretic hormone.

Chapter 5 describes hematologic and immunologic disorders, such as acquired immunodeficiency syndrome, disseminated intravascular coagulation, and organ transplantation.

Chapter 6 examines neurologic problems, including spinal cord injury, cerebral aneurysm and embolism, encephalitis, meningitis, brain abscess, Reye's syndrome, Guillain-Barré syndrome, myasthenia gravis, and seizures.

Chapter 7 investigates disorders associated with the GI system, such as acute abdominal trauma, GI hemorrhage, acute pancreatitis, bowel infarction, obstruction, and perforation, liver failure, and hepatic coma.

Chapter 8 explores problems of the renal system, including acute renal failure, electrolyte imbalances, kidney transplantation, continuous arteriovenous hemofiltration, hemodialysis, and peritoneal dialysis.

Chapter 9 focuses on disorders that affect multiple body systems, such as asphyxia, burns, septic shock, and toxic ingestions.

Numerous charts, tables, and illustrations appear throughout the text to clarify important concepts or highlight key data. Appendix A lists the drugs most commonly used in critical care nursing and summarizes their actions, indications, and nursing implications. Appendix B provides a brief practice test to determine your skill in analyzing arterial blood gas values and identifying their clinical significance.

Two posttests offer further opportunity for study and evaluation before you take the actual examination. Each test contains 50 questions (similar in style and content to the actual test), followed by the correct answers and rationales, and a self-diagnostic profile to guide evaluation of your progress.

A list of selected references offers suggestions for further reading, and a useful index helps locate important topics quickly.

American Nursing Review for Critical Care Nursing Certification contains all the information you need to pass the CCRN examination and can serve as a valuable reference afterward. Good luck on the examination and throughout your nursing career.

Joseph T. Catalano, RN, PhD, CCRN
Professor of Nursing
East Central University
Ada, Okla.

1

Certification examination

Certification is a type of credentialing that has professional but usually not legal status. It is a method of documenting that a health care professional has achieved an advanced level of knowledge and excellence in a particular practice area.

The American Association of Critical Care Nurses (AACN) Certification Corporation administers the certification examination for adult critical care nursing. Through the certification examination, the AACN evaluates and recognizes nurses who have attained specialized knowledge and skills in the care of critically ill patients. One of the primary functions of the AACN credentialing process is to define the knowledge and skills required for the practice of critical care nursing.

A health care professional who takes a certification examination for a specialty area of practice already has the knowledge required by the basic licensure examination. Because the knowledge measured by a certification examination is specialized for the area being tested, the examination is more difficult than NCLEX.

As a critical care nurse, you have mastered complex technical skills related to the care of critically ill patients as well as the theoretical knowledge that underlies these skills. You have developed the ability to make sound nursing judgments in crisis situations that often determine whether a patient lives or dies. Despite this advanced education, skill mastery, and decision-making ability, many critical care nurses experience high levels of test-taking anxiety that may prevent them from seeking certification as a critical care registered nurse (CCRN). The purpose of this book is to alleviate test-taking anxiety by providing a thorough review of the subject matter contained in the CCRN certification examination.

Eligibility and application

The AACN establishes criteria for eligibility to take the CCRN certification examination (see *Certification eligibility requirements for CCRN candidacy*, pages 2 and 3). Because requirements can change, you should obtain the latest criteria before applying for certification. To obtain this information, you can contact the AACN by mail (101 Columbia, Aliso Viejo, CA 92656-1491) or by phone (1-800-899-AACN, 714-362-2000, or 714-362-2020 [facsimile]).

Once you have decided to take the examination, you should request a CCRN examination application from the AACN; use the same address and phone numbers as above.

To apply for the CCRN examination, you must complete the examination application form, the verification of critical care practice form (signed by a registered nurse supervisor), the validation of RN licensure form, and a validation of critical care practice form. All these forms are included in the application book-

Certification eligibility requirements for CCRN candidacy

The eligibility criteria established by the American Association of Critical Care Nurses (AACN) for certification in adult critical care nursing, in effect as of 1992, are listed below. The eligibility requirements consist of two components, with the second one being subdivided, as shown below.
1. Current RN licensure in the United States or any of its territories that use the NCLEX examination as the basis for determining RN licensure
2. Clinical Practice Requirement composed of two parts: hours and experiences

Hours
—One (1) year of experience in critical care nursing practice as a registered nurse.
—One year is defined as **1,750 hours** within the 2 years preceding application, with 875 of those hours accrued in the most recent year preceding application.

Experiences
Provide bedside care to critically ill adults whose condition required any or all of the following interventions. Applicants must have performed, at least once, 17 (65%) of the interventions listed below in order to meet the experience requirement.
Hemodynamic instability that required:
1) arterial pressure monitoring
2) central venous pressure monitoring
3) pulmonary artery pressure monitoring
4) invasive cardiac output or cardiac index determination
5) direct right atrial, left atrial, or pulmonary artery pressure monitoring
6) administration of I.V. vasoactive agents
Life-threatening conditions that required:
1) emergency drug administration (for example, epinephrine or atropine)
Compromised air exchange that required:
1) continuous respiratory monitors
2) an endotracheal tube
3) a newly inserted tracheostomy tube
4) nasal or facial continuous positive airway pressure
5) conventional mechanical ventilation
Cardiac dysfunction that required:
1) continuous ECG monitoring
2) a temporary pacemaker
3) elective cardioversion
4) 12-lead ECG interpretation
5) a transcutaneous (external) pacemaker
6) a newly inserted permanent pacemaker
7) administration of I.V. antiarrhythmic agents
8) administration of I.V. thrombolytic agents
9) defibrillation
10) administration of I.V. phosphodiesterase inhibitors (for example, amrinone)
11) mediastinal chest tube(s)

Certification eligibility requirements for CCRN candidacy *(continued)*

Physiologic alterations that required:
1) administration of I.V. paralytic agents
2) continuous I.V. insulin infusion
3) administration of I.V. push anticonvulsant agents

• Clinical practice hours accrued in a student role are not acceptable.
• Clinical practice hours and experiences obtained while supervising student nurses at the bedside are acceptable as long as verification is provided by the unit clinical supervisor.
• Additional eligibility requirements may be adopted by the AACN Certification Corporation in its sole discretion from time to time. Any such requirements will be designed to establish, for the purposes of critical care registered nurse certification, the adequacy of a candidate's knowledge and experience in caring for the critically ill.

let sent by the AACN. The clinical practice experience required for CCRN certification must be obtained in an intensive care unit, a cardiac care unit, a postanesthesia care unit, an emergency department, or a telemetry unit. If your experience was not obtained in one of these areas, additional documentation of clinical practice is required.

Pay careful attention to all steps in the application process, particularly the deadlines. The AACN adheres strictly to its initial and final postmark deadlines for application. Fees for the computer-based test (CBT) change periodically and range from $220 (for an AACN member who files by the initial deadline) to $295 (for a nonmember who files after the initial deadline but before the final deadline).

The examination is administered at approximately 80 Sylvan Learning Centers across the country. Once you have selected a test site on the application form, it cannot be changed later. Special arrangements can be made for handicapped candidates if documentation of the disability is sent along with the application form.

Certification test plan

The CCRN examination contains 200 multiple-choice questions, some of which are preceded by a brief clinical situation. Each question carries equal weight toward the final score, and every question must be answered. Candidates have 4 hours to complete the test.

The AACN develops the certification examination based on the task statements identified in its Role Delineation/CCRN Validation study. This study determines the skills and knowledge most commonly used by critical care nurses; the examination tests the critical care nurse's grasp of these skills and concepts. The three components of the CCRN examination test plan are categories of content; levels of cognitive ability; and professional tasks.

Categories of content

The categories of content component is organized around the major body systems affected when a patient is critically ill. About 39% of the test questions on the CCRN examination pertain to the cardiovascular system. The other areas covered in the examination are the pulmonary system (22% of questions), neurologic system (8%), renal system (5%), GI system (8%), endocrine system (4%), hematologic and immunologic system (4%), and multisystemic disorders (10%).

Levels of cognitive ability

The levels of cognitive ability component measures how knowledge has been learned and how it is used by the nurse. For the CCRN examination, knowledge is tested at three levels.

Level 1 consists of knowledge and comprehension questions; they compose 36% of the test. These questions involve memory of specific facts and the ability to apply those facts to specific pathophysiologic conditions. Level 1 questions test your knowledge of anatomy and physiology, medication doses and adverse effects, signs and symptoms of diseases, laboratory test results, and the components of certain treatments and interventions.

Here is an example of a Level 1 question:

William Carlton is admitted to the intensive care unit (ICU) with acute respiratory failure. Which of the following is the normal range for the PO_2 value?

A. 10 to 30 mm Hg

B. 35 to 55 mm Hg

C. 10 to 20 cm H_2O

D. 70 to 100 mm Hg

The correct answer is D. As you can see, this question is designed to test your memory of a specific fact.

Level 2 questions ask you to analyze and apply information to specific patient-care situations; they make up 39% of the test. *Analysis* involves the ability to separate information into its basic parts and decide which of those parts is important. *Application* involves the ability to use that information in patient-care decisions. These questions are more difficult to answer because they require you to apply information you have learned. Level 2 questions may assess your ability to interpret electrocardiogram (ECG) strips and arterial blood gas (ABG) values, make a nursing diagnosis based on a set of symptoms, or decide on a course of treatment.

An example of a Level 2 question follows:

William Carlton is becoming progressively short of breath. The results of his ABG studies include a pH of 7.13, PO_2 of 48 mm Hg, PCO_2 of 53 mm Hg, and HCO_3^- of 26 mEq/L. Which problem do these values indicate?

A. Uncompensated metabolic acidosis with moderate hypoxia

B. Respiratory alkalosis with hyperoxia

C. Uncompensated respiratory acidosis with severe hypoxia

D. Compensated respiratory acidosis with normal oxygen

The correct answer is C. Not only must you know the normal values for each of the ABG values given, but you also must use that information to determine the underlying condition.

Level 3 questions, which constitute 25% of the test, involve synthesis and evaluation. Questions at this level ask you to make judgments about patient care. Some questions may be followed by more than one appropriate option, but you must choose the *best* option from those listed. Questions at this level ask about the priority of care to be given, the priority of the formulated nursing diagnosis, how to evaluate the effectiveness of care, and the most appropriate nursing action to take.

An example of a Level 3 question follows:

William Carlton has become cyanotic and is experiencing Cheyne-Stokes respirations. What is the *best* action for the nurse to take at this time?

A. Call a code blue and begin CPR.

B. Call Mr. Carlton's doctor and report the condition.

C. Ensure that Mr. Carlton's airway is open and begin supplemental oxygen.

D. Immediately administer the ordered dose of 200 mg I.V. aminophylline by way of push bolus.

The best answer is C. Although answers B and D also are appropriate, opening the airway and oxygenating the patient have the highest priority in this situation. Not only does this type of question require you to know specific facts (definitions of cyanosis and Cheyne-Stokes respirations), but it also requires that you make a decision about the seriousness of the condition (analysis) and select the type of care to be given from several appropriate options (judgment).

Professional tasks

The professional tasks component encompasses the four steps of the nursing process—assessment, planning, intervention and implementation, and evaluation. All questions on the CCRN examination relate to one of these nursing process steps. Most of the questions pertain to assessment (32% of questions) or intervention and implementation (40% of questions). Planning questions comprise 15% of the test, and evaluation questions make up the remaining 13%.

The assessment step establishes the database on which the rest of the nursing process is built. Components of the assessment phase include subjective and objective data about the patient, significant medical history, history of the current illness, signs and symptoms, environmental elements, laboratory test results, and vital signs. The questions frequently ask you to distinguish between appropriate and inappropriate assessment factors.

An example of an assessment-phase question follows:

William Carlton's respiratory status continues to worsen. Which of the following signs and symptoms would best indicate deterioration of his respiratory status?

A. Increased restlessness and changes in level of consciousness

B. Bradycardia and increased blood pressure

C. Complaints of chest pain and shortness of breath

D. Rapidly dropping PCO_2 and pH values

The correct answer is A. The brain is one of the first organs to be affected by decreased oxygenation. Restlessness and changes in level of consciousness reflect this decrease. Choices B, C, and D are signs and symptoms of other conditions.

The planning step of the nursing process involves setting goals for the patient. The planning-phase questions include determination of expected outcomes, development of appropriate nursing diagnoses, prioritization of goals and nursing diagnoses, and anticipation of patient needs based on the nursing assessment.

Here is an example of a planning-phase question:

William Carlton is diagnosed with acute respiratory failure and connected to a positive pressure, volume-cycled ventilator with positive end-expiratory pressure (PEEP) set at 10 cm H_2O. Which of the following nursing diagnoses would have the highest priority for this patient?

A. Impaired skin integrity related to immobility

B. Decreased cardiac output related to changes in intrathoracic pressure

C. Ineffective individual coping related to anxiety

D. Impaired gas exchange related to decreased lung compliance

The correct answer is B. A patient placed on a ventilator with PEEP typically experiences a dramatic decrease in cardiac output because of the alterations in normal chest pressure produced by the ventilator. When asked to select the goal or nursing diagnosis with the highest priority, you should remember Maslow's hierarchy of needs—the patient's physiologic and safety needs must be met before higher needs, such as love and belonging, can be fulfilled.

The intervention, or implementation, step of the nursing process involves identifying the nursing actions required to meet the goals stated in the planning phase. The intervention phase includes providing nursing care based on the defined goals, preventing injury or spread of disease, administering medications, giving treatments, carrying out procedures, monitoring changes in the patient's condition, documentation (charting and record-keeping), and teaching the patient and family about health care.

An example of an intervention-phase question follows:

William Carlton has been on the ventilator for 3 days. He suddenly becomes extremely restless, and the pressure alarm sounds with each ventilator-initiated inspiration. Which of the following would be an appropriate initial nursing action?

A. Disconnect the ventilator and call a code.

B. Disconnect the ventilator and manually oxygenate the patient for a few minutes with a handheld ventilator.

C. Increase the ventilator pressure limit to 50 mm Hg.

D. Remove the endotracheal tube and reintubate the patient with a tube one size larger.

The correct answer is B. When the pressure alarm sounds, it typically indicates an increase in airway resistance from some cause. Evaluating the amount of airway resistance with a manual ventilator may help determine the source of the problem. Other appropriate nursing actions include suctioning the patient's airway, administering sedatives, assessing ventilator function, and using calming measures to reduce the patient's anxiety. Choices A, C, and D are not appropriate in this situation.

The evaluation phase of the nursing process determines whether the goals stated in the planning phase were met by the nurse's interventions. The evaluation phase also ties the nursing process together. If the goals were met, the patient no longer has a problem. If the goals were not met, you must determine where the difficulty lies. Were the assessment data inadequate? Were the goals defective, or was there a deficiency in the implementation? Questions pertaining to the evaluation phase include comparison of actual outcomes with expected outcomes, verification of assessment data, evaluation of nursing actions and patient responses, and evaluation of the patient's level of knowledge and understanding.

Here's an example of an evaluation-phase question:

William Carlton has been extubated and transferred to the step-down unit and is now being prepared for discharge. He needs to take oral theophylline at home for his lung disease. Which response indicates that William has understood the nurse's instructions about how to take theophylline?

A. "I can stop taking this medication when I feel better."

B. "If I have difficulty swallowing the timed-release capsules, I can crush or chew them."

C. "If I become very sleepy when I take this medication, I need to cut back on the dosage."

D. "I need to avoid drinking coffee and soft drinks while I'm taking this medication."

The correct answer is D. The patient must be taught to avoid excessive amounts of caffeine because it increases the adverse effects of theophylline. Choices A and C are incorrect because patients should never suddenly stop taking the medication. Choice B is incorrect because timed-release capsules should never be crushed or chewed; also, theophylline should be taken with a glass of water and a small amount of food. The patient also must understand that theophylline may interact with certain over-the-counter medications.

Computerized CCRN examination

In 1997, the AACN began offering the CCRN examination in a computer format. As of 1998, the examination is offered only on computer.

Candidates with little or no computer experience will be relieved to discover that the test does not require extensive computer skills. After the candidate types in his or her name, address, and identification number, the only two keys used are the space bar (to move among the four options) and the enter key (to select and confirm an option). All other keys are locked out.

In the CCRN examination, no question is ever repeated, and the candidate cannot change an answer once it has been selected.

The examination is graded on a pass-fail basis. A candidate who fails the examination must retake the entire examination. There is no waiting period for retaking the examination. Test results usually are returned within 2 weeks after completion of the examination.

Study strategies

You can prepare for the certification examination in a number of ways. You may want to use some or all of the following study strategies, depending on your knowledge level, years of experience, and individual study requirements. Carefully directed study and preparation will significantly increase your chances of passing the examination.

You have already begun to prepare for certification by purchasing this review book, which covers the key material on the CCRN examination and closely follows the CCRN test plan. But a review book is just that—it reviews the material you should already know. Reviewing is an important step in reinforcing learning and recalling old or unused information. However, review books are not designed to present new information. If you are completely unfamiliar with the material in a particular section of this book, you should read a more complete textbook on the subject.

A review book also can point out your weak areas. As you go through this book, if you find sections that seem to contain new material, you should review that subject in more detail.

Group study can be an effective method of preparing for the certification examination. To optimize the results of group study sessions, several rules should be followed:

• Be selective about the members of the study group. They all should have a similar attitude toward preparing for the CCRN examination. An ideal study group consists of four to six persons; groups larger than six become difficult to work with. After the group has been formed and has begun its study sessions, it may be necessary to ask an individual to leave the group if he or she does not prepare assigned material, disrupts the study process, or displays a negative attitude toward the examination.

• Have each person prepare a particular section of the study topic before the group meets, which may be as often as once or twice a week. For example, if the next study topic is the endocrine system, assign one group member to discuss the anatomy and physiology of the system, another to review the pathologic conditions of the endocrine system, a third to cover the medications used for treatments, and a fourth to review the key elements of nursing care. Each person then presents the section worked on at the next group study session. This type of preparation prevents the "What are we going to study tonight?" syndrome that plagues many group study sessions.

• Limit the duration of each study session to 2 hours. Sessions that run longer tend to wander off the topic and foster a negative attitude toward the examination.

• Avoid turning group study sessions into a party. A few snacks and refreshments may be helpful in maintaining the energy level of the group; however, a party atmosphere will detract significantly from the effectiveness of the study session.

No matter which other study strategies you use, individual preparation for the CCRN examination is a must. This preparation can take several forms.

As mentioned earlier, this review book can help you pinpoint areas in which your knowledge needs improvement. You can then concentrate on reviewing material in those areas.

Reading and studying critical care nursing textbooks and study guides also can be helpful. As you read the material, mentally organize the information into a format similar to that of the CCRN examination. After reading a page, ask yourself three or four multiple-choice questions about that information. These questions can be asked mentally or actually written out. Ask yourself, "How might the certification examination test my knowledge of this material?"

An extremely effective method of individual study is to answer practice questions similar to those on the test. You may increase your score by as much as 10% using this study strategy. By answering practice questions, you become more familiar and comfortable with the format of the examination. Answering practice questions also reinforces the information you have studied.

Answering practice questions also can quickly identify areas that require further study. It is easy to tell yourself "I know the renal system pretty well" but much more difficult to answer 10 to 15 questions about that system correctly. If you answer most practice questions on a particular subject correctly, you can move on to the next topic. If you answer several questions incorrectly, you'll need to review that subject in more detail.

Using practice questions as a study method helps you organize your thoughts into the question-and-answer format found in the CCRN examination. After working with multiple-choice questions long enough, you will begin to think of everything you read in that format. You can find practice questions in various sources. This review book, for example, contains two 50-question practice tests (see pages 260 to 305).

To obtain the optimal benefit from practice questions, spend 30 to 45 minutes each day answering 10 to 20 questions rather than trying to answer 100 questions on your day off. After you answer the questions, compare your answers with the correct answers; also review the rationales provided for correct and incorrect answers. If you have answered some questions incorrectly and are not sure why, return to the textbook or review book to find the rationale.

Although the AACN does not directly endorse or sponsor any review courses for the CCRN examination, local chapters of the AACN frequently conduct reviews 1 month or so before the examination date. These reviews range from 2 to 5 days and cover the information found in this review book. The review sessions can be expensive, especially if you do not belong to the local AACN chapter. The quality of the CCRN review courses can vary, depending primarily on the skills of the instructor presenting the material.

Test-taking strategies

Multiple-choice questions are one of the most commonly used test formats for such standardized tests as the CCRN examination. You may have noticed that some people do well on such tests, whereas others have problems with this format. The people who do well are not necessarily smarter. More likely, they have intuitively mastered some of the strategies needed to do well on multiple-choice tests. Once you have mastered the following test-taking strategies, you also will be able to score better on multiple-choice tests.

Read the patient situation, the question, and the answer choices carefully. Many mistakes are made because the test-taker did not read all parts of the question carefully. As you read the question and the answer choices, try to determine what kind of knowledge the question is testing.

Treat each question individually. Use only the information provided for that particular question. Also avoid reading into a question information that is not provided. You may have a tendency to think of exceptions or atypical patients encountered in your practice. Most questions on the CCRN examination test textbook-type knowledge of the material.

Monitor the time as you take the examination. You will have approximately 70 seconds per question. Most test-takers average 45 seconds per question, so you may finish well before the time limit. Be sure to complete the entire examination. Your score is based on the number of questions you answer correctly out of a total of 200 questions. If you have time to finish only 100 questions and answered all of them correctly, your score would be only 50%. Practice answering questions at the rate of one question per minute.

Take a watch with you to the examination. You should at least be to question 50 by the end of the first hour; to question 100 by the end of the second hour; and to question 150 by the end of the third hour. If you fall behind by 10 or more questions during any hour, make a conscious effort to speed up. If you spend more than 2 minutes on a question, choose an answer and move on.

Keep in mind that there is no penalty for guessing. An educated guess is better than no answer—an incomplete answer is graded as incorrect. If you cannot decide on a correct answer, just select one and move on. You have a one-in-four chance of selecting the correct answer.

You can use the process of elimination to narrow down your choices. You usually can identify one or more answers as incorrect. By eliminating these answers from the possible choices, you can focus your attention on the answers that may be correct (and improve your chances of answering the question correctly). Reread the question and try to determine exactly what type of information is being tested. If you are still unable to make a decision, select one of the possible correct choices and move on to the next question.

Look for the answer that has a broader focus. If you can narrow down the possible correct choices to two, examine the answers to determine whether one answer may include the other. The answer that is broader (that is, the one that includes the other answer) is probably the correct one.

An example of this type of question follows:

Billy Black is diagnosed with Wolff-Parkinson-White syndrome. When evaluating his ECG, the nurse should note which of the following characteristics of this condition?

A. PR interval less than 0.12 second and wide QRS complex

B. PR interval greater than 0.20 second and normal QRS complex

C. Delta wave present in a positively deflected QRS complex in lead V_1 and PR interval less than 0.12 second

D. Delta wave present in a positively deflected QRS complex in lead V_6 and PR interval greater than 0.20 second

The correct answer is C. Answer A also may be correct, but answer C includes the information in answer A and adds additional information. Again, reading all the answer choices carefully is essential. Selecting answer A without reading the other answers would have led to an incorrect choice.

You cannot change your answers. You need to trust your intuition. The first time you read a question and then read the answer choices, an intuitive connection is made between the right and left lobes of your brain, with the end result that your first answer usually is the best one. Studies of test-taking habits have shown that test-takers who change an answer on a multiple-choice examination usually change it from a correct answer to an incorrect one or from one incorrect answer to another incorrect answer. Seldom do they change from an incorrect to a correct answer.

Look for qualifying words in the question. Such words as *first, best, most, initial, better,* and *highest priority* can help you determine what type of information is called for in the answer. When you see one of these words, your task is to make a judgment about the priority of the answers and select the one answer that has the highest priority.

An example of a judgment question follows:

Roger Redman, age 62, has a history of coronary heart disease. He is brought to the emergency department (ED) complaining of chest pain. What is the *first* action the nurse should take?

A. Give the patient sublingual nitroglycerin gr 1/150.
B. Call the patient's cardiologist about his admission.
C. Place the patient in high-Fowler's position after loosening his shirt.
D. Check the patient's blood pressure and note the location and degree of chest pain.

The correct choice is D. When a question asks for a first or an initial action, think of the nursing process. The first step in the nursing process is assessment. If no choice includes the assessment step, look for a choice involving the planning process, and so forth. In this particular situation, the nurse needs to assess the patient's chest pain first to determine whether it is cardiac in nature. (Many other conditions also cause chest pain.)

Here's another example of a judgment question:

Mr. Redman is connected to an ECG monitor. He was given sublingual nitroglycerin 5 minutes ago but still is experiencing chest pain. The nurse notices that he is beginning to have frequent premature ventricular contractions (PVCs) and short runs of ventricular tachycardia. What is the *most* appropriate nursing intervention?

A. Administer another dose of nitroglycerin.
B. Administer an I.V. bolus of lidocaine and start a lidocaine infusion.
C. Evaluate the patient's mental and circulatory status.
D. Notify the ED doctor.

The correct answer is B. All four choices should be done at some point, but the most appropriate action at this time is to control the PVCs and tachycardia with lidocaine.

Look for negative words in the question. Negative words or prefixes will change how you look for the correct answer. Some common negatives include *not, least, unlikely, inappropriate, unrealistic, lowest priority, contraindicated, false, except, inconsistent, untoward, all but, atypical,* and *incorrect.* In general, when you are asked a negative question, three of the choices are appropriate actions and one is not appropriate. You are being asked to select the inappropriate choice as your answer. When you see a negative question, ask yourself, "What is it that they don't want me to do in this situation?"

An example of a negative question follows:

Mr. Redman is admitted to the ICU. He is still experiencing mild chest pain. Which of the following medications would be inappropriate for relief of Mr. Redman's chest pain?

A. Diltiazem (Cardizem)

B. Propranolol (Inderal)

C. Digoxin (Lanoxin)

D. Meperidine (Demerol)

The correct answer is C. Digoxin is a positive inotropic drug that increases the contractility and oxygen demands of the heart. This medication may increase chest pain in this patient. The other three medications relieve chest pain by means of different mechanisms. If you did not read the question carefully and missed the *in-* prefix of *inappropriate,* you would not have selected choice C.

Avoid selecting answers that contain absolute words; they usually are incorrect. Absolute words include *always, every, only, all, never,* and *none.*

Here's an example of this type of question:

Which of the following is an accurate statement about cardiac chest pain?

A. This pain always is caused by constriction or blockage of the coronary arteries by fatty plaques or blood clots.

B. True cardiac pain never is relieved without treatment.

C. This type of pain is relieved only by nitroglycerin.

D. Patients generally attribute the pain to indigestion.

The correct answer is D. Choice A is incorrect because coronary-type chest pain also may be caused by coronary artery spasm, as in variant (Prinzmetal's) angina. Answer B is incorrect because sometimes chest pain goes away by itself, although it probably will return. A number of other medications also relieve chest pain, thus making choice C incorrect.

Avoid selecting answers that refer the patient to a doctor. The CCRN examination is for nurses and includes conditions and problems that nurses should be able to solve independently. An answer that refers a patient to the doctor usually is incorrect and can be eliminated from consideration.

Avoid looking for a pattern in the selection of answers. The questions and answers on the examination are arranged in random order. Treat each question individually and avoid looking over previous answers for a pattern.

Do not panic if you encounter a question that you do not understand. The CCRN examination is designed so that it is difficult to answer all the questions correctly. As a result, some questions may refer to disease processes, medications, or laboratory tests that you are unfamiliar with.

When test-takers encounter difficult questions about material they do not understand, they have a tendency to select an answer they do not understand. Avoid this practice. Remember that nursing care is similar in many situations, even though the disease processes may be quite different. If you encounter a question you do not understand, select the answer that seems logical and involves general nursing care. Common sense can go a long way on this type of examination.

An example of this type of question follows:

George Green, age 33, is diagnosed as having a pheochromocytoma. Appropriate initial nursing care would involve:

A. Administering large doses of xylometazoline to help control the symptoms of the disease.

B. Closely monitoring Mr. Green's vital signs, particularly his blood pressure.

C. Preparing Mr. Green and his family for imminent death.

D. Having the family discuss the condition with the doctor before informing Mr. Green about the disease because of the protracted recovery period after treatment.

The correct answer is B. A pheochromocytoma is a tumor of the adrenal medulla that causes an increase in the secretion of epinephrine or norepinephrine. This type of tumor can trigger a hypertensive crisis in some patients. Monitoring blood pressure is an important nursing care measure and fits well with the qualifying word *initial* used in the question.

If you do not know what a pheochromocytoma is, you might select choice A if you also do not know what xylometazoline is. This medication is used to relieve nasal congestion. Answer C is not a good choice because preparing a patient for death usually is not an initial nursing action. Choice D could be eliminated because it is overly long and refers the family to a doctor for a nursing care measure.

Remember, if you encounter a question like this on the CCRN examination, do not spend a great deal of time on it. You either know the answer or you don't. If you do not know the answer, try to eliminate some of the choices using the strategies discussed earlier. If you still have no idea, make an educated guess and move on to the next question.

When answers are grouped by similar concepts, activities, or situations, select the one that is different. If three of the four choices have a common element and the fourth answer lacks this element, the different answer probably is correct.

Here's an example of this type of question:

For several years, Karen Cooper has been treated for severe chronic emphysema with bronchodilating agents and relatively high doses of prednisone (Deltasone). Which activity poses the least risk for triggering an adverse effect of prednisone therapy in this patient?

A. Shopping at the mall on a Saturday afternoon

B. Cleaning her two-story house

C. Attending Sunday morning church services

D. Serving refreshments at her 6-year-old son's school play

The correct answer is B. In choices A, C, and D, the common element is that Mrs. Cooper would encounter a group of strangers. Because steroids suppress the immune system, patients taking these medications must avoid exposure to potential infections. Cleaning her house, although strenuous, results in the least exposure to infection.

Think positively about the examination. People who have a positive attitude score higher than those who have a negative attitude. Try repeating these phrases to yourself: "I am an intelligent person. I will do well on the CCRN examination. I have prepared for the examination and will receive a high score. I deserve to pass this examination. I know I can do this!"

Preparing for the certification examination

Being prepared to take the CCRN examination involves not only intellectual preparation but physical and emotional preparation as well. Before the day of the examination, drive to the test site to familiarize yourself with the parking facilities and to locate the test room. Knowing where to go will greatly decrease your anxiety on the day of the examination. Try to follow as normal a schedule as possible on the day before the examination. If you need to travel to the examination site and stay away from home overnight, try to follow your usual nightly routine and avoid the urge to do something different.

The night before the examination, avoid drinking alcoholic beverages. Alcohol is a central nervous system (CNS) depressant that interferes with your ability to concentrate; a hangover also will affect your concentration. Also avoid eating foods you have never eaten before because this may cause adverse GI activity the day of the examination. Do not stay up late to study; this will make you tired during the test, which will decrease your ability to concentrate. Avoid taking medications you have never taken before to help you sleep. Like alcohol, most sleep aids are CNS depressants; some produce a hangover effect, whereas others produce drowsiness for an extended period.

By the night before the examination, you probably are as prepared as you can be. Do not begin major study efforts now. Review formulas, charts, or lists of information for no more than 1 hour. Then relax, perhaps by watching television or reading a magazine or book. These activities will help decrease your anxiety. To keep your biorhythms as regular as possible and help you in your performance on the examination, go to bed at your usual time.

On the morning of the examination, do not attempt a major review of the material. The likelihood of learning something new is slim, and intensive study may only increase your anxiety.

Also avoid drinking excessive amounts of coffee, tea, or caffeine-containing beverages before the test. The caffeine in these beverages will increase your nervousness and stimulate your renal system. Rest room visits are permitted during the examination; the total amount of time allowed for the test is not extended, however, if you leave the room during the examination.

Eat breakfast, even if you usually do not, and include foods that are high in glucose and protein. Glucose will help you maintain your energy level for 1 to $1\frac{1}{2}$ hours. A protein source is required to maintain your energy level throughout the examination. Do not eat greasy, heavy foods. They tend to form an uncomfortable knot in your stomach and may decrease your ability to concentrate. Bring mints or hard candy to the test room to relieve dry mouth.

Dress in comfortable, layered clothing that can be taken off easily. Jogging suits are popular. Many rooms are air-conditioned in the summer and may be cool even if it is hot outside. Be prepared by taking a sweater or sweatshirt.

Arrive at the test site 30 to 45 minutes early, and make sure you have the required papers and documents for admittance to the test room.

Think positively about how you will do on the examination. Taking the CCRN examination shows confidence in your knowledge of critical care nursing. When you receive your passing results, plan to celebrate your success. It is a significant achievement in your life and deserves to be rewarded.

2 Cardiovascular disorders

I. **Anatomy**
   A. Layers of the heart
      1. Pericardium
         a. The pericardium is a double-walled (a fibrous outer wall and a serous inner wall) sac that surrounds the heart and roots of the great vessels
         b. It functions as a barrier against infection, holds the heart in a fixed position, and shields the heart from trauma
         c. The pericardium normally contains 10 to 30 ml of pericardial fluid, which serves as a lubricant, and can hold up to 300 ml of fluid without compromising cardiac function; in chronic disease states, the pericardial space can hold up to 1 L of fluid
      2. Epicardium
         a. The epicardium is the outer, visceral layer of the heart
         b. It forms the inner layer of the pericardium and sometimes is called the visceral pericardium
      3. Myocardium
         a. The myocardium is a thick, muscular layer that contains the muscle fibers needed for contraction
         b. The cardiac muscle cells that make up the myocardium contain myosin, actin, and sarcoplasmic reticulum
            (1) Myosin is a thick contractile protein with tiny projections that interact with actin to form cross-bridges
            (2) Actin is a thin contractile protein that is connected to Z bands on one end and the myosin cross-bridges on the other; the Z bands act as an anchor, allowing the muscle fibers to slide over one another in one direction
            (3) Sarcoplasmic reticulum stores calcium ions and releases calcium after depolarization; this allows the cross-bridges on the myosin filaments to effect cell contraction
      4. Endocardium
         a. The endocardium is a thin layer of endothelium and connective tissue that lines the heart
         b. It is continuous with the blood vessels, papillary muscles, and valves
         c. Disruptions in the endocardium can predispose the patient to infection

B. Position of the heart
  1. The heart lies in the anterior thoracic cavity, just behind the sternum
  2. It is anterior to the esophagus, aorta, vena cava, and vertebral column
  3. The right ventricle constitutes the majority of the inferior and anterior surfaces
  4. The left ventricle constitutes the anterolateral and posterior surfaces
  5. The base of the heart is the superior surface; the apex is the inferior surface
C. Normal size and weight
  1. The normal heart is 4.7″ (12 cm) long and 3.1″ to 3.5″ (8 to 9 cm) wide
  2. The adult male heart weighs 10.2 to 11.5 oz (290 to 325 g); the heart of an adult female weighs 8.1 to 9.3 oz (230 to 265 g)
D. Chambers of the heart
  1. Atria
    a. The atria are thin-walled, low-pressure chambers that receive blood from the vena cava and pulmonary veins
    b. The atria act as a conduit between the venous system and the ventricles
    c. Atrial contractions contribute up to 30% of ventricular filling; this is known as atrial kick
  2. Ventricles
    a. The right ventricle, which is approximately 3 mm thick, pumps blood into low-pressured pulmonary circulation
    b. The left ventricle, which is approximately 10 to 13 mm thick, ejects blood into the high-pressured aorta; the left ventricle is considered the major pump of the heart
E. Cardiac valves
  1. Description
    a. The valves in the heart consist of flexible fibrous tissue thinly covered by endocardium
      (1) The chordae tendineae are avascular structures covered by a thin layer of endocardium that connect the papillary muscles to the valve
      (2) The papillary muscles connect the chordae tendineae to the floor of the ventricular wall and help prevent the valve cusps from everting during systole
    b. The valves permit blood to flow in only one direction; their opening and closing is a passive process
  2. Atrioventricular valves
    a. The atrioventricular (AV) valves are located between the atria and the ventricles
    b. AV valves prevent the backflow of blood into the atria during ventricular contraction

      c. There are two types of AV valves

        (1) The tricuspid valve has three cusps and is located between the right atrium and the right ventricle

        (2) The mitral (bicuspid) valve has two cusps and is located between the left atrium and the left ventricle

   3. Semilunar valves

      a. The semilunar valves have three main cuplike cusps that separate the ventricles from the aorta and the pulmonary arteries

      b. The semilunar valves open during ventricular systole

F. Coronary blood supply

   1. Coronary veins

      a. The coronary veins return deoxygenated blood from the heart to the right atrium by way of the coronary sinus

      b. The thebesian vessels empty deoxygenated blood into all four chambers of the heart

   2. Coronary arteries

      a. The coronary arteries supply the heart with oxygenated blood

      b. They arise at the base of the aorta immediately after the aortic valve and run along the outside of the heart in natural grooves called sulci

      c. Branches of the main coronary arteries penetrate the muscular wall of the heart and nourish the endocardium

      d. During ventricular contraction, no blood flows to cardiac tissue

      e. Two types of coronary arteries are found in the heart

        (1) The right coronary artery supplies blood to the right atrium and right ventricle, the sinoatrial (SA) and AV nodes (in more than 50% of the population), the inferior wall of the left ventricle, the posterior wall of the septum, the posterior papillary muscle, and the posterior (inferior) division of the left bundle branch; occlusion of the right coronary artery can result in posterior or inferior wall myocardial infarction (MI)

        (2) The left coronary artery branches into the left anterior descending artery and the circumflex artery

          (a) The left anterior descending coronary artery supplies blood to the anterior portion of the ventricle, the anterior papillary muscle, the anterior division of the septum, the anterior (superior) division of the left bundle branch, and the right bundle branch

          (b) The circumflex coronary artery supplies blood to the left atrium, posterior surfaces of the left ventricle, and the posterior aspect of the septum

          (c) Occlusion of the left coronary artery can result in anterior or lateral MI

G. Conduction system

   1. Definitions

   a. *Excitability* is the ability of a cell or tissue to depolarize in response to a given stimulus
   b. *Conductivity* is the ability of cardiac cells to transmit a stimulus from cell to cell
   c. *Automaticity* is the ability of certain cells to spontaneously depolarize (that is, these cells have pacemaker potential)
   d. *Rhythmicity* is automaticity that is generated at a regular rate
   e. *Contractility* is the ability of the cardiac myofibrils to shorten in response to an electrical stimulus
   f. *Refractoriness* is the state of a cell or tissue during repolarization when the cell or tissue either cannot depolarize (regardless of the intensity of the stimulus) or requires a much greater stimulus than normal

2. Sinoatrial node
   a. The SA node is the natural pacemaker of the heart and has the highest degree of automaticity in all the cardiac cells
   b. Located in the upper portion of the right atrium near the mouth of the superior vena cava, the SA node has an intrinsic rate of 60 to 100 beats/minute
   c. Once the SA node depolarizes, atrial depolarization occurs by way of three internodal tracts that carry the electrical impulse from the SA node through the right atrium to the AV node; Bachmann's bundle carries the electrical impulse from the SA node to the left atrium

3. Atrioventricular node
   a. The AV node is located posteriorly on the right side of the interatrial septum
   b. It conducts all electrical impulses from the atria to the ventricles; its intrinsic rate is 40 to 60 beats/minute
   c. The electrical impulse from the SA node depolarizes the AV node
   d. The AV node then slows conduction of the electrical impulse to allow for optimal ventricular filling from the atrial contraction; the delay normally is 0.04 second
   e. The AV node delay limits the number of impulses that are transmitted to the ventricles
   f. The AV node also can conduct impulses in a retrograde manner that are initiated in or below the AV node, as in junctional ectopic beats and ventricular ectopic beats

4. Bundle of His
   a. The bundle of His conducts electrical impulses in the ventricles; its intrinsic rate is 40 to 60 beats/minute
   b. The bundle of His is divided into the right bundle branch and the left bundle branch
      (1) The right bundle branch continues down the right side of the interventricular septum toward the right apex; its conduction velocity is slower than that of the left bundle branch

   (2) The left bundle branch continues down the left side of the interventricular septum and divides into two branches: the anterior (superior) branch and the posterior (inferior) branch

  c. The Purkinje fibers are the smallest divisions of the right bundle branch and left bundle branch; they have the fastest conduction velocity of all heart tissue, and their intrinsic rate is 15 to 40 beats/minute

II. Physiology

 A. Refractory period

  1. The absolute refractory period is the time during which the myocardium cannot respond to even a strong stimulus

  2. The relative refractory period is the time during which the myocardium responds to a strong stimulus or a normal stimulus with delayed conduction

 B. Cardiac cycle

  1. Diastole

   a. Diastole is the period during which the chambers of the heart relax

   b. Electrical diastole is the resting phase of the electrical cardiac cycle

  2. Systole

   a. Systole, or ejection, is the period during which the chambers of the heart contract

   b. Systole begins as soon as the ventricles fill with blood

   c. As the systolic pressure rises, the AV valves are forced to close; this is the source of the first heart sound (S_1)

   d. When the ventricular pressure is greater than the aortic pressure, the semilunar valves open and blood is ejected into the aorta and the pulmonary artery

   e. As the ejection phase ends, the ventricles relax and intraventricular pressure decreases, causing reversal of the blood flow in the aorta and forcing the semilunar valves to close (this is the source of the second heart sound, S_2); the end of the ejection phase is reflected by a dicrotic notch on the aorta's pressure waveform (graphic representation of the cardiac cycle when an arterial line is used to monitor hemodynamic variables)

   f. Ventricular pressure falls quickly after the semilunar valves close; the atrial tracing on the electrocardiogram (ECG) shows a V wave, which denotes the period during which the ventricles relax and blood enters the atria

 C. Cardiac function

  1. The measurement of several hemodynamic variables are used to monitor cardiac function (for information about the normal values and formulas used to determine some of these variables, see *Hemodynamic values obtained by means of a pulmonary artery catheter,* page 21, and *Computed hemodynamic values,* page 22)

Hemodynamic values obtained by means of a pulmonary artery catheter

Pulmonary artery catheters allow the direct measurement of certain hemodynamic values; the chart below lists the ones more commonly used in critical care nursing. These values are used in the calculation of other indicators of cardiac function, such as cardiac index.

HEMODYNAMIC VALUE	NORMAL RANGE
Central venous pressure (CVP)	1 to 7 mm Hg
Right atrial pressure (RAP)	1 to 7 mm Hg
Pulmonary artery pressure (PAP)	15 mm Hg
Pulmonary artery wedge pressure (PAWP); also called pulmonary capillary wedge pressure (PCWP) or pulmonary artery occlusion (PAO)	8 to 12 mm Hg
Cardiac output (CO)	4 to 8 L/minute

2. Cardiac output is defined as the volume of blood that is ejected from the heart in 1 minute
   a. The determinants of cardiac output (CO) are heart rate (HR), in units of beats/minute, and stroke volume (SV), in units of ml/beat, as shown in the following equation: $CO = SV \times HR$
   b. Normal cardiac output is 4 to 8 L/minute
3. The cardiac index is the cardiac output indexed to body surface area
   a. The following equation shows how cardiac output and body surface area (BSA) are related to cardiac index (CI): $CI = \frac{CO}{BSA}$
   b. Normal cardiac index is 2.5 to 4.0 L/minute/m^2
4. SV refers to the difference between the diastolic volume in the left ventricle and the residual volume of blood in that ventricle after systole; the determinants of SV are preload, afterload, and contractility (see *Factors that influence cardiac workload,* page 23)
   a. Preload is the volume of blood in the left ventricle coupled with the ability of the ventricle to stretch at the end of diastole; if the intravascular volume exceeds the stretch limit, cardiac output diminishes
      (1) Preload is best measured hemodynamically by the pulmonary artery wedge pressure (PAWP) in the left side of the heart and the right atrial pressure or central venous pressure (CVP) in the right side of the heart
      (2) Venous return, total blood volume, and atrial kick affect the volume aspect of preload; the stiffness and thickness of the cardiac muscle wall affect compliance of the ventricle
   b. Afterload is the ventricular wall tension or stress during systolic ejection

Computed hemodynamic values

Certain hemodynamic values cannot be measured directly; they need to be calculated from other hemodynamic measurements. The chart below lists indicators of cardiac function and the formulas used to derive them. Note the following abbreviations: BSA = body surface area; CO = cardiac output; DBP = diastolic blood pressure; HR = heart rate; MPAP = mean pulmonary artery pressure; PAWP = pulmonary artery wedge pressure; RAP = right atrial pressure; SBP = systolic blood pressure.

HEMODYNAMIC VARIABLE	NORMAL RANGE	FORMULA
Stroke volume (SV)	40 to 80 ml	$SV = CO \div HR$
Cardiac index (CI)	2.5 to 4.0 L/minute/m²	$CI = CO \div BSA$
Pulmonary vascular resistance (PVR)	50 to 150 dynes $\times$ seconds $\times$ cm⁻⁵	$PVR = (MPAP - PAWP) \div CO$
Mean arterial pressure (MAP)	70 to 100 mm Hg	$MAP = \dfrac{SBP + (2\ DBP)}{3}$
Systemic vascular resistance (SVR)	800 to 1,500 dynes $\times$ seconds $\times$ cm⁻⁵	$SVR = \dfrac{MAP - RAP}{CO \times 80}$

(1) Afterload is best measured hemodynamically by the systemic vascular resistance in the left side of the heart and the pulmonary vascular resistance in the right side of the heart

(2) Afterload is increased by factors that oppose ejection, such as arteriosclerotic disease, hypervolemia, and aortic stenosis

c. Contractility, or the heart's contractile force, can be increased by the Starling mechanism (in which the heart increases output by increasing preload) and the sympathetic nervous system; sympathomimetic and adrenergic medications can affect contractility greatly

5. Heart rate is regulated by nervous control and intrinsic regulation

a. Nervous control is divided into parasympathetic control and sympathetic control

(1) Parasympathetic fibers (in the vagus nerve) are concentrated near SA and AV conduction tissue; stimulation of these tissues causes bradycardia

(2) Sympathetic nerve fibers parallel the coronary circulation before penetrating the myocardium; stimulation of these fibers causes acceleration and increased contractility (this is known as the fight-or-flight response)

b. Intrinsic regulation is produced by baroceptors and chemoreceptors

(1) Baroceptors, which are located in the carotid sinus and aortic arch, sense changes in pressure and activate the autonomic nervous system to raise or lower the heart rate

Factors that influence cardiac workload

Drugs as well as certain conditions can alter cardiac workload. The table below lists factors that increase and decrease cardiac workload. An alteration in the cardiac workload in turn influences stroke volume, stroke volume index, cardiac output, cardiac index, right ventricular stroke work index, and left ventricular stroke work index.

Factors that increase cardiac workload	Factors that decrease cardiac workload
Drugs (increased contractility)	*Drugs (decreased contractility)*
Amrinone	Atenolol
Digitoxin	Metoprolol
Digoxin	Nadolol
Dobutamine	Propranolol
Dopamine	Timolol
Epinephrine	
Isoproterenol	*Abnormal conditions*
	Heart failure
	Hypovolemia
Abnormal conditions	Increased vascular resistance
Decreased vascular resistance	Myocardial infarction
Hyperthermia	Pulmonary emboli
Hypervolemia	Septic shock (late stages)
Septic shock (early stages)	
	Hyperinflation of lungs
	Continuous positive airway pressure
	Mechanical ventilation
	Positive end-expiratory pressure

       (2) Chemoreceptors, which are located in the bifurcation of the aortic arch, sense changes in oxygen tension, pH, and carbon dioxide tension; they trigger increases in respiratory rate and depth

III. Cardiovascular assessment
    A. Noninvasive assessment techniques
        1. Patient history
           a. The patient's presenting symptoms or complaints provide the starting point for obtaining the patient history
           b. The patient history should include past medical history, family history, current medications, and past diagnostic studies
        2. Physical examination
           a. Inspection focuses on the general appearance of the patient's face, extremities, neck, thorax, and abdomen
           (1) During the physical examination, note the patient's weight and whether the patient is overweight or underweight

(2) Note the patient's skin color (whether it is pale or flushed) and body position; also observe for diaphoresis, confusion, and lethargy

(3) Examine the patient's nails for cyanosis and clubbing, and assess hair distribution, skin condition, skin color, edema, and varicosities of the extremities

(4) Check for distention of the external jugular vein by having the patient sit at a 30- to 45-degree angle and assessing the fullness of the jugular vein at the end of exhalation

   (a) Fullness more than 3 cm above the sternal angle is evidence of increased CVP

   (b) The higher the sitting angle of the patient when jugular vein distention is discovered, the higher the CVP

(5) Assess for right-sided heart failure by checking the hepatojugular reflex

   (a) Observe the pulsation of the internal jugular vein as you press firmly over the right upper quadrant of the patient's abdomen for 30 seconds

   (b) The hepatojugular reflex test is considered positive if the amount of distention in the vein is more than 1 cm above baseline after the pressure is removed

(6) Check the thorax and abdomen for scars, skeletal deformities, bruises, and wounds

(7) Assess for apical impulse (the point of maximal impulse [PMI]), which normally is at the fifth intercostal space just to the left midclavicular line in an adult patient

b. Palpation is used to assess pulses, capillary refill, presence of edema, and skin temperature

(1) Assess pulses separately and compare bilaterally

   (a) Check the carotid, brachial, radial, ulnar, popliteal, dorsalis pedis, and posterior tibial pulses

   (b) Use Allen's test to assess adequate blood flow to the hand through the ulnar artery before the radial artery is punctured (such as for drawing arterial blood gas [ABG] samples or insertion of an arterial line)

(2) To assess capillary refill (which measures arterial circulation to the extremity), compress the nails for a few seconds and release quickly; normal color should return within 3 seconds

(3) To determine if pitting edema (a sign that fluid has accumulated in the extravascular space) is present, press the skin to the underlying bone

   (a) If an impression remains when pressure is removed, the patient has pitting edema

   (b) Measure the amount of pitting in millimeters

(4) Assess for thrombophlebitis using Homans' sign, in which the knee is flexed and the foot is abruptly dorsiflexed

Auscultation of the cardiovascular system

Although heart sounds may vary from patient to patient, the ones listed below are the most common ones. The heart sounds are grouped according to where they are best heard.

Aortic area
- S_2 loud
- Aortic systolic murmur

Pulmonic area
- S_2 loud and split with inhalation
- Pulmonic valve murmurs

Erb's point
- S_2 split with inhalation
- Aortic diastolic murmur
- Pericardial friction rub

Tricuspid area
- S_1 split
- Right ventricular S_3 and S_4
- Tricuspid valve murmurs
- Murmur of ventricular septal defect

Mitral area
- S_1 loud
- Left ventricular S_3 and S_4
- Mitral valve murmurs

      (a) If the patient experiences pain in the popliteal region or calf, Homans' sign is positive and the patient has thrombophlebitis

      (b) Homans' sign is not as reliable in the identification of thrombophlebitis as is the observation of erythema, low-grade fever, edema, and pain in the extremity

    (5) Palpate the PMI, which should be less than 2 cm in diameter

c. Auscultation is used to measure blood pressure, detect bruits, and assess heart sounds (see *Auscultation of the cardiovascular system*)

    (1) Check for bruits (extracardiac high-pitched "sh-sh" sounds) by placing the bell of the stethoscope over the carotid or femoral artery; the presence of a bruit indicates a tortuous or partially occluded vessel or increased blood flow through a vessel

    (2) Assess heart sounds using the stethoscope

      (a) S_1 is produced by the rapid deceleration of blood flow when the AV valves close at the start of systole; the S_1 heart sound is best heard over the mitral and tricuspid areas

      (b) S_2 is produced by the closing of the semilunar valves at the end of systole; it is best heard over the aortic and pulmonic areas

      (c) S_3 is related to diastolic motion and rapid filling of the ventricles in early diastole; this soft, low-pitched sound is best heard at the apex of the heart; it is normal in patients under age 40 but signals heart failure in older patients

         (d) S_4 is heard at the end of diastole and is associated with atrial contraction; this soft, low-pitched sound is best heard at the apex of the heart; it is a pathologic condition produced by increased resistance to ventricular filling

      (3) Use the stethoscope to listen for murmurs, which are prolonged extra heart sounds heard during systole or diastole

         (a) Murmurs are caused by an increased rate of blood flow through cardiac structures, blood flowing across a partial obstruction or irregularity, shunting of blood through an abnormal passage from a high-pressure to a low-pressure area, or backflow of blood through an incompetent valve

         (b) New murmurs associated with an acute MI may be caused by papillary muscle dysfunction or rupture, ventricular septal defect, or ventricular rupture; these emergency situations may require surgical intervention

      (4) Assess for pericardial friction rub (a high-pitched sound) at Erb's point; this may occur secondary to pericarditis, after an MI has occurred, or after the patient has undergone cardiac surgery; occasionally, it is the presenting symptom

    d. Percussion is not used in cardiovascular assessment

B. Noninvasive diagnostic testing

  1. A standard 12-lead ECG shows electrical activity of the heart at 12 locations: 6 on the chest and 6 on the limbs; in addition to detecting abnormal transmission of impulses, the 12-lead ECG provides information on the heart's axis (electrical position) and the size of the cardiac chambers

  2. A Holter monitor is a portable device that produces a continuous ECG and is used for 12, 24, or 48 hours

    a. The Holter monitor is used to detect arrhythmias, to evaluate the effectiveness of antiarrhythmic medications, to evaluate pacemaker function, and to diagnose dizziness, syncope, palpitations, and episodes of chest pain

    b. The patient keeps a diary of activities and symptoms while wearing the Holter monitor; this correlates with the Holter monitor's data

  3. The exercise stress test evaluates the patient's cardiac response to physical stress; ECG activity, blood pressure, and physical symptoms are monitored during the test

  4. Echocardiography is used to evaluate the internal structures and motions of the heart and great vessels

C. Invasive assessment techniques

  1. Cardiac catheterization and angiography are used to visualize the heart's chambers, valves, great vessels, and coronary arteries; these techniques also are useful for obtaining pressure measurements (right and left sides of the heart) to evaluate cardiac function and valve patency

     a. In right-sided cardiac catheterization, the catheter is inserted through the basilic or femoral vein; this allows for continuous hemodynamic monitoring, determination of cardiac output and heart pressures on the right side, shunt studies, oximetry, and angiography (of the right atrium, right ventricle, tricuspid and pulmonic valves, and pulmonary artery)

     b. In left-sided cardiac catheterization, the catheter is inserted through the femoral or brachial artery, thereby allowing visualization of the coronary arteries, aortic root, and right ventricle; pressures are obtained from the aorta and heart chambers on the left side, thereby providing information on left ventricular function, mitral and aortic function, and shunting

   2. Electrophysiologic studies are used to evaluate the heart's electrical conduction system

   3. Hemodynamic monitoring requires placement of a multipurpose catheter in the right side of the heart through the pulmonic valve and into the pulmonary artery

     a. Hemodynamic monitoring allows measurement of pulmonary artery pressure (PAP), PAWP, right atrial pressure, and cardiac output

     b. These pressures are used to assess the patient's progress, to monitor the patient's response to fluids and medications, and to adjust medication dosages

   4. Intra-arterial pressure monitoring, in which a catheter is placed in a major artery (usually the radial, femoral, or brachial artery) and connected to a transducer, allows continuous monitoring of blood pressure and provides ready access for arterial blood sampling

D. Normal laboratory values

   1. Sodium (Na^+): 135 to 145 mEq/L

   2. Potassium (K^+): 3.5 to 5.0 mEq/L

   3. Calcium (Ca^{+2}): 8.5 to 10.0 mg/dl

   4. Magnesium (Mg^{+2}): 1.5 to 2.5 mEq/L

   5. Chloride (Cl^-): 98 to 106 mg/dl

   6. Cardiac enzymes (see page 37)

IV. Arrhythmias

A. ECG components

   1. A normal ECG waveform includes the P wave, PR interval, QRS complex, ST segment, J point, T wave, QT interval and sometimes, the U wave

   2. A P wave, which usually is rounded and upright, precedes each QRS complex; the P wave indicates atrial depolarization and impulse origination in the SA node, atria, or AV junctional tissue

     a. Peaked P waves are seen in right atrial hypertrophy

     b. Broad, notched P waves are seen in left atrial hypertrophy

     c. Inverted P waves are caused by retrograde conduction from the AV junction

d. Varying P waves originate from various sites in the atrium
3. The PR interval measures electrical activity from the start of atrial depolarization to the start of ventricular depolarization; the duration of the PR interval normally is 0.12 to 0.20 second (measured from the beginning of the P wave to the beginning of the QRS complex)
   a. A PR interval less than 0.12 second indicates that the electrical impulse originated in an area other than the SA node
   b. A PR interval greater than 0.20 second indicates that the impulse is delayed as it passes through the AV node
4. The QRS complex follows the PR interval and reflects ventricular depolarization
   a. The Q wave is the first negative deflection, the R wave is the first positive deflection, and the S wave is the negative deflection after the R wave; the duration of the QRS complex normally is 0.06 to 0.10 second (measured from the beginning of the Q wave to the end of the S wave)
   b. A widened QRS complex (greater than 0.12 second) can occur when impulse conduction to one ventricle is slowed or when the impulse originates in the ventricles
   c. QRS complexes of varying size and shape may indicate the occurrence of ectopic or aberrantly conducted impulses
   d. A missing QRS complex may denote a block or complete ventricular standstill
5. The ST segment measures the end of ventricular depolarization and the beginning of ventricular repolarization; it extends from the end of the S wave to the beginning of the T wave; a normal ST segment usually is isoelectric and does not vary more than 1 mm
   a. An ST-segment elevation of 2 mm or more above the baseline value may indicate myocardial injury
   b. ST-segment depression may indicate myocardial injury or ischemia
   c. ST-segment changes may occur in patients with pericarditis, myocarditis, left ventricular hypertrophy, pulmonary embolism, or electrolyte disturbances
6. The J point marks the end of the QRS complex and the beginning of the ST segment; it is important in determining ST-segment elevation or depression
7. The T wave follows the S wave; typically rounded and smooth, the T wave reflects ventricular repolarization
   a. The T wave usually is positive in leads I, II, V_3, V_4, V_5, and V_6
   b. Inverted T waves in leads I, II, V_3, V_4, V_5, or V_6 may indicate myocardial ischemia
   c. Peaked T waves commonly occur in patients with hyperkalemia
   d. Heavily notched T waves may indicate pericarditis in adult patients

Normal sinus rhythm

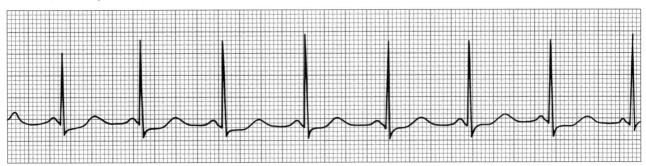

e. Variations in T-wave amplitude may result from an electrolyte imbalance
8. The QT interval represents the time needed for ventricular depolarization and repolarization; the duration of the QT interval normally is 0.36 to 0.44 second (measured from the beginning of the QRS complex to the end of the T wave)
   a. A prolonged QT interval indicates a prolonged relative refractory period, which may be caused by certain medications or may be congenital
   b. A shortened QT interval may be caused by hypercalcemia or digitalis glycoside toxicity
9. The U wave reflects repolarization of the His-Purkinje system; when present, the U wave follows the T wave and appears as an upright deflection
   a. A prominent U wave may occur in patients with hypokalemia
   b. An inverted U wave may occur in patients with heart disease
B. Analysis of ECGs
   1. Determine the rhythm (regular or irregular)
   2. Determine the rate
   3. Evaluate the P wave
   4. Determine the duration of the PR interval
   5. Determine the duration of the QRS complex
   6. Evaluate the T wave
   7. Determine the duration of the QT interval
   8. Evaluate the other components of the ECG
C. Normal sinus rhythm
   1. A normal sinus rhythm is the most common rhythm seen on an ECG strip (for a sample ECG rhythm strip, see *Normal sinus rhythm*)
   2. In a normal sinus rhythm, the atrial and ventricular rhythms are regular and the atrial and ventricular rates are between 60 and 100 beats/minute

Premature ventricular contractions

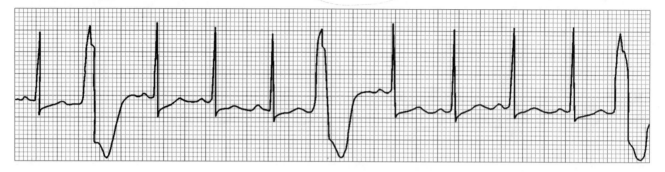

3. The P waves are normal, upright, and similar to one another, and there is one P wave for each QRS complex
4. The T waves are normal, and the PR interval, QRS complex, and QT interval are within normal limits
5. No ectopic or aberrantly conducted beats are present

   D. Premature ventricular contractions

      1. Description

         a. Premature ventricular contractions (PVCs) can occur in healthy and diseased hearts; they may occur singly or in pairs, on every second beat (this is called bigeminy) or on every third beat (this is called trigeminy), or they fall on the T wave (the R-on-T phenomenon; for a sample ECG rhythm strip, see *Premature ventricular contractions*)

         b. PVCs signal danger when two or more occur in a row, when they are multiform or occur on every second beat, or when the R-on-T phenomenon is present

         c. PVCs result from the firing of an ectopic focus in the ventricle, which causes the QRS complex to occur early

            (1) In a patient with PVCs, the duration of the QRS complex is greater than 0.12 second; the configuration is bizarre and usually followed by a compensatory pause

            (2) The T wave usually is deflected in the opposite direction of the QRS complex

            (3) Uniform (unifocal) PVCs look alike and originate from the same ectopic focus

         d. PVCs may result from drug administration (such as digitalis glycosides and sympathomimetic agents), electrolyte imbalances (hypokalemia and hypocalcemia), stimulants (exercise, caffeine, or tobacco), or other factors (alcohol, hypercapnia, hypoxia, myocardial ischemia, or myocardial irritation by pacemaker electrodes)

      2. Clinical signs and symptoms

         a. Irregular pulse during PVCs

Ventricular tachycardia

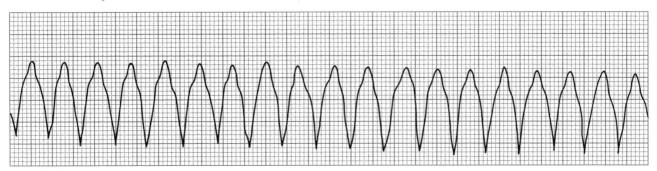

      b. Complaints of palpitations

      c. Hypotension, syncope, and blurred vision if decreased cardiac output is uncompensated

   3. Medical management

      a. Correct the underlying cause

      b. Administer I.V. lidocaine if the patient has an underlying cardiac problem

      c. Administer I.V. atropine for symptomatic bradycardia

   4. Nursing management

      a. Assess the patient's level of consciousness and changes in ECG, heart rate, and blood pressure; changes in clinical status may indicate low cardiac output

      b. Maintain continuous ECG monitoring to identify arrhythmias

      c. Administer antiarrhythmic medications, as prescribed, and monitor the patient's response to maintain therapeutic drug levels and prevent toxicity

      d. Administer oxygen, as prescribed, to treat hypoxia, which could lead to myocardial ischemia and life-threatening arrhythmias

      e. If a life-threatening arrhythmia occurs, initiate prompt treatment, including cardiopulmonary resuscitation (CPR), defibrillation, I.V. drug therapy, and preparation for pacemaker insertion

      f. Maintain a patent I.V. line to ensure access if emergency medications must be administered

 E. Ventricular tachycardia

   1. Description

      a. Ventricular tachycardia is defined as the occurrence of three or more PVCs in a row with a ventricular rate more than 100 beats/minute; it can be paroxysmal or sustained (for a sample ECG rhythm strip, see *Ventricular tachycardia*)

      b. A rapid ventricular rate without the atrial kick reduces the effective ventricular filling time and decreases cardiac output

Ventricular fibrillation

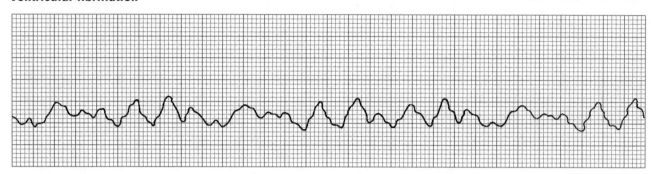

    c. Ventricular tachycardia usually is caused by myocardial irritability related to cardiac conditions, including acute MI, coronary artery disease, rheumatic heart disease, mitral valve prolapse, heart failure, and cardiomyopathy; it also may be caused by the R-on-T phenomenon

    d. Noncardiac conditions that can trigger ventricular tachycardia include pulmonary embolism, hypokalemia, severe hypoxemia, and drug toxicity resulting from digitalis, procainamide, quinidine, or epinephrine therapy

  2. Clinical signs and symptoms

    a. Nonpalpable pulse or palpable with a fast rate

    b. No symptoms or mild symptoms if cardiac output is compensated

    c. Signs and symptoms of decreased cardiac output and unresponsiveness

  3. Medical and nursing management

    a. If the patient is conscious and stable, administer lidocaine followed by procainamide or bretylium; if drugs are ineffective, synchronized cardioversion may be necessary

    b. If the patient has no pulse, use defibrillation; initiate CPR if a defibrillator is not immediately available

F. Ventricular fibrillation

  1. Description

    a. Ventricular fibrillation is characterized by coarse fibrillating waves on the ECG, which indicate increased electrical activity (for a sample ECG rhythm strip, see *Ventricular fibrillation*); coarse fibrillating waves are easier to convert to a normal sinus rhythm than fine fibrillating waves, which indicate acidosis and hypoxemia

    b. During ventricular fibrillation, ventricular muscle fibers rapidly depolarize in a disorganized way; because the ventricles quiver rather than contract, cardiac output is nonexistent

Asystole

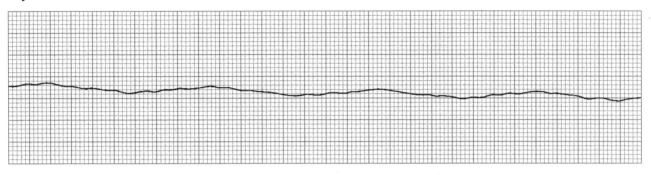

    c. Ventricular fibrillation is caused by ischemia secondary to acute MI, untreated ventricular tachycardia, the R-on-T phenomenon, hypokalemia, hyperkalemia, hypercalcemia, severe hypoxemia, acid-base imbalances, epinephrine or quinidine toxicity, electric shock, or hypothermia

  2. Clinical signs and symptoms

    a. Pulselessness and unresponsiveness

    b. Complete cardiopulmonary arrest

  3. Medical and nursing management

    a. Initiate CPR and continue until a defibrillator is available

    b. Administer epinephrine and antiarrhythmic medications

    c. Administer magnesium sulfate to suppress ventricles

G. Asystole

  1. Description

    a. In asystole, there is no electrical activity in the ventricles and no cardiac output, and the ECG shows a flat line; however, if P waves are present on an ECG, it is called ventricular standstill (for a sample ECG rhythm strip, see *Asystole*)

    b. Asystole can be triggered by any condition that causes inadequate blood flow (such as pulmonary embolism, air embolism, or hemorrhage) or ineffective cardiac contractility (such as heart failure, heart rupture, MI, or cardiac tamponade)

    c. It also can result from insufficient conduction caused by hypoxemia, hypokalemia, severe acidosis, electric shock, ventricular arrhythmias, AV block, or cocaine overdose and from electromechanical dissociation (separation of the heart's electrical and mechanical activities in which evidence of electrical activity is seen on the monitor but a pulse or blood pressure cannot be obtained)

  2. Clinical signs and symptoms

    a. Pulseless electrical activity and unresponsiveness

    b. Complete cardiopulmonary arrest

Telltale ECG findings: The three I's of an acute MI

Ischemia, injury, and infarction (the three I's of an acute MI) produce characteristic ECG changes.

Ischemia temporarily interrupts blood supply to myocardial tissue but generally does not cause cell death. ECG changes: T-wave inversion, resulting from altered tissue repolarization. (See waveform at top right.)

Injury results from prolonged blood supply interruption, causing further cell injury. ECG changes: elevated ST segment, resulting from altered depolarization. Consider an elevation greater than 1 mm significant. (See middle waveform.)

Infarction ensues from complete lack of blood reaching the cell. This causes myocardial cell death (necrosis). ECG changes: pathologic Q wave, resulting from abnormal depolarization or from scar tissue that cannot depolarize. Look for Q wave duration of 0.04 second or more or an amplitude measuring at least one-third of the QRS complex. (See waveform at bottom right.)

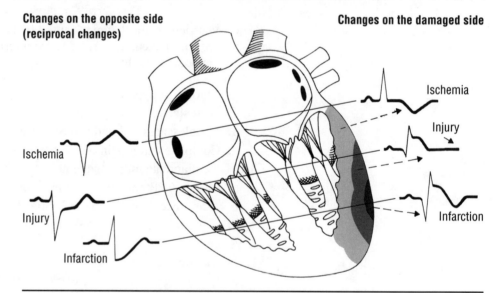

Changes on the opposite side (reciprocal changes)

Changes on the damaged side

Ischemia

Injury

Infarction

Ischemia

Injury

Infarction

3. Medical and nursing management
   a. Initiate CPR
   b. Administer epinephrine and atropine
   c. Consider cardiac pacing

V. Acute myocardial infarction
   A. Description
   1. An acute MI produces zones of infarction, ischemia, and injury (see *Telltale ECG findings: The three I's of an acute MI*)
   2. An infarction is an area of cell death and muscle necrosis
      a. Evidence of infarction on the ECG is seen by pathologic Q waves (the Q wave is wider than 0.04 second and its height is between one-fourth and one-third the height of the R wave), which reflect the inability of the dead tissue to depolarize
      b. As healing occurs, the necrotic cells are replaced by scar tissue

3. Injured tissue surrounds the infarcted zone
   a. Injured cells do not completely repolarize because the blood supply is deficient
   b. An area of injury is recorded on the ECG as an elevated ST segment
4. Ischemia, an area consisting of viable cells, surrounds the injured zone
   a. Repolarization in the ischemic area is impaired but eventually returns to normal
   b. An area of ischemia is recorded on the ECG as a T-wave inversion
   c. An ischemic zone is the point of origin of many arrhythmias associated with acute MI that are caused by impaired repolarization
B. Classification
1. A transmural acute MI affects all three muscle layers of the heart and is associated with a higher incidence of left ventricular dysfunction
   a. During depolarization, the ECG shows the appearance of new Q waves
   b. In the acute phase of repolarization, the ST segment is elevated in the leads overlying the involved surface, with reciprocal ST changes in the leads overlying the surface opposite the involved site
2. A subendocardial acute MI affects the endocardium and the myocardium
   a. It is the most common nontransmural infarction
   b. The ECG shows ST-segment depression and T-wave inversion
C. Location
1. The location and extent of damage caused by an acute MI depends on the site and severity of coronary artery narrowing; the presence, site, and severity of coronary artery spasm; the size of the vascular bed perfused by the compromised vessels; the extent of the collateral blood vessels; and the oxygen needs of the poorly perfused myocardium (see *Identifying the myocardial infarction damage site,* page 36)
2. Anterior wall infarctions are classified as true anterior, anteroseptal, or anterolateral
   a. A true anterior infarction results from occlusion of the left anterior descending coronary artery, resulting in serious left ventricular dysfunction; ECG changes include loss of positive R-wave progression in leads V_1 through V_6, ST-segment elevation in leads V_1 through V_4, and T-wave inversion in leads I, aV_L, and V_3 through V_5

Identifying the myocardial infarction damage site

Use this chart to identify the location of myocardial infarction (MI) damage. Remember that myocardial damage may spread to other areas. (*Note:* ECG changes occurring in the acute phase of a transmural MI include pathologic Q waves, ST-segment elevation, and T-wave inversion.)

Wall affected	Leads	Possible ECG changes	Possible coronary artery involved	Possible reciprocal changes
Inferior (diaphragmatic)	II, III, aV$_F$	Q, ST, T	Right coronary artery	I, aV$_L$
Lateral	I, aV$_L$, V$_5$, V$_6$	Q, ST, T	Circumflex artery, branch of left anterior descending artery	V$_1$, V$_3$
Anterior	V$_1$, V$_2$, V$_3$, V$_4$, I, aV$_L$	Q, ST, T, loss of R-wave progression	Left coronary artery, left anterior descending artery	II, III, aV$_F$
Posterior	V$_1$, V$_2$	R greater than S, ST-segment depression, elevated T wave (mirror change)	Right coronary artery, circumflex artery	
Apical	V$_3$, V$_4$, V$_5$, V$_6$	Q, ST, T, loss of R-wave progression	Left anterior descending artery, right coronary artery	
Anterolateral	I, aV$_L$, V$_4$, V$_5$, V$_6$	Q, ST, T	Left anterior descending artery, circumflex artery	II, III, aV$_F$
Anteroseptal	V$_1$, V$_2$, V$_3$	Q, ST, T, loss of septal R wave in lead V$_1$	Left anterior descending artery	
Subendocardial	Any of the above	ST, T for more than 3 days with cardiac enzyme changes		

b. An anteroseptal infarction results from occlusion of the left anterior descending coronary artery, resulting in serious left ventricular dysfunction; ECG changes include loss of R-wave progression in leads V$_1$ and V$_2$, the presence of Q waves in leads V$_2$ through V$_4$, and ST-segment elevation and T-wave inversion (usually without reciprocal changes) in leads V$_4$ and V$_5$

c. An anterolateral infarction results from occlusion of the circumflex coronary artery; ECG changes include the presence of Q waves, ST-segment changes, and T-wave changes in leads I, aV$_L$, and V$_4$ through V$_6$ as well as reciprocal changes in leads I and aV$_L$

    3. Inferior wall infarctions result from occlusion of the right coronary artery; ECG changes include ST-segment elevation in leads II, III, and aV_F; reciprocal ST-segment depression in leads I and aV_L; and abnormal Q waves in leads II, III, and aV_F

    4. Posterior wall infarctions result from occlusion of the circumflex branch of the left or right coronary artery; ECG changes include tall R waves and ST-segment depression in leads V_1 and V_2

D. Clinical signs and symptoms

    1. Prolonged, severe chest pain lasting 30 minutes or more and usually located in the substernal or left precordial area

        a. The patient may describe the pain as a heaviness or tightness

        b. The pain may radiate to the back, jaw, neck, or left arm and is not relieved by rest or nitrates

    2. Changes in cardiac enzyme levels, especially creatine kinase (CK) and lactate dehydrogenase (LD)

        a. CK, the most sensitive indicator of acute MI, can be detected 4 hours after an acute MI occurs, peaks at 12 to 24 hours, and returns to the baseline value in 72 to 96 hours; the CK-MB isoenzyme is specific to cardiac tissue

        b. LD is detected 8 to 12 hours after an acute MI occurs, peaks at 3 days, and returns to the baseline value in 10 to 14 days; the LD_1 isoenzyme predominates in cardiac muscle tissue after an MI

           (1) In the normal heart, LD_2 levels usually are greater than LD_1 levels

           (2) With cardiac muscle damage, LD_1 levels are greater than LD_2 levels; this reversal in LD levels is characteristic of an acute MI

E. Medical management

    1. Relieve pain with morphine sulfate (morphine also decreases anxiety, restlessness, autonomic nervous system activity, and cardiac preload)

    2. Administer I.V. beta-blocking drugs to reduce infarct size and decrease mortality

    3. Unless contraindicated, initiate thrombolytic therapy during the early stage of an acute MI (0 to 6 hours after onset of chest pain) to prevent or limit myocardial necrosis

    4. Administer oxygen for 24 to 48 hours to prevent or treat hypoxia

    5. Maintain continuous cardiac monitoring to detect ventricular arrhythmias

    6. Maintain the patient on bed rest with bedside commode privileges

    7. Administer stool softeners and antiplatelet agents

    8. Administer nitroglycerin to dilate coronary arteries and to reduce afterload, workload of the heart, and chest pain

F. Nursing management

1. Assess the patient's chest pain on a scale of 1 to 10, noting its type, location, and duration as well as precipitating events and relieving factors
2. Administer medication, as prescribed, and assess the patient's response to pain medication
3. Be prepared to initiate thrombolytic therapy; because 85% of coronary artery occlusions are caused by a blood clot, initiation of thrombolytic treatment (to reestablish perfusion) within 4 to 6 hours after onset of chest pain can significantly reduce mortality
4. Maintain a patent I.V. line to ensure access if emergency medications need to be administered
5. Monitor the patient's use of oxygen for the first 24 to 48 hours, as prescribed; oxygen therapy is used to prevent and treat hypoxia, and the nasal cannula commonly is not worn properly by the patient
6. Maintain continuous cardiac monitoring, especially in the leads showing ST-segment elevation and depression, to detect ventricular arrhythmias and to monitor ST-segment status in the leads that reflect the affected area of heart
7. Explain to the patient that bed rest decreases the heart's workload and myocardial oxygen consumption
8. Make the patient as comfortable as possible; also tell the patient to avoid using the knee gatch on the bed and crossing the legs in bed (these actions slow venous return and increase the risk of thrombus formation)
9. Assess for normal bowel habits and administer stool softeners, as prescribed, to decrease the risk of constipation and straining; if possible, maintain the patient's normal bowel regimen
10. Administer anticoagulants, as prescribed, to decrease the incidence of embolic complications; monitor the patient, as needed, to assess the effectiveness of therapy
    a. Monitor prothrombin time (PT); normal PT is 11 to 12.5 seconds, and the therapeutic range is 1.5 to 2 times the normal range
    b. Monitor partial thromboplastin time (PTT); notify the doctor if it is not within the normal range (35 to 45 seconds)
    c. Monitor the international normalized ratio (INR); the recommended INR target range for a patient on warfarin is 2.5 to 3.5
11. Unless contraindicated, administer antiplatelet agents, as prescribed, to decrease platelet aggregation; antiplatelet medications should be administered at the same time each day to maintain therapeutic drug levels
12. Assess the patient's anxiety level and initiate measures to decrease anxiety, including maintaining a quiet environment, maintaining a calm demeanor, offering reassurance, permitting family members to visit, and providing explanations for all procedures; high anxiety levels contribute to increased myocardial oxygen demands

13. Educate the patient about the atherosclerotic disease process, modification of risk factors, diet and exercise programs, medication regimen, cardiac rehabilitation, and available support groups; increasing the patient's knowledge level can help the patient make informed health care decisions

VI. Acute heart failure

A. Description

1. Acute heart failure has a sudden onset; it occurs secondary to a precipitating factor that causes a decrease in cardiac output
2. Left-sided heart failure is caused by failure of the left ventricle to pump, thereby resulting in pulmonary congestion and edema or decreased cardiac output; it usually is secondary to left ventricular infarction, hypertension, or aortic or mitral valve disease
3. Right-sided heart failure usually is caused by failure of the right ventricle to pump secondary to left-sided heart failure; it also may be caused by a pulmonary embolus or right ventricular infarction
4. In patients with nonacute heart failure, three compensatory mechanisms that enhance cardiac output (by manipulating heart rate, preload, contractility, and afterload) are activated
   a. Increased sympathetic activity in the adrenergic system stimulates the release of epinephrine, resulting in peripheral vasoconstriction, increased venous return, and increased preload
   b. The renin-angiotensin-aldosterone system constricts the renal arterioles, which decreases the glomerular filtration rate, increases the reabsorption of sodium, and promotes fluid retention
   c. The development of ventricular hypertrophy increases the force of each contraction, which helps the ventricles overcome an increase in afterload

B. Clinical signs and symptoms

1. Left-sided heart failure: dyspnea, orthopnea, wheezing, tachypnea, S_3 gallop, nocturnal angina, paroxysmal nocturnal dyspnea, PAWP greater than 20 mm Hg, and moist crackles
2. Right-sided heart failure: systemic venous congestion, jugular venous pressure greater than 8 cm, elevated CVP, hepatomegaly, dependent pitting edema, and peripheral edema

C. Medical management

1. Remove the precipitating cause and correct the underlying cause
2. Reduce cardiac workload by prescribing bed rest, small meals, weight reduction if the patient is overweight, and small doses of sedatives if the patient is anxious
3. Enhance myocardial contractility by administering digitalis glycosides (such as digoxin), sympathomimetic agents (such as dopamine or dobutamine), or other drugs that have a positive inotropic effect (such as amrinone)
4. Control excess fluid retention with a low-sodium diet, diuretic therapy, and vasodilating therapy with nitrates

5. Administer morphine sulfate to effect vasodilation and to decrease the patient's anxiety
6. Administer oxygen therapy
7. Insert a pulmonary artery catheter to monitor left ventricular function
8. Raise the head of the bed or let the patient dangle the legs over the bed with the feet dependent; this helps improve the patient's pulmonary status

D. Nursing management

1. Monitor blood pressure, heart rate, respirations, heart and lung sounds, level of consciousness, and hemodynamic parameters every 1 to 2 hours or as needed to detect signs and symptoms of decreased cardiac output or disease progression or improvement
2. Maintain the patient on bed rest with the head of the bed elevated 30 to 60 degrees, administer oxygen as prescribed, and promote rest by spacing treatments; these interventions can decrease myocardial oxygen demand and facilitate ventilation
3. Administer drugs, as prescribed, and monitor for signs and symptoms of toxicity; vasodilators decrease preload and afterload, inotropic agents improve contractility and renal blood flow, and diuretics decrease circulating volume
4. To detect fluid retention, weigh the patient daily, keep an accurate record of intake and output, and auscultate heart and lung sounds
5. Maintain a patent I.V. line to ensure access if emergency medications need to be administered
6. Restrict dietary sodium and fluid intake to control sodium reabsorption and fluid retention
7. Monitor electrolyte results and report abnormalities to the doctor; loop diuretics typically cause hypokalemia
8. Provide frequent, small meals; patients with heart failure often have a feeling of fullness, experience nausea and vomiting, and have difficulty eating and breathing simultaneously
9. Assess skin integrity and initiate measures to prevent skin breakdown and enhance circulation, including turning the patient every 2 hours, using a turning sheet, and keeping linens clean and free of wrinkles
10. Educate the patient about the disease process, the drug regimen and its adverse effects, and the need for a sodium-restricted diet
11. Tell the patient to weigh self every morning and to report a weight gain of more than 2 lb (0.9 kg) in a 24-hour period
12. Instruct the patient to pace all activities, to rest in the middle of the day, and to rest on weekends if the patient worked during the week

VII. Acute peripheral vascular insufficiency
  A. Description
    1. The incidence of acute peripheral vascular insufficiency increases with age; the chief contributing factors are atherosclerosis, hypertension, and certain cardiac disorders (including mitral valve disease, rheumatic heart disease, atrial fibrillation, left atrial myxoma, and prosthetic valves)
    2. Acute peripheral vascular insufficiency primarily is caused by thrombi resulting from cardiac disorders; in 95% of cases, the lower extremities are involved
      a. Venous thrombosis can be precipitated by injury to the vessel, hypercoagulability, or prolonged immobility
      b. Acute arterial insufficiency can result from thrombosis, embolism, or trauma
    3. An embolus can travel through the systemic circulation and lodge in an arterial branch, thus occluding the blood flow
      a. This blockage causes a secondary thrombus to form along the arterial wall, which compromises collateral circulation
      b. The distal tissues are deprived of oxygen, thereby leading to ischemia, pain, and paresthesia in the affected area
      c. If ischemia is prolonged, cellular damage leads to muscle necrosis
    4. Complications of acute peripheral vascular insufficiency include gangrene and muscle necrosis, with the possible need for limb amputation
  B. Medical management
    1. Perform arteriography with percutaneous transluminal coronary angioplasty if indicated
    2. Administer anticoagulants to maintain the PTT at twice the normal value
    3. Administer fibrinolytic agents
    4. If possible, perform an embolectomy before advanced ischemia occurs
    5. Amputate the limb if advanced ischemia has occurred
  C. Nursing management
    1. Assess arterial pulses distal to the occlusion every 1 to 2 hours to check arterial blood flow to the extremity; use Doppler ultrasonography to evaluate the presence of hard-to-palpate pulses
    2. Check skin color and temperature of the affected extremity, and assess for absence of sensation and level of motor deficit
    3. Monitor vital signs and cardiac rhythm; an arterial embolus commonly is associated with myocardial disease
    4. Maintain the patient on bed rest during the acute phase to reduce the oxygen demand of the extremity
    5. To maintain optimal gravitational blood flow, do not raise the affected extremity above the level of the heart

6. To prevent further embolization, administer anticoagulants as prescribed; monitor PTT results and notify the doctor if they are not within the therapeutic range (that is, twice the normal value)

7. Assess the patient's level of pain, and administer analgesics as prescribed; pain usually is alleviated when the obstruction and ischemia are relieved

8. Use a bed cradle, cotton blankets, or sheepskin as needed to protect the extremity from injury

9. Educate the patient about the disease process and its possible causes and treatment; tell the patient to avoid crossing the legs and sitting or standing for prolonged periods (which can cause pooling or obstruction of blood flow); teach the patient about the importance of anticoagulant therapy and follow-up clotting studies to monitor the effectiveness of anticoagulant therapy; advise the patient to avoid extreme temperatures and to always wear shoes

VIII. Angina

A. Description

1. Angina is a severe, constricting pain that is classified as stable, variant, or unstable

2. Stable angina begins gradually, reaching maximal intensity in a few minutes before dissipating

   a. It is precipitated by activity, tachycardia, systemic hypertension, thyrotoxicosis, sympathomimetic drugs, systemic illness, or anemia

   b. Correction of the precipitating event or the administration of I.V. nitroglycerin usually terminates the episode of angina

3. Variant (Prinzmetal's) angina is a reversible reduction in the diameter of the coronary artery that is caused by coronary artery spasms and results in severe myocardial ischemia

   a. Variant angina often occurs when the patient is not active and has no precipitating factors

   b. Treatment is aimed at decreasing the incidence of spasm with vasodilators or calcium channel blockers

4. Unstable angina is a change in previously stable angina or new onset of severe angina

   a. There is a progressive increase in the frequency and severity of anginal pain, and the pain is induced by less exertion than previously; the pain may last up to 30 minutes and may be only partially relieved by rest or nitrates; pain is not accompanied by cardiac enzyme level changes or ECG changes characteristic of infarction

   b. Precipitating factors include worsening of atherosclerosis in multiple vessels, left main coronary artery disease, increases in localized platelet agglutination, acute or chronic thrombosis, plaque hemorrhage or fissure, acute vasoconstriction, and mechanical problems after acute MI (such as left ventricular aneurysm, ruptured papillary muscle, ventricular septal defect, or left-sided heart failure)

B. Clinical signs and symptoms
   1. Chest pain lasting up to 30 minutes
   2. Transient ECG changes with chest pain
   3. No changes in cardiac enzyme levels

C. Medical management
   1. Administer beta-blocking agents to reduce heart rate, contractility, and blood pressure
   2. Administer nitrates to decrease blood flow to the heart, thereby reducing left ventricular filling pressure; nitrates also dilate coronary arteries and decrease peripheral resistance, which reduces myocardial oxygen consumption
   3. Administer calcium channel blockers to relax the vascular smooth muscle
   4. Control hypertension and heart failure to help relieve angina
   5. Maintain bed rest until the episode of angina is controlled
   6. Administer sedatives to reduce the patient's anxiety
   7. Administer I.V. heparin to prevent thromboembolism formation during bed rest
   8. Administer oxygen to reduce ischemia

D. Nursing management
   1. Assess the patient's anginal pain and his or her activity before the onset of pain to determine precipitating factors
   2. Administer medications, as prescribed, to control pain
      a. Nitrates relieve pain through venous and arterial dilation
      b. Morphine sulfate relieves pain by reducing the autonomic response
   3. Request an immediate ECG while the patient is experiencing chest pain to document if ischemia or infarction exists
   4. To reduce myocardial oxygen demand, restrict the patient's activity until the angina is controlled
   5. Administer nitrates and beta-blocking agents, as prescribed
      a. Nitrates reduce afterload
      b. Beta-blocking agents decrease myocardial ischemia by decreasing contractility and reducing the workload of the heart
   6. Educate the patient about the atherosclerotic disease process, modification of risk factors, diet and exercise programs, drug regimen, cardiac rehabilitation, and available support groups; increasing the patient's knowledge level can help the patient make informed health care decisions

First-degree atrioventricular block

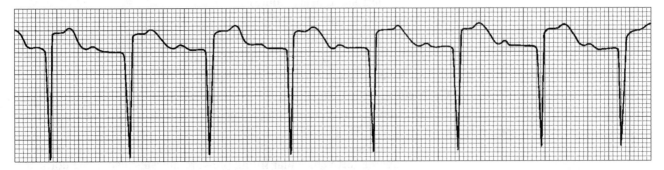

IX. First-degree atrioventricular block

    A. Description

        1. First-degree AV block results when conduction is delayed at the AV node or the His-Purkinje system, causing a prolonged PR interval on the ECG

        2. A first-degree AV block may occur in healthy people; secondary to treatment with antiarrhythmic medications; or in association with rheumatic fever, chronic degenerative disease of the conduction system, hypokalemia, hyperkalemia, hypothyroidism, or inferior wall MI

    B. Defining characteristics

        1. Atrial and ventricular rhythm: regular (for a sample ECG rhythm strip, see *First-degree atrioventricular block*)

        2. Atrial and ventricular rates: usually between 60 and 100 beats/ minute

        3. P wave: normal

        4. PR interval: prolonged but constant

            a. A PR interval of 0.21 to 0.24 second indicates slight block

            b. A PR interval of 0.25 to 0.29 second indicates moderate block

            c. A PR interval of 0.30 second or more indicates severe block

        5. QRS complex: usually within normal limits

        6. T wave: normal

    C. Clinical signs and symptoms

        1. Usually produces no symptoms

        2. Pulse rate slow to normal

    D. Medical management

        1. Treat the underlying cause

        2. Monitor ECG for worsening of AV block

        3. Administer I.V. atropine if symptomatic bradycardia occurs

    E. Nursing management

        1. Maintain continuous ECG monitoring to observe for worsening of AV block

        2. Be prepared to administer I.V. atropine if symptomatic bradycardia develops; atropine is a cholinergic blocker that blocks the action of acetylcholine in the SA and AV nodes

X. **Second-degree atrioventricular block, Mobitz type I**

    A. Description

        1. Second-degree AV block, Mobitz type I, results when diseased AV nodal tissue conducts impulses increasingly earlier in the refractory period until an impulse arrives during the absolute refractory period, when it cannot be conducted

        2. Second-degree AV block, Mobitz type I, may be caused by inferior wall MI, cardiac surgery, acute rheumatic fever, vagal stimulation, digitalis glycoside toxicity, or the use of propranolol, quinidine, or procainamide

        3. The ECG shows a constant P-P interval, a progressively longer PR interval, and a progressively shorter R-R interval; after several cycles, there is a missing QRS complex; the PR interval shortens after the missed beat, then progressively lengthens again; this pattern has the visual effect of "group beating"

    B. Defining characteristics

        1. Atrial rhythm: regular (for a sample ECG rhythm strip, see *Second-degree atrioventricular block, Mobitz type I,* page 46)

        2. Ventricular rhythm: irregular, with the R-R interval shortening until a P wave appears without a QRS complex

        3. Atrial rate: greater than the ventricular rate but usually within normal limits

        4. Ventricular rate: slower than the atrial rate but usually within normal limits

        5. P wave: normal

        6. PR interval: progressively lengthens until a P wave appears without a QRS complex; the PR interval after the nonconducted beat is shorter than the previous beat's PR interval

        7. QRS complex: periodically absent, but within normal limits

        8. T wave: usually normal

    C. Clinical signs and symptoms

        1. Usually produces no symptoms

        2. Pulse rate usually normal, with occasional irregularity

        3. Symptoms of decreased cardiac output if ventricular rate is too slow

    D. Medical management

        1. Treat the underlying cause

        2. Monitor ECG for worsening of AV block

        3. If symptomatic bradycardia occurs, administer I.V. atropine and consider a temporary pacemaker

Second-degree atrioventricular block, Mobitz type I

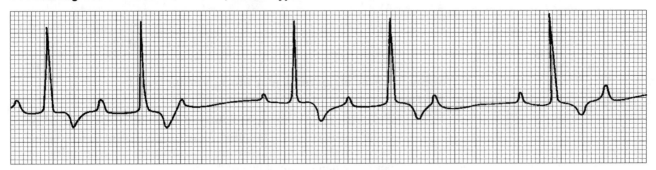

    E. Nursing management
1. Maintain continuous ECG monitoring to observe for worsening of AV block
2. Be prepared to administer I.V. atropine if symptomatic bradycardia develops; atropine is a cholinergic blocker that blocks the action of acetylcholine in the SA and AV nodes

XI. Second-degree atrioventricular block, Mobitz type II
    A. Description
1. Second-degree AV block, Mobitz type II (also called classic second-degree AV block) results when a conduction disturbance in the His-Purkinje system causes an intermittent block
2. Second-degree AV block, Mobitz type II, is caused by organic heart disease, acute anterior wall MI, severe coronary artery disease, and acute myocarditis
3. There is no warning on the ECG before a beat is blocked, and there can be any number of dropped beats before a beat is conducted; the block is referred to by the number of beats dropped, that is, 2:1, 3:1, or 4:1 block

    B. Defining characteristics
1. Atrial rhythm: regular (for a sample ECG rhythm strip, see *Second-degree atrioventricular block, Mobitz type II*)
2. Ventricular rhythm: regular (even if the block is constant) or irregular
3. Atrial rate: usually within normal limits
4. Ventricular rate: normal to slow; may be slower than the atrial rate
5. P wave: normal, with regular P-P interval
6. PR interval: usually within normal limits; always constant when followed by a QRS complex (the PR interval after a nonconducted beat may be shortened slightly)

Second-degree atrioventricular block, Mobitz type II

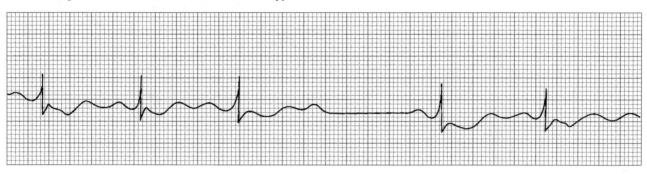

7. QRS complex: within normal limits but absent with nonconducted beat
8. T wave: normal
C. Clinical signs and symptoms
 1. Pulse rate slow to normal
 2. Pulse regular or irregular
 3. Symptoms of decreased cardiac output if pulse rate is too slow
D. Medical management
 1. Monitor ECG continuously for worsening of AV block
 2. If symptoms of decreased cardiac output develop, administer isoproterenol or use an external pacemaker to increase the heart rate
 3. Consider inserting a permanent pacemaker if indicated
E. Nursing management
 1. Monitor ECG continuously for worsening of AV block
 2. Be prepared to administer an I.V. infusion of isoproterenol if symptomatic bradycardia develops
 3. Assess the patient's level of consciousness, heart rate, and blood pressure every 2 hours or as needed to evaluate changes in clinical status that may indicate decreased cardiac output
 4. If symptoms of decreased cardiac output occur, apply an external pacemaker; symptoms of decreased cardiac output usually can be alleviated by increasing the heart rate to within normal limits; the external pacemaker is the treatment of choice if personnel are trained in its use
 5. Assess the patient's level of anxiety and degree of understanding of the problem; remain with patient when he or she is frightened
 6. Explain all procedures and protocols; information usually alleviates anxiety and gives the patient a sense of control
 7. If applicable, educate the patient about permanent pacemaker implantation

XII. Third-degree atrioventricular block

A. Description

    1. Third-degree AV block, or complete heart block, results when no impulses are conducted from the atria to the ventricles

        a. The ventricular rhythm is either junctional escape or ventricular escape, depending on whether it originates in the bundle of His or the Purkinje system, respectively

        b. Ventricular escape rhythms are slower and less stable and place the patient at risk for ventricular standstill and decreased cardiac output

    2. Acute third-degree AV block may be caused by severe digitalis glycoside toxicity or inferior wall MI; it also may occur transiently during cardiac catheterization or angioplasty

    3. Chronic third-degree AV block may be caused by bilateral bundle branch block, congenital abnormalities, rheumatic fever, hypoxia, postoperative complications of mitral valve replacement, Lev's disease, or Lenegre's disease

B. Defining characteristics

    1. Atrial and ventricular rhythms: regular (for a sample ECG rhythm strip, see *Third-degree atrioventricular block*)

    2. Atrial rate: usually within normal limits but faster than the ventricular rate

    3. Ventricular rate: usually 25 to 40 beats/minute

    4. P wave: normal

    5. PR interval: varies

    6. QRS complex: wide, bizarre complex if it originates in the ventricles; normal if it originates in the junction

    7. T wave: normal

    8. QT interval: may be normal

C. Clinical signs and symptoms

    1. Slow, regular pulse

    2. May produce no symptoms

    3. Signs and symptoms of decreased cardiac output if pulse rate is too slow

D. Medical management

    1. Monitor ECG continuously for worsening of AV block

    2. Administer I.V. atropine or isoproterenol if symptomatic bradycardia occurs

    3. Insert a temporary pacemaker and consider a permanent pacemaker if indicated

E. Nursing management

    1. Monitor ECG continuously for worsening of AV block

    2. Be prepared to administer an infusion of I.V. atropine or isoproterenol if symptomatic bradycardia develops

Third-degree atrioventricular block

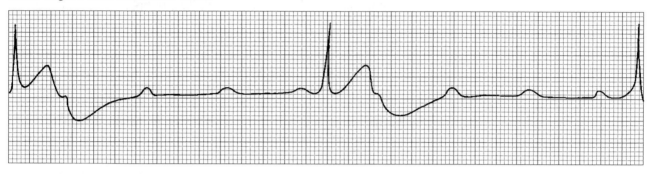

3. Assess the patient's level of consciousness, heart rate, and blood pressure every 2 hours or as needed to evaluate changes in clinical status that may indicate decreased cardiac output

4. If symptoms of decreased cardiac output occur, apply an external pacemaker; symptoms of decreased cardiac output usually can be alleviated by increasing the heart rate to within normal limits; the external pacemaker is the treatment of choice if personnel are trained in its use

5. Assess the patient's level of anxiety and degree of understanding of the problem; remain with patient when he or she is frightened

6. Explain all procedures and protocols; information usually alleviates anxiety and gives the patient a sense of control

7. If applicable, educate the patient about permanent pacemaker implantation

XIII. Aortic aneurysm

A. Description

1. There are two types of aortic aneurysm: saccular and fusiform

a. A saccular aortic aneurysm is a balloonlike dilation produced by a weakened area in the aorta and involves only a portion of the circumference of the aorta

b. A fusiform aortic aneurysm is a diffuse area of weakness that produces a spindle-shaped, balloon-like dilation that affects the total circumference of the aorta

2. Once an aneurysm develops, it worsens according to the principles of Laplace's law—a vicious circle in which the larger the diameter of the vessel, the greater the tension, and the increased tension produces progressive dilation of the aorta

3. The aneurysm expands at an unpredictable rate; the incidence of aortic rupture increases dramatically when the aneurysm reaches 6 cm in diameter

4. Risk factors for aortic aneurysm include atherosclerosis, increasing age, smoking, hypertension, increased triglyceride and low-density lipoprotein levels, decreased high-density lipoprotein levels, aortic necrosis, and trauma

    a. Atherosclerosis, the most common underlying disease, initially affects the intima of the vessel; hemorrhage into the plaque formation may invade the medial layer, causing weakness and generalized dilation of the aorta; the abdominal aorta most commonly is affected by this atherosclerotic process

    b. Increasing age is linked to a reduction in the elastin content within the media aorta, contributing to weakness of the aortic wall

    c. Smoking causes an increase in atherosclerotic plaques, ulceration, and calcification within the aorta

    d. Hypertension increases injury to the endothelium and may accelerate medial degeneration

B. Clinical signs and symptoms

    1. Usually produces no symptoms until the aneurysm begins to leak or reaches a size that impinges on other organs

    2. Ascending aortic aneurysm: commonly produces no symptoms or is associated with dyspnea and chest pain, widened pulse pressure, bounding pulse, aortic murmur, pulsating abdominal mass, and abdominal bruits

    3. Aortic arch aneurysm: dyspnea, stridor, cough, chest pain, distended jugular and arm veins, left vocal cord paralysis, abnormal pulsation of the upper anterior chest, absent breath sounds or dullness on percussion, crackles, and an S_3 heart sound

    4. Descending thoracic aortic aneurysm: intermittent or constant dull pain between the shoulders and in the lower back, abdomen, shoulders, arms, or neck; occasionally, hoarseness caused by pressure on the laryngeal nerve; seldom detected by physical examination

    5. Abdominal aneurysm: dull and constant back pain caused by pressure on the lumbar nerves, abdominal pain and bloating caused by stretching of the duodenum over an enlarged aorta

C. Medical management

    1. Check the size of the aneurysm every 6 months and repair surgically when it reaches 6 cm in diameter

    2. Control risk factors (hypertension, hypercholesterolemia, hyperlipidemia, and smoking) through changes in diet, exercise, medications, and cessation of smoking

D. Nursing management

    1. Assess the patient's level of anxiety and administer sedatives as prescribed, explain procedures and protocols, and remain with the patient and offer realistic assurance as needed; remember that the sympathetic response to anxiety can have detrimental hemodynamic effects in the perioperative period

2. Monitor vital signs, hemodynamic parameters, and level of consciousness every 15 minutes to 1 hour as needed; early recognition of deteriorating hemodynamic status increases the patient's chances of survival

3. Keep in mind that symptoms of hypovolemia will be present if the aneurysm ruptures

4. Maintain the patient on bed rest in the supine position to prevent further decreases in blood pressure

5. Maintain a patent I.V. line to ensure venous access if emergency drugs and fluids need to be administered

6. Administer fluids, as prescribed, to restore circulating blood volume

7. Record intake and output every hour to assess kidney function and circulating fluid volume

8. Educate the patient about the disease process and the importance of controlling blood pressure and adhering to a low-sodium diet; hypertension places added stress on the aneurysm and sodium retention increases blood pressure

9. Teach the patient about signs and symptoms, including back and chest pain (which indicate leakage of the aneurysm), that should be reported to the doctor

XIV. Ruptured aortic aneurysm

A. Description

1. When a weakened aorta ruptures, blood flows freely into the thoracic cavity

2. Extreme tenderness of the mass in the abdominal aorta is symptomatic of imminent rupture

B. Clinical signs and symptoms

1. Unremitting back or abdominal pain

2. Hypovolemia: weakness, light-headedness, nausea, vomiting, low blood pressure, tachycardia, and unconsciousness

C. Medical management

1. Control hypovolemia

2. Apply an external counterpulsation device (such as a pneumatic antishock garment) to minimize leakage

3. Surgically repair the ruptured area by using a synthetic graft to replace the section containing the aneurysm

D. Nursing management

1. Control hypovolemia by administering I.V. fluids, blood, or plasma as ordered

2. Apply an external counterpulsation device (such as a pneumatic antishock garment) to minimize leakage

XV. Aortic dissection

A. Description

1. Aortic dissection primarily results from a longitudinal tearing of the aortic media caused by a dissecting hematoma; blood is propelled through the torn intima into the media

2. Aortic dissection occurs most frequently in the thoracic aorta

3. It is more common in men than in women and typically occurs in people in their 60s and 70s; its mortality rate is 90% for those people who do not receive treatment

4. The underlying pathophysiologic causes of aortic dissection include intimal damage as seen with atherosclerosis, syphilis, infection, or trauma; medial degeneration secondary to Marfan's syndrome, aging, or hypertension; and shearing stress related to the hemodynamic forces of the pulse wave

B. Clinical signs and symptoms

1. Acute chest pain spreading down into the back and abdomen; pain may be intense, sharp, tearing, or stabbing

2. Symptoms indicating compromised circulation to a major artery
   a. Coronary arteries: MI
   b. Aortic valve: systolic or diastolic murmur
   c. Carotid artery: strokelike symptoms
   d. Aortic bifurcation: loss or decrease of femoral pulses
   e. Subclavian artery: blood pressure between the two arms differ significantly
   f. Erosion into esophagus: nausea and vomiting with hematemesis

3. Signs of shock but normal to high blood pressure

C. Medical management

1. Administer nitrates and beta-blocking agents to decrease blood pressure and contractility of the heart

2. Maintain the patient on bed rest

3. Administer morphine sulfate to relieve pain

4. Repair dissected area surgically if indicated

D. Nursing management

1. Monitor blood pressure, cardiac rhythm, CVP, PAP, urine output, and peripheral pulses; changes in hemodynamic pressures may indicate progression of the dissection or aortic rupture, and oliguria may indicate renal artery dissection

2. Assess the location, quality, and radiation of the pain; the location of the pain can help pinpoint the location of the dissection, and pain that increases or subsides and returns may indicate the initiation of a dissection

3. Administer medications as prescribed; opioid analgesics relieve pain; nitrates and beta-blocking agents decrease blood pressure and myocardial contractility, which reduces the shearing effect that causes dissection

4. Auscultate bowel sounds and palpate the abdomen every 2 hours to detect signs of acute abdomen, which may indicate involvement of the mesenteric artery

5. Maintain the patient on bed rest in a quiet environment

6. Assess the patient's anxiety level; institute measures to decrease anxiety to help reduce stimulation and sympathetic response

7. Educate the patient about the disease process and the importance of controlling blood pressure and abstaining from the use of tobacco products; hypertension and smoking increase the risk of aortic dissection

8. Discuss the drug regimen, activity restrictions, and the need to avoid isometric exercises

9. Teach the patient about signs and symptoms, including pain, pallor, paresthesia, paralysis, and pulselessness, that should be reported to the doctor

XVI. Aortic insufficiency *Regurg*

   A. Description

      1. Aortic insufficiency results from incompetency of the aortic valve, which may be caused by rheumatic fever, syphilis, infectious endocarditis, or connective tissue disorders (such as Marfan's syndrome)

      2. Aortic insufficiency causes the left ventricle to become overloaded and hypertrophied

      3. Left ventricular end-diastolic pressure and left atrial pressure increase over time and myocardial contractility diminishes, resulting in heart failure

   B. Clinical signs and symptoms

      1. Dyspnea on exertion, palpitations, orthopnea, chest pain on exertion, bounding pulse, and widened pulse pressure

      2. Decrescendo diastolic murmur (blowing) and high-pitched heart sounds, which are best heard at the base of the heart

      3. Systolic ejection murmur best heard at the base of the heart

   C. Medical management

      1. Intervene surgically at the onset of left ventricular dysfunction and before the development of severe symptoms

      2. Differentiate between aortic insufficiency and aortic stenosis

   D. Nursing management

      1. Prepare the patient for surgical intervention

      2. Differentiate between aortic insufficiency and aortic stenosis

XVII. Aortic stenosis

   A. Description

      1. Aortic stenosis most often is associated with congenital bicuspid or unicuspid valve formation and degenerative changes associated with aging; sometimes it is associated with rheumatic heart disease

2. Degenerative aortic stenosis is caused by thickening and calcification of the aortic cusps in people over age 65
3. In patients with aortic stenosis, increased left ventricular pressure develops; this propels blood across the valve into the aorta and leads to left ventricular hypertrophy

B. Clinical signs and symptoms
1. Fatigue, dyspnea, orthopnea, angina pectoris, dizziness, and syncope
2. Narrowed pulse pressure
3. Crescendo-decrescendo, harsh systolic murmur best heard at the base of the heart

C. Medical management
1. Restrict strenuous physical activity
2. Intervene surgically, including commissural incision into the valve under direct visualization to release the valve flaps and improve blood flow or valve replacement

D. Nursing management
1. Instruct the patient to avoid strenuous physical activity
2. Prepare the patient for surgical intervention

XVIII. Cardiac trauma
A. Penetrating cardiac trauma
1. Description
   a. Fatal in 90% of cases, penetrating cardiac trauma is caused by stab wounds or bullet wounds
   b. Penetrating trauma can lacerate any anatomic part of the heart, causing shunts, fistulas, and valve disruptions that result in murmurs
   c. Pericardial laceration resulting in cardiac tamponade or exsanguination is the most common consequence of penetrating cardiac trauma
   d. If the penetrating wound is small, cardiac tamponade can help reduce the severity of bleeding, thus improving the patient's chances of survival
2. Clinical signs and symptoms
   a. Hypotension secondary to cardiac tamponade or hemorrhage
   b. Penetrating mediastinal wound
   c. X-ray film showing object in or near cardiac silhouette
3. Medical management
   a. Immediately transport patient from the scene to a health care facility
   b. Initiate pericardiocentesis to stabilize cardiac tamponade until an emergency thoracotomy can be performed
   c. Perform immediate emergency thoracotomy to control bleeding (once bleeding is controlled, the recovery rate is about 80%)

4. Nursing management
    a. Maintain continuous ECG monitoring; damage to the heart muscle can cause ventricular arrhythmias and AV block
    b. Assess for symptoms of chest pain, and have the patient rate the pain on a scale of 1 to 10; obtain an immediate ECG to determine nature of chest pain
        (1) Chest pain caused by penetrating trauma is similar to that caused by an acute MI
        (2) An ECG is needed to differentiate among acute MI, myocardial contusion, and pericardial chest pain
    c. Monitor blood pressure, heart rate, and urine output
        (1) Hypotension may signal cardiac injury
        (2) Hypotension with tachycardia may indicate cardiac tamponade or hypovolemia
        (3) Urine output provides an indication of kidney function
    d. Auscultate breath sounds and heart sounds to assess for new murmurs and the onset of heart failure
B. Nonpenetrating cardiac trauma
    1. Description
        a. In nonpenetrating cardiac trauma, or blunt trauma, there may be no evidence of trauma to the chest wall; the severity of the chest wall trauma does not correlate with the likelihood or extent of cardiac injury
        b. Blunt trauma commonly is caused by impact (such as with the steering wheel in a car accident), resulting in injury to the sternum; tearing of the aorta or other great vessels results from the shearing forces associated with sudden deceleration
        c. Other causes of blunt trauma include a hard blow to the chest from sports activities, industrial crush injuries, falls or accidents, and personal assaults
        d. Blunt trauma may result in myocardial contusion, rupture of the ventricle or interventricular septum, pericardial laceration, valve disruption, coronary artery thrombosis, or great vessel rupture
        e. Myocardial contusion (usually in the right ventricle) is the most common blunt injury; chest pain may be masked by musculoskeletal pain, and myocardial necrosis can range from petechiae to transmural necrosis
        f. Myocardial contusion has several consequences
            (1) Arrhythmias may occur, and ventricular tachycardia should be vigorously suppressed; high-grade AV block usually is transient but may require temporary pacing
            (2) Right-sided heart failure may be caused by severe right ventricular injury; it usually is treated with digitalization, maintenance of high right-sided filling pressures, and reduction of elevated pulmonary arterial pressures

(3) Rupture of the myocardium and tearing of the interventricular septum, papillary muscles and chordae tendineae, valve cusps, or aortic annulus usually are treated surgically

(4) Cardiac tamponade typically is treated by pericardiocentesis until the cause can be determined

2. Clinical signs and symptoms
   a. Chest pain (the most common symptom) and hypotension
   b. Ventricular arrhythmia or AV block
   c. ECG changes indicating acute MI or pericarditis
   d. Pericardial rub, murmur, or muffled heart sounds
   e. Symptoms of heart failure

3. Medical management
   a. Perform cardiac catheterization with coronary angiography if cardiac enzyme levels are elevated
   b. Control pain and arrhythmias; do not administer anticoagulants
   c. Perform thoracotomy with surgical intervention if indicated

4. Nursing management
   a. Prepare the patient for cardiac catheterization
   b. Control pain and arrhythmias; do not administer anticoagulants because internal bleeding may occur
   c. Prepare the patient for thoracotomy and surgical intervention if indicated

XIX. Cardiogenic shock

A. Description

1. Cardiogenic shock results from loss of more than 40% of the functional myocardium

2. It may be caused by left ventricular dysfunction (secondary to acute MI), ischemia, inflammatory diseases, papillary muscle rupture, left ventricular free wall rupture, acute ventricular septal defect, end-stage cardiomyopathy, severe valvular dysfunction, myocardial contusion, cardiac tamponade, or left atrial myxoma

3. It also may result from thrombus formation or massive pulmonary embolus formation, which causes hypoperfusion of vital organs; this lack of perfusion results in inadequate cellular oxygen delivery and local accumulation of toxic cellular waste

B. Stages of cardiogenic shock

1. Stage I (initial stage): decreased cardiac output without clinical symptoms

2. Stage II (compensatory stage): decreased cardiac output with early clinical signs and symptoms
   a. Sympathetic compensatory mechanisms are activated, resulting in increased heart rate and increased force of ventricular contraction

      b. Hormonal compensatory mechanisms trigger secretion of renin, angiotensin, and aldosterone, resulting in increased reabsorption of sodium and water

   3. Stage III (progressive stage): compensatory mechanisms become ineffective as cardiac workload and oxygen demand increase

      a. Acidosis allows blood to leak out of the capillary bed, causing fluid to shift into the interstitial space

      b. Sustained vasoconstriction results in cold and pulseless fingers, toes, tip of the nose, and earlobes

   4. Stage IV (refractory stage): shock state is irreversible

C. Clinical signs and symptoms

   1. Systolic blood pressure less than 90 mm Hg or a 30- to 60-mm Hg decrease in systolic pressure in a previously hypertensive patient

   2. Tachycardia with neck vein distention

   3. Increased CVP, PAP, PAWP, and systemic vascular resistance (SVR)

   4. Decreased cardiac output

   5. Oliguria (less than 20 ml/hour) secondary to decreased renal perfusion

   6. Rapid, thready pulse

   7. Rapid, shallow respirations with crackles and rhonchi; may progress to pulmonary edema

   8. Decreased peristalsis, resulting in absent bowel sounds

   9. Restlessness, agitation, confusion, or obtundation

  10. Cool, pale, diaphoretic skin becoming mottled and cyanotic as cardiogenic shock progresses

D. Medical management

   1. Insert an arterial line and a pulmonary artery catheter to monitor arterial pressure, left ventricular filling pressure, and cardiac output

   2. Administer oxygen therapy based on patient's oxygen saturation level

   3. Use intra-aortic balloon counterpulsation to decrease afterload

   4. Administer analgesics to control pain, vasopressors to raise the arterial pressure, crystalloids or diuretics to keep PAWP at less than 20 mm Hg, positive inotropic agents to increase contractility, and venous vasodilators to decrease preload

E. Nursing management

   1. Continuously monitor PAP, PAWP, cardiac output, urine output, skin color and temperature, peripheral pulses, level of consciousness, respiratory status, and bowel sounds; these evaluations are needed to assess tissue and organ perfusion

   2. Administer medications as prescribed; use the smallest amount of solution possible when mixing I.V. infusions and use infusion pumps; keep precise records of intake and output

      a. I.V. drugs are potent medications that must be administered carefully

      b. Fluids commonly are restricted in cardiogenic shock to decrease circulating volume

  3. Implement safety precautions (including monitoring the patient's level of consciousness, reorienting the patient as needed, and decreasing sensory stimulation) and administer oxygen therapy as prescribed; changes in mentation occur secondary to decreased cerebral perfusion or tissue hypoxia

  4. Maintain skin integrity by using heel and elbow protectors, special mattresses, frequent turning, and passive range-of-motion exercises; skin breakdown may result from hypoperfusion

XX. Cardiomyopathies

A. General information

  1. Cardiomyopathies are classified as primary (if the heart is the only organ affected with no involvement of valves or other cardiac structures) or secondary (if the myocardial abnormality is related to another abnormality or condition and other organs are affected)

  2. Cardiomyopathies are further classified by pathophysiologic changes as dilated (congestive), hypertrophic, or restrictive (see *Morphologic and hemodynamic characteristics of cardiomyopathies*)

B. Dilated cardiomyopathy

  1. Description

    a. Dilated cardiomyopathy results from damage to the myofibrils

    b. All four heart chambers are dilated, and contractile function of the ventricles is impaired; thrombus formation occurs most commonly in the ventricles

    c. Cardiomegaly and impairment of systolic pump function leads to heart failure

    d. Cardiac output declines as the disease progresses, with the final result being biventricular pump failure

  2. Clinical signs and symptoms

    a. Dyspnea on exertion that progresses to orthopnea; paroxysmal nocturnal dyspnea; and dyspnea at rest

    b. Fatigue and weakness; symptoms of biventricular failure

    c. Chest pain

    d. Narrowed pulse pressure

    e. Laterally displaced apical pulse

    f. Decreased cardiac output

    g. Increased right atrial pressure (RAP), PAP, PAWP, and SVR

  3. Medical management

    a. Restrict the patient's activity, sodium intake, and fluid intake

    b. Maintain continuous ECG monitoring

    c. Administer oxygen as needed

    d. Monitor hemodynamic parameters to assess left ventricular function and cardiac output

Morphologic and hemodynamic characteristics of cardiomyopathies

	Dilated	Hypertrophic	Restrictive
Morphologic characteristics	Biventricular dilation	Marked hypertrophy of left ventricle and, occasionally, of right ventricle; usually disproportionate hypertrophy of septum	Reduced ventricular compliance; usually caused by infiltration of myocardium (for example, by amyloid or glycogen deposits)
Hemodynamic characteristics			
Cardiac output	Decreased	Normal	Normal to decreased
Stroke volume	Decreased	Normal or increased	Normal or decreased
Ventricular filling pressure	Increased	Normal or increased	Increased
Chamber size	Increased	Normal or decreased	Normal or increased
Ejection fraction	Decreased	Increased	Normal to decreased
Diastolic compliance	Normal or decreased	Decreased	Decreased
Other findings	• May have associated functional mitral or tricuspid insufficiency	• Obstruction may develop between interventricular septum and septal leaflet of mitral valve • Mitral insufficiency may be present	• Characteristic ventricular pressure tracings that resemble those recorded in constrictive pericarditis

    e. Use intra-aortic balloon counterpulsation as needed

    f. Administer digitalis glycosides, diuretics, vasodilators, and antiarrhythmic medications

    g. Consider heart transplantation if indicated

4. Nursing management

    a. Monitor blood pressure, hemodynamic parameters, and intake and output to detect early or progressive signs of low cardiac output

    b. Monitor for excessive fluid volume and increased congestion by weighing the patient daily, recording intake and output, auscultating breath sounds and heart sounds, and checking RAP, PAP, and PAWP; weighing the patient daily can help to determine the response to therapy and the amount of fluid retention

      c. Restrict sodium and fluid intake, as prescribed, to decrease fluid retention

      d. Coordinate care to provide the patient with frequent rest periods; uninterrupted rest can help restore the patient's physical and psychological well-being

      e. Increase the patient's level of activity gradually and help the patient as needed

      f. Assess the patient's level of knowledge about the disease process, and educate him or her about the disease and its treatment

      g. Help the patient develop coping strategies that give the patient a sense of control over the situation

      h. Refer the patient to support groups for people with heart disease; support groups can alleviate feelings of isolation and are a source of information about the disease

      i. Encourage family members to learn CPR; ventricular arrhythmias associated with dilated cardiomyopathy are a common cause of sudden cardiac death; performing CPR can increase the patient's chances of survival

C. Hypertrophic cardiomyopathy

  1. Description

      a. Hypertrophic cardiomyopathy is a disproportionate thickening of the interventricular septum; this overgrowth of muscle makes the ventricular walls rigid, thus obstructing left ventricular outflow and impeding left ventricular ejection during systole

      b. The atria become hypertrophied and dilated as a result of the high resistance to ventricular filling

      c. Hypertrophic cardiomyopathy may be genetically transmitted, occurs equally in men and in women, and is seen in young adults

  2. Clinical signs and symptoms

      a. Dyspnea, shortness of breath, angina, fatigue, palpitations, and syncope

      b. Normal cardiac output with elevated RAP, PAP, PAWP, and SVR

  3. Medical management

      a. Restrict the patient's activity, sodium intake, and fluid intake

      b. Maintain continuous ECG monitoring

      c. Administer oxygen as needed

      d. Monitor hemodynamic parameters to assess left ventricular function and cardiac output

      e. Use intra-aortic balloon counterpulsation as needed

      f. Administer beta-adrenergic blocking agents, calcium channel blockers, and antiarrhythmic medications

      g. Consider myotomy or myectomy if indicated

  4. Nursing management

      a. Same as for dilated cardiomyopathy

      b. Educate the patient about a low-sodium, fluid-restricted diet

D. Restrictive cardiomyopathy
  1. Description
      a. Restrictive cardiomyopathy results in abnormal diastolic filling secondary to excessively rigid ventricular walls
      b. Fibroelastic tissue infiltrates the endocardium or myocardium; contractility is mostly unimpaired, with normal systolic emptying of the ventricles
      c. Hemodynamically, restrictive cardiomyopathy resembles constrictive pericarditis
  2. Clinical signs and symptoms
      a. Fatigue, exercise intolerance, and symptoms of right-sided heart failure
      b. Narrowed pulse pressure
      c. Low cardiac output with increased RAP, PAP, PAWP, and SVR
  3. Medical management
      a. Restrict the patient's activity, sodium intake, and fluid intake
      b. Maintain continuous ECG monitoring
      c. Administer oxygen as needed
      d. Monitor hemodynamic parameters to assess left ventricular function and cardiac output
      e. Use intra-aortic balloon counterpulsation as needed
      f. Administer digitalis glycosides and diuretics
      g. Consider excision of fibrotic endocardium if indicated
  4. Nursing management
      a. Same as for dilated cardiomyopathy
      b. Educate the patient about the proper use of medications and their adverse effects as well as about dietary restrictions

XXI. Hypertensive crisis
  A. Description
  1. A hypertensive crisis is defined as a diastolic blood pressure of 120 mm Hg or higher
  2. It occurs in less than 1% of hypertensive patients and usually in those whose hypertension is poorly controlled or untreated
  3. Although the cause is unknown, hypertensive crisis commonly is associated with preeclampsia, acute or chronic renal disease, acute central nervous system events, and ingestion of foods that contain tyramine by patients taking monoamine oxidase inhibitors
  4. Hypertensive crisis is a life-threatening event that can cause irreversible damage to vital organs
  5. Pathologic changes associated with hypertensive crisis include arterial dilation and contraction resulting in encephalopathy, microangiopathic hemolytic anemia contributing to deterioration of renal function, and arteriolar fibrinoid necrosis

      6. Activation of the renin-angiotensin-aldosterone system in response to decreased renal blood supply caused by hypertensive changes can raise blood pressure even higher

B. Clinical signs and symptoms

      1. Rapid increase in blood pressure, usually above 120 mm Hg diastolic

      2. Grade III or IV retinopathy with or without papilledema

      3. Restlessness, confusion, somnolence, blurred vision, headache, nausea, and vomiting

      4. Proteinuria, hematuria, red blood cell casts, azotemia, oliguria, hemolytic anemia, and epistaxis

      5. Hypertensive encephalopathy with severe headache, vomiting, vision disturbances, seizures, stupor, and coma

C. Medical management

      1. Administer beta-blocking agents and diuretics to reduce blood pressure

      2. Recommend a sodium-restricted diet, exercise program, weight reduction in overweight patients, stress reduction, and smoking cessation

D. Nursing management

      1. Continuously monitor blood pressure, heart rate, and heart rhythm to assess the effects of antihypertensive medications

      2. Maintain a patent I.V. line for administration of antihypertensive medications, and assess the line every 4 hours for infiltration or extravasation, which may cause localized tissue damage

      3. Titrate antihypertensive medications carefully because hypertensive patients can become hypotensive rapidly

      4. Monitor for toxic effects of medications; nitroprusside sodium infusions are associated with bleeding tendencies and may cause agitation and disorientation at toxic doses

      5. Assess urine output, monitor CVP or PAWP if available, and check neurologic function; report trends or changes in the patient's condition to the doctor

      6. Check for symptoms of hypovolemia or hypervolemia

      7. Because uncompensated sensory losses place the patient at risk for physical injury, implement safety precautions, including monitoring the patient's level of consciousness every hour, implementing seizure precautions, reorienting the patient as needed, decreasing sensory stimulation, and applying adequate pressure to puncture sites

      8. Assess the patient's level of pain (patients in hypertensive crisis typically complain of severe headache) and administer analgesics as prescribed; when dressing and immobilizing cannulated areas, be sure to maximize patient movement and comfort

      9. Help the patient change position gradually to reduce the likelihood of orthostatic hypotension

10. Provide the patient with hard candy, ice chips, and good oral care to alleviate dry oral mucosa (an adverse effect of antihypertensive therapy)

11. Assess the patient's level of anxiety and administer sedatives as prescribed; the patient may be anxious because he or she is in an unfamiliar environment, is experiencing a lack of control, and may be fearful of death or the unknown consequences of the crisis

12. Allow family members to visit, and ensure the patient's privacy

XXII. Hypovolemic shock

   A. Description

   1. Hypovolemic shock results when 30% to 40% of blood volume is lost

   2. Hemorrhage and dehydration are the principal causes

      a. Fluid loss may result from diarrhea, diabetes insipidus, vomiting, or overuse of diuretics

      b. Fluid loss into the extravascular compartment is a nonhemorrhagic cause of hypovolemic shock

   3. If the vascular volume is not replaced within 90 minutes, the state of shock may be irreversible

   B. Clinical signs and symptoms

   1. Cool, clammy, mottled skin

   2. Systolic blood pressure less than 90 mm Hg

   3. Agitation, confusion, or obtundation

   4. Urine output less than 30 ml/hour

   C. Medical management

   1. Initiate rapid corrective fluid therapy—including blood, blood products, and plasma expanders—to replace blood loss and crystalloid solutions to replace plasma or fluid losses

   2. Use oxygen therapy to maintain partial pressure of arterial oxygen at 80 mm Hg or above

   3. Monitor hemodynamic parameters to assess fluid status

   4. Monitor ABG values to assess acid-base balance

   5. Monitor urine output

   6. Give nothing by mouth if the patient is unconscious; give ice chips and liquid if the patient can swallow

   7. Maintain the patient on complete bed rest with the head of the bed flat

   8. Treat the underlying cause after the immediate crisis has passed

   D. Nursing management

   1. To facilitate circulation and increase venous return, maintain the patient on complete bed rest with the head of the bed flat and the legs elevated 6″ to 8″ (15 to 20 cm) above the head of the bed

   2. Monitor vital signs, neurologic function, intake and output, and peripheral pulses every 15 minutes to 1 hour as indicated; as the state of shock progresses, vital functions will deteriorate rapidly

3. Monitor for symptoms of decreased cardiac output and report changes to the doctor

4. Administer fluids, as prescribed, to restore blood volume

5. Keep an accurate record of intake and output to assess kidney function

6. Administer oxygen therapy and monitor ABG values, as prescribed, to ensure optimal oxygen delivery and gas exchange

7. Weigh the patient daily to assess overall fluid status

8. Assess skin integrity and initiate measures to prevent skin breakdown and enhance circulation, including turning the patient every 2 hours, using a turning sheet, and keeping linens clean and free of wrinkles

9. Assess the patient's level of anxiety and administer sedatives as prescribed; the patient may be anxious because he or she is in an unfamiliar environment, is experiencing a lack of control, and may be fearful of death or the unknown consequences of the crisis

10. Allow family members to visit, and ensure the patient's privacy

XXIII. Infectious endocarditis

A. Description

1. Endocarditis is caused by a microbial infection (bacteria, fungi, *Rickettsia,* or *Chlamydia*) of the endothelial tissue of the heart valves

   a. Acute infectious endocarditis ordinarily involves the normal heart and is common in I.V. drug abusers

   b. Subacute infectious endocarditis usually involves the abnormal heart

   c. Right-sided endocarditis is most common in I.V. drug abusers but may occur as a result of an infected peripheral or CVP catheter or transvenous pacing wires; it manifests as acute endocarditis with pulmonary infarction and abscess formation

2. Patients at greatest risk for infectious endocarditis are those with preexisting heart disease, including congenital disease involving bicuspid aortic valves, mitral and aortic valves damaged by rheumatic fever, calcified mitral and aortic valves, mitral valve prolapse, prosthetic heart valves, Marfan's syndrome, hypertrophic cardiomyopathy, coarctation of the aorta, arteriovenous shunt, ventricular septal defect, and patent ductus arteriosus

3. Bacteria can seed and proliferate on an abnormal valve

4. As a result, sterile platelet-fibrin thrombi, called vegetations, form on the injured valve leaflets

   a. These vegetations may cause valvular destruction and ulceration associated with valvular insufficiency, obstruct the valve, or become dislodged (thus producing emboli)

   b. Embolism causes infarctions and abscesses in the heart, brain, lungs, kidneys, spleen, and extremities

5. The infection can extend to surrounding structures, causing a mycotic aneurysm, myocardial abscess, or cardiac conduction defect; acute valvular insufficiency may occur if the chordae tendineae rupture

B. Clinical signs and symptoms
1. Acute infective endocarditis: high fever, chills, petechiae, prominent embolic phenomena, Roth's spots, Janeway lesions, and headache
2. Subacute infective endocarditis: low-grade fever with afternoon and evening peaks; night sweats; headache; anorexia and weight loss; malaise; fatigue; weakness; arthralgia; petechiae in the mucosa of the mouth, pharynx, conjunctiva, and upper anterior trunk; Osler's nodes; and symptoms of embolism
3. Right-sided endocarditis: high fever, pleuritic chest pain, hemoptysis and sputum production, dyspnea on exertion, malaise, anorexia, and fatigability

C. Medical management
1. Obtain blood samples to determine the causative organism
2. Administer bactericidal antibiotics for 2 to 6 weeks; prescribe antipyretic agents for fever and anticoagulants if a large thrombus or atrial fibrillation develops
3. Supplement the patient's regular diet with high-calorie feedings if he or she cannot eat well
4. Consider surgical intervention if indicated

D. Nursing management
1. Monitor the patient's temperature every 1 to 4 hours; elevated temperature is a sign of infection
2. Monitor intake and output every shift, assess for dehydration, weigh the patient daily, and encourage oral fluid intake as tolerated; fever causes a water loss in the tissues, and oral fluids help maintain the fluid balance; daily weigh-ins provide a good indication of fluid balance (1 L of fluid weighs approximately 2.2 lb [1 kg])
3. During every shift, assess for symptoms of embolization, including neurologic changes, splenomegaly, decreased urine output, hematuria, and symptoms of pulmonary embolus
   a. Central nervous system emboli occur in one-third to one-half of all patients with infectious endocarditis; splenic emboli occur in 44% of cases
   b. Renal and pulmonary emboli or pulmonary infarction also may occur
4. Administer antibiotics, as prescribed and according to the dosing schedule, to maintain therapeutic blood levels
5. To prevent parenteral I.V. line sepsis, monitor the I.V. site for redness and signs of infection; change the site according to institutional protocol or as needed

6. Check for signs of malnutrition: weigh the patient daily; monitor the patient's daily food intake; offer small, frequent feedings or supplemental feedings high in calories and protein; consult a dietitian; and allow family members to bring food from home if the doctor approves
   a. The infectious process increases metabolic needs, and chronic illness leads to anorexia
   b. Malnourishment also decreases the body's resistance to infection
7. Provide diversionary activities as needed; as the patient's condition improves, he or she may complain of boredom, depression, or a feeling of being trapped
8. Educate the patient about the disease process and its treatment; discuss precipitating factors for reinfection (such as poor oral hygiene, dental work, GI or genitourinary procedures, vaginal deliveries, furuncles [boils], staphylococcal infections, and surgical procedures), the need to notify doctors and dentists before undergoing procedures, and the importance of antibiotic prophylaxis

XXIV. Mitral stenosis

A. Description
   1. In mitral stenosis, the mitral valve orifice is less than one-half the normal size
      a. As a result, increased left atrial pressure is needed to propel blood from the left atria through the stenotic valve to the left ventricle
      b. The elevated left atrial pressure raises the pulmonary venous and arterial pressures, thereby reducing pulmonary compliance and causing dyspnea on exertion
   2. Usually a result of rheumatic fever, mitral stenosis causes the valve leaflets to thicken with fibrous tissue or calcific deposits; the mitral commissures fuse together, the chordae tendineae fuse together and shorten, and the valvular cusps become rigid, thus leading to a narrowing of the valve
   3. The physiologic changes resulting from mitral stenosis cause a low-pitched, rumbling, diastolic murmur that is best heard at the apex of the heart
B. Clinical signs and symptoms
   1. Mild disease: dyspnea and cough on exertion and when blood flow is increased secondary to stressors
   2. Severe disease: orthopnea, paroxysmal nocturnal dyspnea, pulmonary edema, atrial arrhythmias, hemoptysis, increased incidence of pulmonary infarction and bronchitis, chest pain, and reduced pulmonary compliance
C. Medical management
   1. Administer penicillin prophylaxis for beta-hemolytic streptococcal infections and endocarditis
   2. Restrict the patient's sodium intake and prescribe maintenance doses of oral diuretics

   3. Administer digitalis glycosides for atrial fibrillation and right-sided heart failure
   4. Administer anticoagulants for embolization or intermittent atrial fibrillation
   5. Recommend that the patient avoid physically strenuous occupations
   6. Consider valvulotomy and valve replacement for symptomatic patients

D. Nursing management
   1. Monitor vital signs, heart sounds, and arrhythmias to assess the development of right- or left-sided heart failure
   2. Be prepared to assist with cardioversion of atrial fibrillation; loss of atrial kick can decrease cardiac output by 25% to 30%
   3. Restrict the patient's dietary intake of sodium to minimize sodium retention
   4. Assess the patient's level of consciousness and neurologic status, and administer anticoagulants as prescribed; mitral valve disease, an enlarged left atrium, and atrial fibrillation place the patient at increased risk for embolus formation
   5. Limit the patient's level of activity during the acute phase to conserve energy and decrease myocardial oxygen demand
   6. Educate the patient about the disease process, drug regimen, activity restrictions, diet and fluid restrictions, and appropriate choice of contraception for women; pregnancy severely strains the cardiovascular system and may result in heart failure, valve rupture, or death
   7. Discuss the need for antibiotic prophylaxis to prevent endocarditis; the need to notify the dentist, urologist, and gynecologist of the patient's valvular heart disease; and the need to maintain good oral hygiene with regular visits to the dentist

XXV. **Mitral insufficiency** Regurg
   A. Description
   1. Mitral insufficiency results from rheumatic fever, which causes thickening, scarring, rigidity, and calcification of the valve leaflets; the commissures become fused with the chordae tendineae, causing shortening and retraction of the leaflets and preventing them from completely closing during systole
   2. Mitral insufficiency also may result from malposition of the papillary muscles
   3. Floppy valve syndrome is a loss of the fibrous and elastic tissue of the chordae tendineae, which keep the valve from opening backward; if the chordae tendineae rupture or break, blood flows backward and causes a murmur
   4. Papillary muscle rupture occurs secondary to acute MI, acute myocardial ischemia, or dilation of the left ventricle and displacement of the papillary muscles; these muscles are attached to the chordae tendineae

B. Clinical signs and symptoms
  1. Dyspnea, fatigue, orthopnea, exercise intolerance, and palpitations
  2. Wide splitting of the S_2 heart sound and holosystolic murmur best heard at the apex of the heart
  3. Atrial dilation and enlargement
  4. Hypertrophied left ventricle

C. Medical management
  1. Restrict the patient's level of physical activity
  2. Reduce the patient's sodium intake and prescribe diuretic therapy
  3. Administer digitalis glycosides and anticoagulants
  4. Consider surgical valve replacement
  5. Differentiate between mitral insufficiency and mitral stenosis

D. Nursing management
  1. Restrict the patient's level of physical activity to reduce the workload of the heart
  2. Reduce sodium intake and administer diuretic therapy, as prescribed, to reduce fluid retention
  3. Administer digitalis glycosides and anticoagulants, as prescribed, to increase cardiac output
  4. Prepare the patient for surgical valve replacement if indicated
  5. Differentiate between mitral insufficiency and mitral stenosis

XXVI. Myocarditis

A. Description
  1. Myocarditis is an inflammation of the myocardium caused by bacterial, viral, or autoimmune disease
     a. It may result from exposure to radiation or chemotherapy or the chronic use of cocaine
     b. It also may occur as a complication of rheumatic fever, infectious mononucleosis, polio, mumps, or typhoid fever
  2. Myocardial damage results from invasion by the causative agent, myocardial toxin production, or autoimmunity
  3. Myocarditis may have no residual effects or may lead to acute dilated cardiomyopathy and death
  4. Viral myocarditis may be difficult to treat and requires an extended recovery period

B. Clinical signs and symptoms
  1. Fatigue, dyspnea, and fever
  2. Palpitations, pericardial discomfort and chest pain, tachycardia, nonspecific ECG abnormalities, and pericardial friction rub

C. Medical management
  1. Administer antibiotics for bacterial myocarditis and treat the symptoms of viral infection
  2. Prescribe bed rest with restricted activity during periods of fever, fatigue, and pain

3. Administer oxygen therapy and antipyretic agents
4. Ensure that the patient receives adequate nutrition
5. Restrict fluid and sodium intake and prescribe digoxin therapy if the patient has symptoms of heart failure
6. Consider immunosuppressant therapy with corticosteroids or cyclosporine

D. Nursing management
1. Maintain the patient on bed rest with restricted activity, and plan the patient's care to include periods of rest; bed rest reduces the workload of the heart, decreases residual myocardial damage, and promotes healing
2. To meet the patient's oxygen demands, administer oxygen, as prescribed, and verify that the patient is wearing the oxygen delivery device correctly
3. Administer antipyretic agents as prescribed; fever increases the heart's workload
4. Maintain continuous ECG monitoring to detect and treat arrhythmias
5. Monitor the patient for signs and symptoms of decreased cardiac output, heart failure, heart block, and pulmonary or systemic emboli; these conditions are the most common complications of myocarditis
6. Educate the patient about the disease process and the signs and symptoms that should be reported to the doctor; tell the patient to consult with the doctor before resuming physical activities

XXVII. Pericarditis
A. Description
1. Pericarditis is an inflammation of the pericardium commonly caused by bacterial or viral infections, cardiac injury, uremia, or trauma
2. Pericarditis is categorized as acute (lasting less than 6 weeks), subacute (lasting 6 weeks to 6 months), or chronic (lasting more than 6 months)
3. In constrictive pericarditis, thick scar tissue fuses the visceral and parietal layers of the pericardium, resulting in a stiff pericardium that prevents adequate diastolic filling and leads to heart failure
4. In postmyocardial infarction pericarditis, fibrin is deposited between the pericardial layers at the site of necrosis after a transmural MI
5. Dressler's syndrome (postmyocardial infarction syndrome) usually occurs weeks to months after the MI and causes fever, pleuritis, and pericardial inflammation; this syndrome may have an autoimmune cause
6. Postcardiotomy syndrome usually occurs 2 to 3 weeks after openheart surgery; it is similar to Dressler's syndrome but the irritation to the pericardium is caused by the surgical procedure

B. Clinical signs and symptoms
  1. Sharp, stabbing precordial or substernal chest pain that is exacerbated by deep inspiration, coughing, or swallowing
  2. Pericardial friction rub and atrial fibrillation
  3. Dyspnea, chills, fever, diaphoresis, and pericardial effusion
  4. Elevated erythrocyte sedimentation rate
C. Medical management
  1. Maintain patient on bed rest until fever and pain subside
  2. Administer nonsteroidal anti-inflammatory drugs to relieve pain
  3. Administer short-term corticosteroid therapy
  4. Administer antibiotics for bacterial pericarditis
  5. Treat constrictive pericarditis surgically
  6. Consider pericardiocentesis if indicated
D. Nursing management
  1. Assess the characteristics of the patient's pain to distinguish pericardial pain from myocardial ischemia
  2. Administer medications, as prescribed, and evaluate the effectiveness of pain-relief measures
  3. Encourage bed rest, elevate the head of the bed, and ensure that the patient is comfortable; bed rest can reduce the workload of the heart, alleviate pain, and promote healing
  4. Check for paradoxical pulse, narrowing pulse pressure, and tachycardia—early signs of cardiac tamponade
  5. Maintain continuous ECG monitoring to detect ECG changes and tachycardia
  6. Check for muffled heart sounds, paradoxical pulse, decreased cardiac output, and distended neck veins—signs of pericardial effusion and cardiac tamponade
  7. Provide emotional support to decrease the patient's anxiety
  8. Educate the patient about the disease process and the signs and symptoms of recurring inflammation
  9. Instruct the patient to avoid overexertion and heavy lifting for 2 weeks or more (based on the doctor's preference) and to notify the doctor if symptoms continue or worsen

XXVIII. Pulmonary edema
  A. Description
    1. In pulmonary edema, increased left atrial and left ventricular pressures cause an excessive accumulation of serous or serosanguineous fluid in the interstitial spaces and alveoli of the lungs
      a. In stage I disease, interstitial edema and increased lymphatic flow occur
      b. In stage II disease, the fluid moves from the interstitium into the alveoli

     2. Fluid in the alveoli interferes with the diffusion of oxygen and leads to tissue hypoxia; the resulting feeling of suffocation increases the patient's fear and elevates the heart rate, which decreases ventricular filling and further depresses cardiac function

B. Clinical signs and symptoms

     1. Coughing, extreme shortness of breath, wheezing, intense anxiety, crackles, and tachypnea

     2. Frothy sputum that may be tinged with blood

     3. Sensation of drowning and fear of impending death

     4. Pallid complexion and cold, clammy, cyanotic skin

     5. Pulmonary artery diastolic pressure and PAWP greater than 30 mm Hg

     6. Respiratory alkalosis secondary to hyperventilation in initial stages; respiratory acidosis and hypoxemia as pulmonary edema progresses

     7. Decreased urine output

     8. X-ray film showing pulmonary venous congestion and interstitial edema

C. Medical management

     1. Same as for acute heart failure (see pages 39 and 40)

     2. Short-term intubation and mechanical ventilation may be required

D. Nursing management

     1. Same as for acute heart failure (see page 40)

     2. Closely monitor patient for progression to cardiogenic shock

3 Pulmonary disorders

I. **Anatomy**
   A. Nose
      1. The internal portion of the nose is hollow and separated by the septum into a right and left cavity; the external portion protrudes from the face
      2. The nasal cavity is divided into three passageways: superior, middle, and inferior meatus
      3. Palatine bones form the floor of the nose and the roof of the mouth
      4. Ciliated mucous membrane lines the nose and the respiratory tract
   B. Pharynx
      1. The pharynx, or throat, is a tubelike structure approximately 9.8″ (25 cm) long in an adult
      2. Constructed of muscle and lined with mucous membrane, the pharynx extends from the base of the skull to the esophagus
      3. The pharynx consists of three parts: the nasopharynx, oropharynx, and laryngopharynx
   C. Larynx
      1. Located at the upper end of the trachea, the larynx, or voice box, is constructed of nine pieces of cartilage, of which the thyroid cartilage is the largest
      2. Stretched across the hollow interior of the larynx are fibrous bands called true vocal cords
   D. Trachea
      1. The trachea is composed of smooth muscle embedded with C-shaped cartilage rings
      2. The adult trachea is approximately 7.8″ (20 cm) long and 2.0″ (5 cm) in diameter
      3. During swallowing, the epiglottis closes over the trachea
   E. Primary bronchi
      1. The right bronchus is slightly larger and more vertical than the left bronchus; the left bronchus is smaller and more horizontal than the right bronchus
      2. Before the bronchi enter the lungs, the bronchial walls are composed of incomplete cartilaginous rings; the rings are complete after the bronchi enter the lungs
   F. Secondary bronchi
      1. Just after they enter the lungs, the primary bronchi are divided into secondary bronchi

    2. The secondary bronchi in turn are divided into small bronchioles, which are divided further into smaller alveolar ducts

G. Alveoli

    1. The alveoli are small, grapelike sacs surrounded by a network of capillaries

    2. The walls of the alveoli are composed of a single layer of squamous epithelial cells

    3. A healthy adult has approximately 300 million alveoli

H. Lungs

    1. The lungs are cone-shaped organs that fill the pleural portion of the thoracic cavity

    2. The bronchi enter the lungs through the hilum, a slit on the medial surface of the lungs

    3. At their base, the lungs are broad and rest on the diaphragm; at the apex in the upper part of the chest cavity, the lungs are pointed

    4. The left lung has two lobes (upper and lower); the right lung has three lobes (superior, middle, and inferior)

I. Thorax

    1. The thorax, or chest, is encased by the ribs

    2. Parietal pleura lines the entire thoracic cavity; visceral pleura covers and adheres to the outer surface of the lungs; a small amount of pleural fluid is contained between these layers to reduce friction and maintain negative pressure

    3. The diaphragm, the principal muscle of ventilation, lies outside the pleura

    4. The intercostal muscles, which aid in ventilation, lie between the ribs

II. Physiology

A. Upper airways

    1. Air reaches the lungs through the upper airways; air passing through the upper airways also produces the voice

    2. The upper airways heat, filter, and humidify the air before it enters the lungs

    3. They also protect the lungs from foreign objects and liquids

B. Lower airways

    1. The bronchioles and alveoli compose the lower airways

    2. Diffusion of gases between the air and the blood takes place in the lower airways; oxygen and carbon dioxide move easily across the thin membranes of the alveoli and capillaries

    3. The exchange of gases is called respiration

        a. External respiration is the exchange of gases in the lungs

        b. Internal respiration is the exchange of gases at the cellular level between the blood and the cells of the organs and muscles

4. The movement of air into and out of the lungs is called ventilation
   a. Air moves into and out of the lungs because of a pressure gradient
   b. Inhalation (inspiration) creates a negative pressure in the chest cavity compared with the atmosphere, and air moves into the lungs; inhalation is an active process and requires the use of the respiratory muscles
   c. Exhalation (expiration) creates a positive pressure in the chest cavity compared with the atmosphere, and air moves out of the lungs; exhalation is a passive process and occurs when the muscles of respiration relax

C. Physical principles that affect gas exchange
   1. Dalton's law (the law of partial pressure) states that in a mixture of gases, each gas exerts its own partial pressure according to the amount of the gas in the mixture
   2. The partial pressure of a gas in a liquid is directly determined by the amount of that gas dissolved in the liquid
   3. Many laboratory test measurements use partial pressure, which is designated by the capital letter P

D. Control of respirations
   1. The carbon dioxide level in the blood is the primary and most powerful stimulant of respiration; when the carbon dioxide level increases above normal (45 mm Hg), the respiratory center in the brain stem is stimulated and the respiratory muscles contract
   2. The oxygen level in the blood is a backup control for respiration; it does not stimulate respiration as long as the carbon dioxide level remains normal; when the oxygen level falls below normal (70 mm Hg), combined with a high carbon dioxide level, respirations are stimulated
   3. Arterial blood pressure helps to control respirations through a pressure-reflex mechanism
      a. A sudden rise in blood pressure slows respirations
      b. A sudden drop in blood pressure increases the rate and depth of respirations
   4. Hering-Breuer reflexes control the depth and regularity of normal respirations at rest
   5. The pneumotaxic center in the pons regulates the rhythmicity of respirations by ending inspirations
   6. The cerebral cortex can override automatic respiratory functions, allowing the rate and depth of respirations to be voluntarily increased or decreased within limits
   7. The buildup of certain substances in the body, particularly those that affect blood pH, can affect respirations

III. Acute pulmonary embolism

    A. Description

        1. Acute pulmonary embolism is caused by the movement of a clot from its site of origin through the right side of the heart, where it lodges in a branch of the pulmonary circulation

            a. The degree of patient compromise caused by pulmonary embolism depends on the extent of the vascular occlusion and the degree of preexisting cardiopulmonary disease

            b. Massive pulmonary embolism can result in a sudden shocklike state; death usually follows within a few minutes unless therapy is promptly initiated

        2. Pulmonary embolism produces an area in the lung that is ventilated but underperfused, thus increasing physiologic dead-space ventilation

        3. Reflex bronchoconstriction occurs in the affected area of the lung and is thought to result from the release of histamine or serotonin from the clot

            a. Reflex bronchoconstriction is considered to be compensatory in the occluded area because it reduces the unevenness of ventilation and perfusion

            b. In adjacent areas, reflex bronchospasm may result in considerable hypoxemia

        4. In some situations, the dual circulation (pulmonary and bronchial) in the lungs may provide adequate circulation distal to the occlusion; if the pulmonary vascular bed is sufficiently reduced by a large embolus or by recurrent multiple emboli, pulmonary hypertension can result, although two-thirds of the vascular bed must be obliterated before this occurs

        5. The absence or altered activity of surfactant associated with pulmonary emboli contributes to alveolar collapse and atelectasis

        6. Nearly 95% of all pulmonary emboli arise from thrombi in the deep veins of the legs; pulmonary emboli of nonthrombolic origin are uncommon but include obstruction caused by air, fat, malignant cells, amniotic fluid, parasites, vegetations, and foreign material

        7. Thromboembolic disease describes the relation between thrombosis, blood clot formation, and the ever-present risk of embolization; pulmonary embolism often is the first sign of venous thrombosis

            a. The principal contributing factors (Virchow's triad) of venous thrombosis are stasis of blood flow, endothelial injury or vessel wall abnormalities, and hypercoagulability

            b. Other risk factors for thrombosis include a history of thrombosis, immobility, chronic heart failure, cancer, use of estrogen contraceptives, blood dyscrasias, advancing age, leg or pelvic trauma or surgery, obesity, and postoperative status

            c. Thrombus formation also can result from heart failure, atrial fibrillation, endocarditis, and myocardial infarction (MI)

8. Deep vein thrombosis (DVT) is an insidious problem that can lead to pulmonary embolism; in some patients with DVT, secondary arterial compromise may occur with massive venous thrombosis as a result of vascular compression or spasm; diminished arterial pulses and pallor may result

   a. The most reliable sign of DVT is swelling of the involved extremity; although unilateral swelling is typical, iliofemoral obstruction can produce bilateral swelling

   b. The most common symptom of DVT is pain, which typically is described as aching or throbbing and may be severe

   c. Calf tenderness on dorsiflexion of the foot (Homans' sign) is not a reliable indicator of DVT

   d. Calf or thigh pain with inflation of an air-filled cuff around the extremity (Lowenberg's sign) is a more reliable indicator of DVT

   e. Other signs of DVT include increased tissue turgor with swelling, increased skin temperature with dilation of the superficial veins, mottling and cyanosis caused by stagnant blood flow, increased oxygen extraction, and reduced hemoglobin level

B. Clinical signs and symptoms

   1. In a patient with signs of thrombophlebitis in leg veins: sudden onset of unexplained dyspnea, tachypnea, tachycardia, and restlessness

   2. In a patient on bed rest: sudden onset of tachypnea, tachycardia, and hypoxemia

   3. In a patient with massive pulmonary embolism: tachycardia, hypotension, cyanosis, stupor, and syncope

   4. Elevated temperature (most often associated with pulmonary infarction)

   5. Pleuritic pain, friction rub, hemoptysis, and fever if pulmonary infarction occurs

   6. Arterial blood gas (ABG) levels indicating respiratory alkalosis (caused by hyperventilation) and hypoxemia; possibly increased A-a gradient

   7. S_3 heart sound, S_4 gallop, or increased pulmonic S_2

   8. Crackles present on auscultation

C. Diagnostic tests

   1. Pulmonary angiography is the definitive diagnostic test for pulmonary embolism

   2. A lung ventilation or perfusion scan is not definitive but suggestive of pulmonary embolism; it also is less risky than angiography

   3. A chest X-ray is nonspecific and frequently normal

   4. An electrocardiogram (ECG) is nonspecific but may show ventricular arrhythmias (in response to hypoxemia) or sinus tachycardia

D. Medical management

   1. Initiate cardiorespiratory support

2. Treat hypoxemia with supplemental oxygen therapy to keep the partial pressure of arterial oxygen (PaO_2) greater than 60 mm Hg

3. Intubate and mechanically ventilate the patient if indicated; a patient with massive pulmonary emboli may experience hypoxemia and hypercapnia and require mechanical ventilation

4. Initiate intravascular volume expansion
   a. Pulmonary emboli reduce blood flow to the left side of the heart, consequently reducing cardiac output and arterial blood pressure
   b. The pulmonary vasculature triggers systemic arteriolar vasodilation, which produces a relative volume depletion

5. Administer anticoagulants to prevent further clot formation; anticoagulants are beneficial as prophylactic therapy to prevent thrombus formation and recurrent embolization in patients with emboli

6. Administer heparin, which impedes clotting by interfering with fibrin formation
   a. Although heparin does not dissolve emboli, it can prevent the formation of new thrombi and enhances fibrinolytic activity on fresh thrombi; heparin blocks platelet-thrombin interactions on the embolus that lead to the release of chemical mediators associated with bronchospasm and hypotension
   b. Typically, a bolus dose of 5,000 to 15,000 units of I.V. heparin is given to achieve therapeutic blood level; the bolus dose is followed by a continuous heparin infusion of 500 to 3,000 units per hour (continuous I.V. therapy prevents the uneven anticoagulation seen with intermittent heparin therapy); I.V. heparin is administered for 7 to 10 days to maintain the partial thromboplastin time at 1.5 times normal (generally 55 to 85 seconds)
   c. The effects of heparin can be reversed with protamine; 1 mg of protamine neutralizes the effect of approximately 100 units of heparin (90 U of beef-lung heparin, 115 U of intestinal mucosa-derived heparin, or 100 U of calcium heparin); a protamine loading dose of 25 to 50 mg may be given by slow I.V. push, with the remaining dose given as a continuous infusion over 8 to 16 hours

7. Administer oral anticoagulants, such as warfarin sodium (Coumadin)
   a. Before the patient is weaned from the heparin infusion, he or she may be started on oral anticoagulant therapy
   b. Warfarin is administered for 6 or more weeks to maintain the prothrombin time at 1.5 times normal (generally 16 to 18 seconds)
   c. The effects of warfarin can be reversed with vitamin K

8. Administer thrombolytic therapy; streptokinase, urokinase, and tissue plasminogen activator can be used to dissolve the clot

9. In patients with recurrent emboli, consider surgical placement of a filter in the vena cava

10. In patients with massive emboli, determine whether embolectomy is indicated

E. Nursing management

1. Maintain the patient on bed rest to reduce the workload of the heart and lungs and to decrease the likelihood of embolus movement

2. Administer stool softeners and mild cathartics as needed; the act of defecation increases the potential for pulmonary embolus in patients with DVT

3. Monitor the patient for complications of pulmonary emboli, which include pulmonary infarction, pneumonia, pulmonary abscess, adult respiratory distress syndrome (ARDS), MI, arrhythmias, and shock

IV. **Acute respiratory failure**

A. Description

1. Acute respiratory failure is characterized by the inability of the lungs to maintain adequate oxygen delivery (PaO_2) and removal of carbon dioxide (partial pressure of arterial carbon dioxide [$PaCO_2$])

2. Respiratory failure is defined as the presence of the following abnormalities when breathing room air at a pressure equal to that of sea level (760 mm Hg):

   a. pH less than 7.25

   b. PaO_2 less than 50 mm Hg

   c. $PaCO_2$ greater than 50 mm Hg

   d. Arterial oxygen saturation (SaO_2) less than 90 mm Hg

3. In diagnosing respiratory failure, the patient's preexisting ABG values are taken into consideration as well as the rapidness of the onset of signs and symptoms (minutes to days)

4. Two broadly defined types of respiratory failure exist

   a. Hypoxemic (type I) respiratory failure is defined as a PaO_2 less than 50 mm Hg and a $PaCO_2$ that is normal or low; type I respiratory failure (hypoxemia without hypercapnia) can be caused by bronchitis, emphysema, pneumonia, pulmonary edema, pulmonary fibrosis, bronchial asthma, atelectasis, ARDS, cardiogenic shock, obesity, chest injury, or pulmonary embolism

   b. Hypercapnic (type II) respiratory failure is defined as a $PaCO_2$ greater than 50 mm Hg and a pH less than 7.25 and generally is accompanied by a low PaO_2; type II respiratory failure (hypoxemia with hypercapnia) can be caused by chronic bronchitis, emphysema, bronchial asthma, crushed chest injury, opioid overdose, obstructive sleep apnea, myasthenia gravis, tetanus, spinal cord and head injuries, poliomyelitis, near drowning, and hypothermia

5. The primary conditions associated with acute respiratory failure are hypoventilation, ventilation-perfusion mismatching, right-to-left pulmonary shunting, and impaired diffusion

    a. *Alveolar hypoventilation* is indicated by an increased $PaCO_2$

      (1) It is caused by a decrease in total minute ventilation or an increase in dead-space ventilation

      (2) A C4 or higher spinal cord injury impairs movement of the diaphragm and intercostal nerves; T4 to C4 spinal cord injuries cause paralysis of the abdominal wall and lower intercostal muscles, resulting in paradoxical chest and abdominal wall movements and reducing the patient's ability to breathe

      (3) Neck and cardiac surgery can cause paralysis of the phrenic nerve (which enervates the diaphragm) and reduce the patient's ability to breathe

    b. *Ventilation-perfusion mismatching* occurs when the lungs are adequately ventilated but inadequately perfused or vice versa

      (1) In a high ventilation–low perfusion condition, the lungs compensate for a low $PaCO_2$ by contracting the airway smooth muscles, which increases airway resistance and decreases ventilation to the area

      (2) In a low ventilation–high perfusion condition, the lungs respond to a high $PaCO_2$ by relaxing the airway smooth muscles, which decreases airway resistance and increases ventilation to the area

      (3) Ventilation-perfusion mismatching can be caused by pulmonary emboli, left-sided heart failure, pulmonary infection, atelectasis, or chronic obstructive pulmonary disease

    c. *Right-to-left pulmonary shunting* is a common cause of hypoxemic pulmonary disease

      (1) It occurs when blood passes by nonventilated alveoli; the subsequent return of unoxygenated blood to the left atrium results in a decreased PaO_2

      (2) Conditions that cause right-to-left pulmonary shunting include ARDS, pneumonia, atelectasis, and oxygen toxicity

    d. *Impaired diffusion* is caused by a physical alteration in the alveolocapillary membrane

      (1) Because oxygen diffuses about 20 times more slowly than carbon dioxide, impaired diffusion is most commonly indicated by a decreased PaO_2 and oxygen saturation level than by an elevated $PaCO_2$

      (2) The signs and symptoms of impaired diffusion are those of hypoxemia, hypercapnia, and the underlying disorder; they include anxiety, restlessness, tachycardia, central cyanosis, cool and dry skin, weakness, fatigue, disorientation, somnolence, coma, decreased blood pressure, and an increased rate and depth of respiration

B. Medical management

  1. Maintain or enhance the delivery of oxygen and the removal of carbon dioxide

    a. Adequate oxygenation is evidenced by a PaO_2 greater than 60 mm Hg

    b. Adequate oxygen saturation is evidenced by an SaO_2 greater than 90 mm Hg

    c. Adequate numbers of red blood cells are evidenced by a hemoglobin level greater than 12 g/dl or a hematocrit greater than 36%

    d. Adequate cardiac index is 2.5 to 4 L/minute

    e. Adequate carbon dioxide elimination is evidenced by a pH of 7.35 to 7.45

2. Manage hypoxemia with supplemental oxygen therapy; administer oxygen with caution to patients with underlying pulmonary disease because oxygen can suppress the hypoxic respiratory drive

3. In conditions characterized by right-to-left shunting, determine whether mechanical ventilation with positive end-expiratory pressure (PEEP) is needed to maintain adequate oxygenation of tissues

4. If hypoventilation is related to drug use, administer an antidote or treat the patient's symptoms until the effects of the drug wear off

5. Encourage coughing, deep breathing, and turning, and prescribe chest physiotherapy to help the patient expectorate retained pulmonary secretions

6. Keep in mind that ventilation of patients with type II respiratory failure can result in metabolic alkalosis

    a. Metabolic alkalosis increases minute ventilation, PaO_2, and mixed venous oxygen tension and decreases oxygen consumption

    b. Metabolic alkalosis can be reversed by correcting fluid and electrolyte abnormalities and administering acetazolamide, ammonium chloride, hydrochloric acid, or arginine hydrochloride

C. Nursing management

1. Assess breath sounds every 1 to 4 hours and note wheezes, crackles, and rhonchi; acute respiratory failure always causes some degree of pulmonary congestion and bronchospasm; frequent auscultation is helpful in determining whether the patient's condition is worsening

2. Monitor the patient's respiratory rate; tachypnea with rapid, shallow, ineffective respirations often is present

3. Encourage and assist with abdominal respirations, pursed-lip breathing, and respiratory therapy; these measure help to control dyspnea, reduce air trapping, and open blocked or constricted bronchi

4. Increase the patient's fluid intake to 2,000 ml/day, and provide warm liquids; hydration helps to decrease the viscosity of secretions and facilitates expectoration, and warm fluids decrease bronchospasms

5. Encourage expectoration of sputum and suction the patient as necessary; secretions in the respiratory tract are a prime source of impaired gas exchange
6. Monitor serial ABG values; changes in ABG values provide an indication of the effectiveness of treatments

V. **Acute respiratory tract infection**
  A. Description
    1. The principal acute respiratory tract infection is pneumonia, which, despite antibiotic therapy, remains the fifth leading cause of death in the United States
    2. Pneumonia is caused when infectious organisms enter the sterile lower respiratory tract, overcome host defenses, and multiply
    3. Pneumonia can be caused by bacteria, viruses, or fungi
      a. Bacterial pathogens include *Legionella pneumophila, Moraxella* (formerly *Branhamella*) *catarrhalis, Staphylococcus, Haemophilus influenzae, Streptococcus pneumoniae* (pneumococcus), *Enterobacter, Escherichia coli, Proteus,* and *Pseudomonas*
      b. Viral pathogens include influenza virus, adenovirus, cytomegalovirus, and herpesvirus
      c. Fungal pathogens include *Aspergillus, Candida, Cryptococcus, Nocardia, Mycoplasma* (a common cause in young, healthy people), and *Pneumocystis carinii*
        (1) *P. carinii* is transmitted by droplets or airborne currents; it settles diffusely throughout the alveoli, forming cysts that adhere to the alveolar walls and lodge in the interstitial spaces; *P. carinii* organisms seldom migrate outside the pulmonary system
        (2) *P. carinii* pneumonia produces a ventilation-perfusion mismatch and decrease in pulmonary compliance
        (3) *P. carinii* pneumonia most commonly occurs in patients whose CD4+ cell count is less than 200 cells/mm^3
        (4) Lung scans with gallium 67 citrate are highly sensitive for *P. carinii* pneumonia; when lung uptake exceeds liver uptake, *P. carinii* infection is likely
    4. Bacterial pneumonia is much more common than viral pneumonia; hospital-acquired (nosocomial) respiratory tract infections often are caused by gram-negative enteric bacteria
    5. The sterility of the airway below the glottis is maintained through several protective mechanisms
      a. Aerodynamic energy comprises sneezing and coughing, which aid in the expectoration of large particles; air also is warmed and filtered by the nasal turbinates
      b. Mucociliary action propels large particles upward
      c. Mucous membranes secrete antibodies when bacteria are present

      d. Phagocytic cells engulf pathogenic microorganisms; as a result of phagocytosis, macrophages display an antigen marker on their surface that summons helper T cells

      e. Lymphatic response produces and releases antibodies specific to the invading organism

  6. Infectious organisms can enter the respiratory tract through inhalation or aspiration

      a. The most common cause of pneumonia is aspiration of bacteria that have colonized the upper airway

      b. Most critical care patients have gram-negative bacteria in their mouths

      c. Infiltrates seen on a chest X-ray can persist for an extended period after resolution of the pneumonia

  7. Respiratory tract infection produces inflammation with or without exudate

      a. Inflammation of the lung parenchyma is characterized by the influx of polymorphonuclear leukocytes, fluid, and fibrin into the alveolar spaces

      b. Inflammation leads to a ventilation-perfusion abnormality and hypoxemia; right-to-left shunting also can occur

B. Clinical signs and symptoms

  1. Dyspnea, fever, hyperpnea, and tachycardia

  2. Bacterial pneumonia: productive cough, with yellow-green or rust-colored sputum

  3. Viral pneumonia: nonproductive cough and low-grade or absent fever

  4. *P. carinii* pneumonia: nonproductive cough

  5. Pleuritic pain caused by inflammation of the pleural surface

  6. Crackles and wheezes over the affected area on auscultation; with frank consolidation, an increase in vocal fremitus may occur

  7. Dullness on percussion of the affected area

  8. Elevated white blood cell (WBC) count with the shift to the left (characterized by an increased number of immature neutrophils) in bacterial pneumonia; a normal or depressed WBC count in the presence of pneumonia suggests an overwhelming infection

C. Medical management

  1. Support the patient's respiratory function

  2. Culture sputum and blood specimens to guide the choice of antibiotic therapy; a saline mist treatment with an ultrasonic nebulizer may be helpful in obtaining a sputum specimen

  3. Prescribe empiric antibiotic therapy until Gram stain and culture results are available

  4. Institute appropriate antibiotic therapy for patients with *P. carinii* pneumonia

a. The two most commonly used drugs for this type of pneumonia are co-trimoxazole (Bactrim or Septra) and pentamidine isethionate (Pentam)

   (1) Co-trimoxazole can be given I.V. or orally; it can cause thrombocytopenia, neutropenia, hepatitis, Stevens-Johnson syndrome, and abnormal liver function test results

   (2) Pentamidine isethionate generally is given in the inhaled form

     (a) I.V. administration can cause severe hypotension in some patients; I.M. administration is associated with sterile abscess formation

     (b) Pentamidine isethionate can cause neutropenia, thrombocytopenia, nephrotoxicity, hepatotoxicity, hypoglycemia, and diabetes mellitus

   (3) The incidence of adverse effects with both co-trimoxazole and pentamidine isethionate is greater than 60%

b. Steroids may be prescribed for patients with *P. carinii* pneumonia to decrease the inflammatory response

D. Nursing management

  1. Institute chest physiotherapy, including postural drainage, percussion, and vibration

  2. To facilitate lung expansion, encourage coughing and deep breathing; this helps expectorate sputum

  3. When only one lung is involved, position the patient on the unaffected side to decrease the ventilation-perfusion imbalance

  4. Closely monitor fluids in patients with *P. carinii* pneumonia; the increased alveolocapillary membrane permeability causes fluids to build up in the alveoli

  5. Control fever with tepid sponge baths and prescribed antipyretics

VI. Adult respiratory distress syndrome

A. Description

  1. Adult respiratory distress syndrome is a common form of respiratory failure that occurs in response to a systemic insult

   a. The systemic injury causes an increase in pulmonary capillary wall permeability, resulting in tremendous loss of fluid from the vascular space into the pulmonary interstitial spaces

   b. The drainage capability of the pulmonary lymphatic system becomes overwhelmed, flooding the alveoli

   c. These responses produce the severe hypoxemia that is the hallmark of ARDS

  2. Various conditions can lead to ARDS (see *Conditions leading to adult respiratory distress syndrome,* page 84)

  3. Mortality from ARDS is between 50% and 70%; mortality rates increase significantly when organ failure occurs

  4. No single common mechanism causing ARDS has been found (see *Pathogenesis of adult respiratory distress syndrome,* page 85)

Conditions leading to adult respiratory distress syndrome

A common form of respiratory failure, adult respiratory distress syndrome occurs in response to a direct or indirect systemic insult, such as those listed below.

DIRECT PULMONARY INJURY

Aspiration of gastric contents or other toxic substances
Near drowning
Inhalation of toxic substances
Diffuse viral pneumonia
Diffuse mycoplasmal pneumonia
Diffuse rickettsial pneumonia
Pulmonary contusion, secondary trauma
Drugs: heroin, panaquat, salicylates
Embolism: fat, air, amniotic fluid

INDIRECT PULMONARY INJURY

Sepsis—especially gram-negative
Severe pancreatitis
Multiple emergency blood transfusions
Multiple trauma
Disseminated intravascular coagulation
Shock from any cause
Neurogenic states: head trauma, increased intracranial pressure
Nonpulmonary systemic diseases
Postcardiopulmonary bypass
Anaphylaxis

5. Pulmonary mechanisms associated with ARDS include defects of the alveolar epithelium, interstitial lung edema, and microthrombosis
   a. Defects of the alveolar epithelium cause loss of vascular proteins from the capillaries to the pulmonary interstitial spaces
      (1) As a result, large amounts of fluid enter the pulmonary interstitial spaces, overwhelming the pulmonary lymphatic drainage system
      (2) The increased hydrostatic pressure eventually collapses the terminal bronchioles, causing hypoxemia
      (3) Fluids subsequently enter the alveoli, decreasing surfactant activity and promoting alveolar collapse, which increases pulmonary shunting; this results in marked reduction of gas exchange and pronounced hypoxemia
      (4) This chain of events increases pulmonary shunting, which results in significant reduction of gas exchange and marked hypoxemia
   b. Interstitial lung edema is classified as noncarcinogenic pulmonary edema; the protein-rich fluid that enters the pulmonary interstitial spaces forms hyaline membranes that further decrease compliance, widen the A-a gradient, and result in refractory hypoxemia
   c. Microthrombosis often is a result of ARDS and can be a complicating factor
B. Clinical signs and symptoms
   1. In early phases of ARDS: hypoxemia, hyperventilation, tachypnea, and tachycardia
   2. Shortness of breath, anxiety, and orthopnea

Pathogenesis of adult respiratory distress syndrome

Adult respiratory distress syndrome typically follows the basic progression detailed here, regardless of the cause.

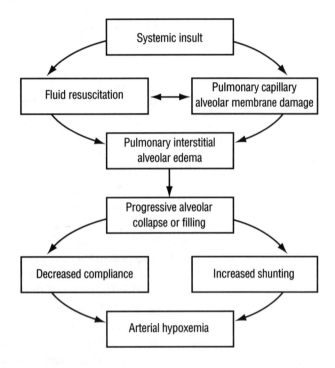

From "Pathogenesis and pathophysiology of ARDS" in Dossey, B.M., Guzzetta, C.E., and Kenner, C.V. *Essentials of Critical Care Nursing: Body-Mind-Spirit* (3rd ed.). Philadelphia: J.B. Lippincott, 1992. Used with permission.

3. PaO_2 greater than 60 mm Hg; SaO_2 less than 90 mm Hg
4. Pulmonary artery wedge pressure (PAWP) less than 18 mm Hg; high wedge pressures are seen in patients with left-sided heart failure
5. Respiratory rate greater than 30 breaths/minute, intercostal retractions, and use of accessory muscles
6. Diffuse crackles and rhonchi on auscultation
7. Dullness on percussion and increased vocal fremitus, which result from the increased density caused by pulmonary edema

C. Diagnostic tests
   1. Chest X-ray findings vary from diffuse patchy infiltrates to a "white out" of the lung
   2. Pulmonary function tests may indicate large right-to-left shunting, increased A-a gradient, and reduced compliance

D. Medical management

   1. Administer supplemental oxygen therapy; the lung can tolerate oxygen concentrations of 40% to 50% indefinitely, but higher concentrations can cause increasing alveolar collapse, type II granular pneumocyte dysfunction, and impaired mucociliary clearance within 3 to 4 days

   2. Use mechanical ventilation to maintain or restore an adequate PaO_2

     a. The tidal volume usually is set at 10 to 15 ml/kg

     b. Forced inspiratory oxygen (FIO_2) is set to maintain a PaO_2 greater than 70 mm Hg

     c. Rate of ventilation is set to maintain a $PaCO_2$ of 35 to 45 mm Hg

   3. Use PEEP, if indicated, to maintain adequate oxygenation; PEEP often is useful for maintaining alveolar air flow during expiration

     a. Closely monitor the patient's cardiovascular status as PEEP is increased

     b. The increased intrathoracic pressure caused by PEEP can decrease cardiac output; high levels of PEEP also predispose the patient to pneumothorax

     c. PEEP greater than 15 cm H_2O generally is not recommended

   4. Use pressure-controlled inverse ratio ventilation (PC-IRV), a mode of ventilation that reverses the conventional inspiratory-expiratory ratio (I:E ratio), if indicated

     a. PC-IRV delivers each breath at a set pressure rather than a set tidal volume and at an I:E ratio of 1:1, 2:1, or higher

     b. The effects of PC-IRV include reduced peak inspiratory pressure, decreased mean airway pressure, increased compliance, reduced minute ventilation, and improved oxygenation with a lower delivered FIO_2

   5. Do not use high-frequency ventilators; although useful during upper airway surgery and in patients with a bronchopleural fistula, these devices are not advantageous in the management of patients with ARDS

E. Nursing management

   1. Use a closed suction system when suctioning the patient

     a. Hypoxemia can rapidly develop when patients are disconnected from the ventilator; a closed system would maintain oxygenation

     b. A closed system also prevents the loss of PEEP, which may result when the ventilator is disconnected

   2. Reposition the patient at regular intervals and note changes in oxygenation; the prone position improves oxygenation, possibly by increasing perfusion of the anterior apical regions; if the prone position is not feasible, use a semiprone position

   3. Implement measures to decrease oxygen consumption, which is necessary for adequate perfusion of vital organs; methods of decreasing oxygen consumption range from anxiety reduction and pain control to pharmacologic paralysis of a restless patient

4. Keep in mind that inotropic support may be required to maintain adequate cardiac output; because dobutamine decreases the PAWP, this inotropic agent is more useful than dopamine in the treatment of ARDS

5. Administer fluid therapy to maintain the PAWP between 10 and 12 mm Hg
   a. Weight gain of more than 0.5 kg/day is indicative of fluid retention
   b. PEEP greater than 10 cm H_2O can interfere with cardiac output, lowering blood pressure and causing increased antidiuretic hormone secretion and fluid retention

6. Use venoarterial or veno-venous extracorporeal membrane oxygenation (ECMO); ECMO facilitates gas exchange and rests the lungs of patients with severe reversible respiratory failure

VII. Flail chest

A. Description
   1. Flail chest is a chest injury in which three or more adjacent ribs are fractured in two or more places, causing a segment of the ribs and chest wall to work paradoxically with respiration
   2. The flail segment moves inward with inspiration and outward with expiration, causing diminished movement of air that leads to hypoxia; a decreased cough mechanism results in retained secretions
   3. The larger the flail, the less effective the exchange of gases
   4. Interstitial and intra-alveolar edema and hemorrhage are caused by the underlying pulmonary contusion; sternal fractures also are frequently associated with myocardial injuries
   5. Flail chest often is associated with hemopneumothorax

B. Clinical signs and symptoms
   1. Hypoxia according to the size of the flail
   2. Cyanosis, dyspnea, apprehension, and anxiety
   3. Diminished breath sounds
   4. Signs of decreased venous return to the heart: distended neck veins, elevated central venous pressure, and decreasing blood pressure

C. Medical management
   1. Maintain airway, breathing, and circulation
   2. Use an intercostal nerve block to reduce pain and splint simple rib fractures
   3. Use mechanical ventilation with PEEP, if indicated; PEEP provides internal stabilization of the flail segment

D. Nursing management
   1. Monitor patient's respiration status, vital signs, and capillary refill time
   2. Administer appropriate pain medication, as prescribed, to aid in respiratory expansion
   3. Frequently assess patient for complications of mechanical ventilation, PEEP, and bed rest

VIII. Hemothorax
  A. Description
    1. Hemothorax refers to a condition in which blood is trapped in the pleural space, resulting in impaired respirations and hypovolemia
    2. The chest cavity can hold up to 4 L of blood
    3. The source of bleeding in hemothorax generally is the pulmonary parenchyma and vessels, the intercostal and internal mammary arteries, or the mediastinum (heart, aorta, and great vessels)
  B. Clinical signs and symptoms
    1. Hypovolemia (shock)
    2. Diminished breath sounds on the affected side
    3. Marked dullness to percussion on the affected side
    4. Mediastinal shift away from the affected side with an accumulation of more than 1,500 ml of blood
    5. Pain that may radiate to the neck, shoulder, and upper abdomen
  C. Medical management
    1. Keep in mind that a small hemothorax may resolve spontaneously because of low pulmonary system pressures and thromboplastin in the lungs
    2. Use thoracentesis or placement of a chest tube for a large hemothorax if indicated
    3. Replace blood volume with volume expanders and blood products as indicated
  D. Nursing management
    1. Frequently assess respiratory status for changes in pleural drainage
    2. Prepare the patient with a large hemothorax for thoracentesis or placement of a chest tube if indicated
    3. Administer blood products as prescribed
    4. Monitor chest tube drainage system for proper functioning

IX. Pneumothorax
  A. Description
    1. A pneumothorax is a defect in the visceral pleura that allows air to enter the pleural space
      a. A simple pneumothorax is one in which the defect does not continue to enlarge
      b. A tension pneumothorax is one in which the defect acts as a one-way valve, allowing air to enter the pleural space on inspiration but preventing it from exiting on expiration
    2. A pneumothorax causes the lung to collapse to a varying extent as the normal negative intrapleural pressure that counteracts elastic recoil is lost
    3. Air enters the pleural cavity through the chest wall or the parietal pleura

4. Pleural causes of pneumothorax include rupture of a subpleural air pocket (bleb or bulla) and necrosis of adjacent lung parenchyma (necrotizing pneumonia or neoplasm); iatrogenic causes include accidental puncture during insertion of a subclavian catheter, tracheostomy, thoracentesis, and mechanical ventilation with PEEP

B. Clinical signs and symptoms
1. Acute onset of dyspnea or chest pain
2. Respiratory distress and hypoxemia (extent varies according to the size of the pneumothorax)
3. Decreased breath sounds on the affected side
4. Hyperresonance and diminished breath sounds on the affected side; decreased tactile fremitus and egophonies in the air-filled pleural space muffle sounds
5. Tracheal deviation away from the affected side
6. Chest wall asymmetry or crepitus (subcutaneous emphysema)
7. Distended neck veins
8. Hypotension secondary to impaired venous return (venous return is impaired by the rising positive intrathoracic pressure)
9. Cyanosis (a late, ominous sign)

C. Medical management
1. Perform emergency needle thoracentesis
2. Insert a pleural chest tube at approximately the second intercostal space
   a. If the pneumothorax is less than 20% of the total lung area, a chest tube may not be necessary unless the patient is to undergo surgery
   b. The size of the air leak is determined at the time of the insult

D. Nursing management
1. Prepare the patient for emergency needle thoracentesis
2. Monitor respiratory status for worsening of condition
3. Monitor chest tube drainage system for proper functioning
4. Encourage coughing and deep breathing to facilitate lung expansion

X. Pulmonary aspiration

A. Description
1. Aspiration is a situation in which solids or fluids from the oropharynx or GI tract enter the tracheobronchial tree
   a. Vomiting is an active mechanism by which gastric contents are ejected out of the stomach
   b. Regurgitation is a passive process by which gastric contents are expelled from the stomach; it can occur even in the presence of paralyzed muscles
2. Large particles, when aspirated, can obstruct the trachea or bronchi and cause asphyxia, which can lead to death
3. When the material aspirated has a pH less than 2.5, it causes a chemical burn to the lung, thus increasing the severity of the injury

a. When acidic material is aspirated, type II alveolar cells are destroyed and alveolocapillary membrane permeability is increased, thereby causing extravasation of fluid into the interstitium and alveoli

b. The accumulation of blood and fluid diminishes functional residual capacity and compliance

c. Alveolar ventilation decreases, leading to intrapulmonary shunting and hypoxia

d. Bronchospasm results from irritation of the airways by the acidic aspirate; this irritation leads to epithelial injury and disruption of the alveolar membrane

e. Peribronchial hemorrhage, pulmonary edema, and necrosis also can occur

4. When the material aspirated is clear and nonacidic, the extent of the damage varies according to the volume of fluid aspirated; such situations as near drowning, reflex airway closure, pulmonary edema, and alterations in surfactant lead to hypoxia

5. Aspiration of small, solid particles can produce a severe, subacute, inflammatory reaction with extensive hemorrhage

6. Aspiration of oropharyngeal secretions contaminates the sterile respiratory tract with resident flora

a. Gram-negative aerobes are the most common organisms isolated from pulmonary aspirates of hospitalized patients

b. Anaerobes are most common in pulmonary aspirates from nonhospitalized patients

7. The significant intrapulmonary shunting caused by pulmonary aspiration can lead to severe hypoxemia

a. Within 6 hours after aspiration, hemorrhagic pneumonia occurs

b. $PaCO_2$ usually is much higher after the aspiration of food

8. The outcome of an aspiration event depends on the patient's preexisting physical state and the amount, type, and distribution of the aspirate in the lungs; silent aspiration is especially common in patients with altered levels of consciousness

9. There are several risk factors for pulmonary aspiration

a. Altered level of consciousness caused by drugs, anesthesia, seizures, or central nervous system disorders

b. Compromised glottic closure

c. Depressed cough or gag reflex

d. Presence of an endotracheal, a tracheostomy, or a nasogastric (NG) tube

e. Tracheoesophageal fistula

f. Cardiopulmonary resuscitation

g. Tube feedings

h. Decreased GI motility, intestinal obstruction, or protracted vomiting

i. Facial, oral, or neck surgery or trauma

B. Clinical signs and symptoms
   1. Dyspnea, cough, and wheezing with aspiration of foreign bodies
   2. Respiratory distress with gastric acid aspiration
   3. Cough with pink, frothy exudate
   4. Fever and elevated WBC count if bacterial infection is present
   5. Tachycardia and tachypnea
   6. Hypotension
   7. Inspiratory stridor if the airway is obstructed
      a. Decreased vocal fremitus is present if a foreign body obstructs a large bronchus
      b. If the airway is completely obstructed, breath sounds distal to the obstruction are absent
   8. Dullness on percussion of areas of atelectasis and infiltrates
   9. Aspiration of gastric contents in pulmonary secretions
C. Diagnostic tests
   1. A chest X-ray may show patchy alveolar infiltrates in portions of the lung
   2. The most common areas of involvement are the lower right and left lobes and the right middle lobe; the patient's position at the time of aspiration influences the pattern of lung involvement
D. Medical management
   1. Use an abdominal thrust when the airway is obstructed by large particles; bronchoscopy can be used to retrieve solid particles
   2. Prevent esophageal reflux; the presence of an NG tube prevents closure of the esophageal sphincter
E. Nursing management
   1. If the patient is unconscious, place him or her in a supine or side-lying position to prevent aspiration and gastric reflux
   2. Elevate the head of the bed 30 to 45 degrees in patients receiving tube feedings to facilitate passage of gastric contents across the pylorus and to prevent reflux and aspiration; if elevation of the head of the bed is contraindicated, place the patient in a right lateral decubitus position
   3. Check NG tube placement at regular intervals to detect migration of the tube
   4. Add food coloring to tube feedings to help in identifying gastric contents in the lungs
   5. Use glucose oxidase reagent strips to detect the abnormal presence of glucose in the sputum; keep in mind that a false-positive reading may be caused by blood in the sputum
   6. Monitor gastric residuals at regular intervals (every 2 to 4 hours); if the residual is greater than 20% of the hourly rate or greater than 100 ml in a patient receiving intermittent feedings, discontinue the tube feeding until the cause of the excess residuals is determined and corrected

7. Measure the patient's abdominal girth to assess gastric distention; an increase in abdominal girth of 3.1″ (8 cm) or more may indicate gastric distention and, possibly, retention of the tube feeding

8. Maintain the patency and functioning of the gastric suctioning system; the presence of an NG tube increases the risk of aspiration

9. Treat nausea promptly to prevent vomiting and reduce the risk of aspiration

10. Administer metoclopramide (Reglan) as prescribed; this medication increases upper GI motility and gastric sphincter tone

11. Monitor gastric pH to ensure a pH greater than 2.5; an alkaline pH in the stomach promotes overgrowth of gram-negative organisms

12. Administer histamine$_2$-receptor antagonists as prescribed; these medications increase gastric pH, thereby limiting the chemical burn to pulmonary tissue if aspiration occurs

13. Avoid using a syringe to introduce fluids into the patient's mouth; use of a syringe increases the risk of aspiration by bypassing the tongue and interfering with the swallowing response

14. Encourage patients with reasonable swallowing competence to eat semisolid foods, such as ice cream or pudding; semisolid foods are more easily swallowed than liquids or solids

15. For patients with an endotracheal or a tracheostomy tube, monitor cuff pressures to maintain proper inflation; this action reduces the possibility of aspiration of oropharyngeal secretions

16. Suction the oropharynx at regular intervals to control the accumulation of oropharyngeal secretions above a cuffed endotracheal tube

17. Administer supplemental oxygen, ranging from nasal prongs to mechanical ventilation, to prevent hypoxemia

18. Monitor the patient closely for signs of infection, a primary complication of pulmonary aspiration; prophylactic antibiotic therapy may be prescribed

19. Administer corticosteroids, as prescribed, after aspiration of acidic material; these medications decrease the inflammatory response, but their use is controversial

20. Avoid pulmonary lavage, which can disseminate the aspirate and increase pulmonary damage

XI. **Pulmonary contusion**

A. Description

1. Approximately 75% of patients with blunt chest trauma, especially those with rib fractures, also have pulmonary contusion

2. Signs and symptoms of pulmonary contusion may not develop until 4 to 24 hours after the injury

3. Direct blunt trauma causes alveolar congestion and atelectasis

4. The resulting decrease in intrathoracic pressure and expansion of the lung parenchyma under pressure ruptures capillaries and produces localized edema and hemorrhage

5. The localized edema and hemorrhage increase pulmonary vascular resistance, which decreases pulmonary blood flow

6. Reduced chest wall motion caused by trauma can lead to an inability to cough, with the resultant development of atelectasis; this in turn leads to shunting and alterations in ventilation and perfusion, which manifest as hypoxemia, hypercapnia, and metabolic acidosis and can lead to ARDS (see *Progression of pulmonary contusion,* page 94)

B. Clinical signs and symptoms
1. Ecchymosis on the chest wall at the site of impact
2. Gradual onset of hypoxemia
3. Coughing and expectoration of bloody sputum
4. Tachycardia and tachypnea
5. Diminished breath sounds or crackles on the affected side
6. Dullness on percussion of the involved area
7. Decreased PaO_2 and $PaCO_2$
8. Increased A-a gradient caused by decreasing pulmonary diffusion capacity
9. Localized, patchy, poorly defined areas of increased parenchymal density on chest X-ray, which reflect intra-alveolar hemorrhage

C. Medical management
1. Institute pulmonary care to mobilize secretions
2. Maintain a patent airway and adequate oxygenation
3. Use intubation and mechanical ventilation with PEEP, if indicated, to maintain oxygenation in severe cases
4. Manage fluid intake carefully to minimize vascular fluid leakage into the lung tissue; PAWP should be kept at 10 to 12 mm Hg

D. Nursing management
1. Position patients with the uninjured side down to enhance ventilation and perfusion
2. Place patients with bilateral disease in the right lateral decubitus position, which places a larger surface area in the dependent position and may increase oxygenation; use a rotating bed to prevent pulmonary stasis
3. Elevate the head of the bed to decrease the pressure of abdominal contents on the diaphragm

XII. **Rib fracture**
A. Description
1. Simple rib fractures can cause a patient to avoid movement to prevent pain and to hypoventilate for prolonged periods; shallow breathing and ineffective cough can lead to atelectasis and pneumonia, which in turn may progress to respiratory failure
2. Fracture of the first rib is uncommon; when it occurs, it may indicate severe underlying thoracic injuries, including brachial plexus injury, pneumothorax, aortic rupture, and thoracic outlet syndrome

Progression of pulmonary contusion

Typical steps in the progression of pulmonary contusion are listed below.

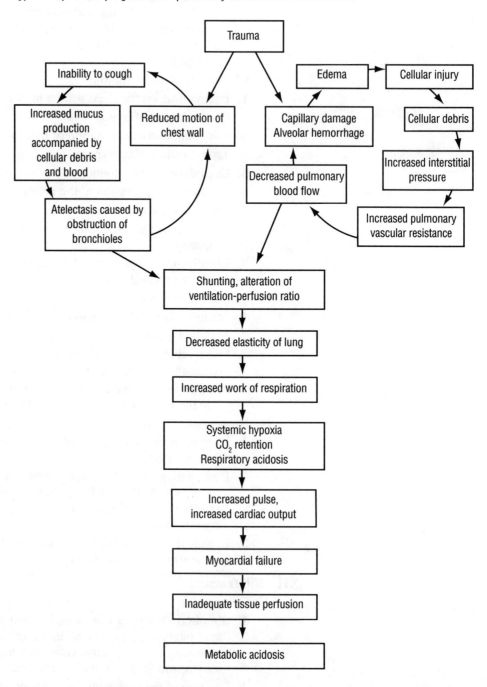

3. The most commonly fractured ribs are the third to eighth ribs; in a single, simple rib fracture, the ribs above and below the fracture site stabilize the broken rib

4. Any rib fracture below the seventh rib is also considered abdominal trauma; lower rib fractures in particular are associated with laceration or tear of the liver or spleen

B. Clinical signs and symptoms

1. Chest pain
2. Pneumothorax
3. Diminished breath sounds and shallow respirations
4. Abnormal ABG values

C. Medical management

1. Provide adequate analgesia, including an intercostal nerve block if necessary; a patient who has a tidal volume less than 5 ml/kg despite adequate pain control generally should be admitted to the hospital

2. Do not use binders, which decrease chest excursion

D. Nursing management

1. Encourage coughing and deep breathing, using bronchial hygiene and chest physiotherapy techniques; these actions keep the airways open and prevent the buildup of secretions

2. Frequently monitor respiratory status, noting changes indicative of pneumothorax

XIII. Status asthmaticus

A. Description

1. Asthma is a state of increased airway responsiveness (hyperreactivity) that produces reversible episodes of bronchoconstriction

2. Asthma is characterized by bronchoconstriction, mucosal edema, and excessive production of thick, tenacious mucus, which increases the work of breathing and impairs gas exchange

    a. Bronchoconstriction and mucus plugging cause trapping of air, which results in hyperinflation of the lungs

    b. The bronchial walls hypertrophy, leading to bronchiolar obstruction, which reduces alveolar ventilation and causes hyperinflation of the alveoli

3. Pathologic airway changes associated with asthma include hypertrophy of the smooth muscle, thickening of the respiratory epithelial basement membrane, hypertrophy and hyperplasia of mucus glands, and proliferation of goblet cells

4. A commonality in many patients with asthma and those with allergies is the tendency to form immunoglobulin E antibodies

5. Many asthmatic patients show decreased responsiveness to $beta_2$ receptors and increased responsiveness to alpha receptors and cholinergic receptors

6. The mortality rate from asthma has risen in the past decade, with the greatest increase occurring in patients older than age 65

7. Status asthmaticus is a severe attack of asthma that does not respond to conventional therapy; hypoxemia and a widened A-a gradient are signs of status asthmaticus

8. The most common causes of status asthmaticus are exposure to allergens, noncompliance with the medication regimen, inappropriate bronchodilator use, and respiratory tract infections

9. Other causes of status asthmaticus include emotional stress, exposure to drastic temperature changes or inhalation of cold air, exposure to cigarette smoke or dust, exercise, and use of aspirin, nonsteroidal anti-inflammatory drugs, or nonselective beta-blocking medications (such as propranolol [Inderal])

B. Clinical signs and symptoms

1. Dyspnea, chest tightness, restlessness, and anxiety

2. Pursed-lip breathing, nasal flaring, and intercostal bulging on expiration

3. Minimal chest expansion on inspiration and decreased vocal fremitus caused by hyperinflation of the lungs

4. Cough that may produce thick, tenacious mucus

5. Inspiratory or expiratory wheezes caused by bronchoconstriction; decreased or absent breath sounds (silent chest) are ominous signs

6. Prolonged expiratory phase of the respiratory cycle as the patient attempts to exhale trapped air

7. Impaired diaphragmatic excursion caused by trapped air

8. Tachypnea or hyperpnea

9. Tachycardia

10. Use of accessory muscles of respiration

11. $PaCO_2$ less than 30 mm Hg (indicating hyperventilation), PaO_2 less than 60 mm Hg (indicating hypoxemia), and pH greater than 7.45 (indicating respiratory alkalosis); a rising $PaCO_2$ is a sign of impending respiratory failure

C. Diagnostic tests

1. The WBC count may indicate eosinophilia in response to allergens

2. The chest X-ray may show hyperinflation of the lungs

3. Pulmonary function tests may show a peak expiratory flow less than 60 L/minute, an FEV_1 (forced expiratory volume in first second) less than 600 ml, and an FVC (forced vital capacity) less than 1 L

D. Medical management

1. Rehydrate the patient with oral or I.V. fluids to liquefy pulmonary secretions

2. Initiate bronchodilator therapy to relieve bronchospasm; bronchodilating agents include sympathomimetics, epinephrine, isoproterenol, metaproterenol, terbutaline, methylxanthines, theophylline, aminophylline, anticholinergic agents, atropine, and ipratropium bromide

   a. Theophylline generally is given by continuous infusion

      b. Methylxanthines and sympathomimetics increase intracellular levels of cyclic adenosine monophosphate in bronchial smooth muscle cells and mast cells

      c. Anticholinergic agents block parasympathetic innervation at cholinergic receptor sites in the airways

  3. Prescribe corticosteroids to reduce the inflammatory response in the lungs

      a. Beclomethasone dipropionate (Beclovent, Vanceril) is administered as an inhaled agent

      b. Hydrocortisone sodium succinate (Solu-Cortef) or methylprednisolone (Solu-Medrol) is administered I.V.; prednisone can be administered orally

      c. Cromolyn sodium, which coats mast cells and prevents the release of the chemical mediators that cause bronchoconstriction, is ineffective if an attack is occurring and usually is not administered to patients with status asthmaticus

  4. Administer sedatives with extreme caution, if at all

  5. Administer supplemental oxygen, ranging from nasal prongs to mechanical ventilation, to prevent hypoxemia

  6. Prescribe antibiotics, including cephalosporins, aminoglycosides, and penicillins, to eradicate respiratory tract infections

E. Nursing management

  1. Position the patient sitting up with the shoulder girdle elevated (for example, with the hands over the head or leaning on a bedside table); this position lessens the feeling of air hunger

  2. Implement chest physiotherapy, including postural drainage with percussion and vibration as well as coughing and deep breathing in conjunction with bronchodilator therapy, to remove retained pulmonary secretions

  3. Implement interventions similar to those for patients with acute respiratory failure (see pages 78 to 81)

4 Endocrine disorders

I. **Anatomy**
   A. Pituitary gland
      1. Located in the sella turcica of the sphenoid bone, the pituitary gland weighs .02 oz (0.5 g)
      2. The pituitary gland is composed of two lobes: the anterior pituitary (adenohypophysis) and the posterior pituitary (neurohypophysis)
   B. Thyroid gland
      1. The thyroid gland is located immediately below the larynx on either side of and anterior to the trachea; it is approximately 1.6″ (4 cm) wide
      2. The two lobes of the thyroid gland are connected by an isthmus
      3. The right lobe of the thyroid gland may be 25% larger than the left lobe
   C. Parathyroid glands
      1. The parathyroid glands are four small glands that are located on the posterior surface of the thyroid gland at the upper and lower ends of each lobe
      2. They receive their blood supply from the thyroid gland and are often damaged by thyroid surgery
   D. Adrenal glands
      1. The adrenal glands are located on the upper lobes of each kidney
      2. They are composed of two separate tissues: the adrenal cortex (outer layer, or covering) and the adrenal medulla (inner layer)
   E. Pancreas
      1. The pancreas is located transversely in the left upper abdominal quadrant, behind the peritoneum and the stomach
      2. It contains specialized cells called alpha, beta, and delta cells

II. **Physiology**
   A. Pituitary gland
      1. The secretion of most pituitary hormones is controlled by the hypothalamus, which secretes releasing and inhibiting factors
      2. The term hypothalamic-pituitary-adrenocortical axis refers to the complex interrelationship between the central nervous system (CNS) and the pituitary gland
      3. Pituitary hormones regulate several other endocrine glands and affect many diverse body functions; most of the hormones produced by the anterior pituitary gland stimulate the secretion of other hormones

Principal hormones of the endocrine glands

Gland	Hormones
Thyroid	Calcitonin
	Thyroxine
	Triiodothyronine
Adrenal	Adrenal androgens
	Aldosterone
	Catecholamines
	Cortisol
Ovary	Estrogen
	Progesterone
Testes	Testosterone
Parathyroid	Parathyroid hormone
Pancreas	Insulin
	Glucagon
Anterior pituitary	Corticotropin (also known as adrenocorticotropic hormone)
	Follicle-stimulating hormone
	Growth hormone
	Luteinizing hormone
	Melanocyte-stimulating hormone
	Prolactin
	Thyroid-stimulating hormone
Posterior pituitary	Oxytocin
	Vasopressin (also known as antidiuretic hormone)

(handwritten annotations: T3 T4 next to thyroid hormones; ACTH, FSH, GH, LH, TSH next to anterior pituitary; Oxytocin, ADH next to posterior pituitary)

(handwritten: ANT PIT → ACTH regulates horm in Adrenal Cortex)

4. The anterior pituitary gland produces several hormones (for a complete listing of the primary hormones, see *Principal hormones of the endocrine glands*)

   a. Thyroid-stimulating hormone regulates thyroid production of hormones

   b. Corticotropin, also known as adrenocorticotropic hormone, regulates hormones produced in the adrenal cortex

   c. Luteinizing hormone and follicle-stimulating hormone stimulate ovulation, progesterone secretion, and spermatogenesis

   d. Prolactin regulates lactation

   e. Growth hormone (GH) regulates growth, metabolism, and secretion of growth-promoting peptides in the liver

   f. Melanocyte-stimulating hormone regulates skin pigmentation

5. The posterior pituitary gland also produces hormones
   a. Antidiuretic hormone (ADH), also known as vasopressin, regulates homeostatic fluid balance by controlling plasma osmolality
      (1) Antidiuretic hormone acts to increase the permeability of the distal renal tubules
      (2) The increased renal permeability leads to an increase in water reabsorption and the production of more concentrated urine
   b. Oxytocin regulates uterine contractions and lactation in pregnant women

B. Thyroid gland
   1. The thyroid gland produces three hormones: triiodothyronine (T_3), thyroxine (T_4), and calcitonin
   2. These three hormones regulate the body's metabolic rate and influence growth and development

C. Parathyroid glands
   1. The parathyroid glands produce parathyroid hormone (PTH)
   2. Also called parahormone, PTH regulates calcium and phosphorus metabolism

D. Adrenal glands
   1. The adrenal glands produce hormones specific to the adrenal cortex and the adrenal medulla
   2. The adrenal cortex produces three hormones
      a. Aldosterone, the major mineralocorticoid, helps regulate electrolyte balance by promoting sodium retention and potassium loss
      b. Cortisol, the major glucocorticoid, influences carbohydrate storage, exerts anti-inflammatory effects, suppresses corticotropin secretion, and increases protein catabolism
      c. Adrenal androgens and estrogens play an important role in the development of secondary sex characteristics and reproduction
   3. The adrenal medulla produces the following catecholamines: epinephrine, a positive inotropic agent, and norepinephrine, a potent peripheral vasoconstrictor

E. Pancreas
   1. The pancreas produces three hormones: insulin, glucagon, and gastrin
   2. Insulin is produced by the beta cells in the islets of Langerhans; the overall effect of insulin release is a decrease in the blood glucose level
      a. Insulin promotes the synthesis of proteins, carbohydrates, lipids, and nucleic acids
      b. It facilitates the transport of glucose across the cell membrane
      c. It increases glucose uptake in the liver and stimulates synthesis of glycogen and fatty acids in the liver

     d. It inhibits hepatic gluconeogenesis (glucose formation), glycogenolysis (splitting of glycogen to form glucose), and ketogenesis (formation of ketones from fats)

     e. It facilitates the intracellular transport of potassium

     f. In muscle, insulin increases uptake of glucose and amino acids, increases glycogen synthesis, stimulates protein synthesis, and inhibits protein breakdown (proteolysis)

     g. In adipose tissue, insulin increases glucose uptake, stimulates fat synthesis, and inhibits fat breakdown (lipolysis); the net effect of insulin in these tissues is to stimulate cellular metabolism

   3. Glucagon, which is secreted by the alpha cells in the islets of Langerhans, stimulates glucose production in the liver and is an insulin antagonist

   4. Gastrin, which is secreted by the delta cells in the islets of Langerhans, regulates the secretion of hydrochloric acid

III. Endocrine assessment

  A. Noninvasive assessment techniques

    1. Inspect the patient's general appearance, noting height, fat distribution, striae, neck scars or nodules, hair distribution and texture, and growth and developmental level; check for medical identification information

    2. Palpate the skin for tissue turgor and diaphoresis and the neck for enlarged or nodular goiter

    3. Percuss for abnormal deep tendon reflexes

    4. Auscultate the neck for bruits over the thyroid and the heart for remote or S_3 heart sounds

    5. Check blood pressure for orthostasis and hypotension

    6. Check heart rate and rhythm for presence of tachycardia, bradycardia, or arrhythmias

    7. Assess the patient's respiratory pattern for tachypnea and Kussmaul's respirations

    8. Check for hypoactive bowel sounds

  B. Invasive assessment techniques

    1. The water deprivation test measures a patient's ability to concentrate urine; it is used when diabetes insipidus is suspected

     a. In a patient with neurogenic diabetes insipidus, a 9% increase in urine osmolality occurs after the administration of vasopressin

     b. In a patient with nephrogenic diabetes insipidus, urine osmolality is unaffected after vasopressin administration

    2. The water loading test measures a patient's ability to increase urine output in response to a large fluid challenge; this test is used to diagnose syndrome of inappropriate antidiuretic hormone secretion (SIADH)

  C. Key laboratory values

    1. Sodium (normal value: 135 to 145 mEq/L)

a. Sodium imbalance may result from a loss of sodium, a gain of sodium, or a change in water volume

b. Hypernatremia (serum sodium level greater than 145 mEq/L) may be caused by excessive sodium intake, insufficient water intake, water loss exceeding sodium intake (which may result from diabetes insipidus, impaired renal function, or prolonged vomiting and diarrhea), or sodium retention secondary to aldosteronism

c. Hypernatremia associated with hypovolemia manifests as increased serum sodium level results from dehydration; this condition is seen in such disorders as diabetic ketoacidosis (DKA), hyperosmolar hyperglycemic nonketotic syndrome (HHNS), and diabetes insipidus

d. Hyponatremia (serum sodium level less than 135 mEq/L) may result from inadequate sodium intake, excessive sodium loss secondary to profuse sweating, gastric suctioning, diuretic therapy, diarrhea, vomiting, adrenal insufficiency, burns, or chronic renal insufficiency with acidosis; in SIADH, hyponatremia is caused by a dilutional sodium decrease

2. Potassium (normal value: 3.5 to 5.5 mEq/L)

a. A reciprocal relationship exists between sodium and potassium; a substantial increase in one substance usually causes a corresponding decrease in the other

b. Because the kidneys have no efficient method for conserving potassium, potassium deficiency can develop rapidly and is quite common

c. Hyperkalemia (potassium level greater than 5.5 mEq/L) is common in patients with DKA or HHNS, which are conditions in which excessive cellular potassium enters the extracellular compartment

d. Hypokalemia (potassium level less than 3.5 mEq/L) may be present in the severe dehydration states associated with DKA or HHNS; hypokalemia is indicative of severe, prolonged dehydration

3. Serum phosphate (normal value: 2.5 to 4.5 mEq/L)

a. Hyperphosphatemia (serum phosphate level greater than 4.5 mEq/L) may result from hypoparathyroidism, DKA, or renal failure

b. Hypophosphatemia (serum phosphate level less than 2.5 mEq/L) may result from chronic alcoholism, hyperparathyroidism, renal tubular acidosis, or the treatment of DKA with glucose

4. Anion gap (normal value: 8 to 14 mEq/L)

a. The anion gap reflects the serum anion-cation balance and can be used to differentiate among types of metabolic acidosis

b. An anion gap greater than 15 mEq/L suggests an acidosis characterized by excessive organic or inorganic acids, such as lactic acidosis or DKA

[Handwritten margin notes:]
↓ Serum Osmo < 280
hypervolemic SIADH

↑ Serum Osmo
DI DKA > 295
HHNS > 350

↑ UOsmo
SIADH
↓ UOsma - DI

    c. A normal anion gap (between 8 and 14 mEq/L) occurs in hyperchloremic acidosis and renal tubular acidosis

  5. Osmolality

    a. Serum osmolality (normal value: 280 to 295 mOsm/kg) is a measure of the number of particles in serum

      (1) Elevated serum osmolality (greater than 295 mOsm/kg) is found in conditions that are produced by osmotic diuresis (such as diabetes insipidus and DKA); HHNS results in an extremely high serum osmolality (usually greater than 350 mOsm/kg)

      (2) Decreased serum osmolality (less than 280 mOsm/kg) is found in certain hypervolemic conditions, such as SIADH

    b. Urine osmolality (normal range: 50 to 1,400 mOsm/kg; average range: 500 to 800 mOsm/kg) is a measure of the number of particles in urine

      (1) Elevated urine osmolality is seen in SIADH

      (2) Decreased urine osmolality is seen in diabetes insipidus

  6. Glucose (normal value for fasting specimen: 70 to 110 mg/dl)

    a. The glucose level can provide a rapid assessment of metabolic status

    b. A glucose level greater than 300 mg/dl indicates DKA; in patients with HHNS, the glucose level may be 600 mg/dl or higher

    c. A glucose level less than 50 mg/dl usually indicates hypoglycemia

    d. Glycosylated hemoglobin is a measurement of the glucose level within erythrocytes; it is a much stabler measurement than plasma glucose, which is affected by metabolic processes; glycosylated hemoglobin is useful for determining control of diabetes up to 4 months before hospital admission

D. Diagnostic tests

  1. Radiologic studies can help to identify the precipitating factor in an endocrine disorder

    a. X-rays of the skull, chest, and abdomen may identify tumors responsible for increased, inhibited, or ectopic secretion of hormones, such as ADH and insulin

    b. The radioactive iodine uptake test may identify abnormal uptake of iodine; a scan of the parathyroid gland may identify abnormal uptake of calcium

  2. Electrocardiograms (ECGs) can identify the arrhythmias associated with a metabolic disturbance, such as an elevated potassium level, and the tachyarrhythmias associated with dehydration; continuous ECG monitoring is recommended for a patient experiencing a metabolic disturbance related to endocrine dysfunction

  3. Arterial blood gas (ABG) analysis can be used to determine the extent and physiologic basis of acidosis or alkalosis; metabolic acidosis (pH less than 7.35) is associated with DKA

IV. Acute hypoglycemia

A. Description

1. Acute hypoglycemia is characterized as a glucose level less than 50 mg/dl, arising from endogenous, exogenous, or functional causes

2. Also called insulin reaction or insulin shock, acute hypoglycemia most often occurs in patients with insulin-dependent diabetes, although it also can occur in those with non-insulin-dependent diabetes

3. Predisposing factors for the development of acute hypoglycemia fall into three categories

   a. Exogenous hypoglycemia is caused by insulin excess, oral hypoglycemic agents, and the use of alcohol or other drugs (for example, salicylates and pentamidine)

   b. Endogenous hypoglycemia is caused by pancreatic and other tumors and inborn errors of metabolism

   c. Functional hypoglycemia is caused by dumping syndrome, spontaneous reactive hypoglycemia, other endocrine deficiency states, and prolonged muscular exercise

4. In acute hypoglycemia, glucose production—by means of food intake or liver gluconeogenesis—lags behind glucose utilization

5. Because glucose is the preferred fuel of the CNS, hypoglycemia produces changes in the level of consciousness and increases the levels of insulin antagonists, such as glucagon, epinephrine, cortisol, and GH

6. In exogenous hypoglycemia and functional hypoglycemia, symptoms generally follow a pattern related to eating, exercise, and administration of insulin or oral hypoglycemic agents; in endogenous hypoglycemia, such as insulinoma, the onset of hypoglycemic events is not precipitated by any factors

B. Clinical signs and symptoms

1. Tachycardia
2. Diaphoresis
3. Fatigue and irritability
4. Tremor, nervousness, and weakness
5. Nausea

C. Laboratory values

1. Serum glucose less than 50 mg/dl
2. Abnormal electrolyte levels, osmolality, urine specific gravity, and ABG values if the patient has been unresponsive for a prolonged period

D. Medical management

1. Administer glucose

   a. Infuse dextrose 10% in water until the serum glucose level reaches 100 to 200 mg/dl

   b. In an unresponsive patient with severe hypoglycemia, administer dextrose 50% in water I.V.

      c. In a conscious patient, administer oral glucose

   2. Inject 1 mg glucagon S.C.

   3. Obtain a fingerstick or plasma glucose sample 20 to 30 minutes after administration of glucose or glucagon

  E. Nursing management

   1. Inspect for cool, clammy, pale skin; assess the patient's level of consciousness and sensory and motor function; check for tremors and seizure activity (adrenergic stimulation is a compensatory reaction that produces the neurologic and cardiovascular changes associated with hypoglycemia)

   2. Check for medical identification information, which may indicate that the patient uses insulin or oral hypoglycemic agents; acute hypoglycemia is seen most often in diabetic patients, and medical identification information can help identify hypoglycemia in an unconscious patient

   3. Palpate and auscultate for tachycardia, tachyarrhythmias, and low blood pressure; these cardiac indicators provide clues about the level of shock the patient may be experiencing and the level of adrenergic stimulation

   4. Monitor the patient's neurologic and cardiovascular status closely; hypoglycemia can cause arrhythmias, extend infarcts, and produce seizures

   5. Use a diabetic flow sheet to record all glucose administration, responses to treatment, and plasma-capillary glucose values; accurate assessment of the trends during recovery or relapse is essential in preventing further hypoglycemic or hyperglycemic complications

   6. Institute seizure precautions to prevent injury: have suction equipment available at the bedside, place an oral airway at the head of the bed, keep padded side rails of the bed upright, and ensure that an oxygen source is readily available

   7. Compare the patient's neurologic status against fingerstick blood glucose level measurements; a rapid, dramatic return to alertness should occur when the glucose level is corrected; if the patient remains unresponsive, suspect cerebral edema

   8. When the patient is stabilized, educate him or her about medication administration, hypoglycemic symptoms, and diet therapy; knowledge of the overall treatment regimen can facilitate self-care and help prevent future complications

   9. Tell the patient to carry a rapid-acting sugar source (such as hard candy) at all times and to wear medical identification; these actions will help ensure prompt treatment if a hypoglycemic episode occurs again

V. Diabetes insipidus

  A. Description

   1. Patients with diabetes insipidus are unable to concentrate urine because of insufficient or impaired ADH production or activity

2. Two types of diabetes insipidus exist

    a. Neurogenic, or central, diabetes insipidus results from organic brain lesions that cause insufficient amounts of ADH to be synthesized, transported, or released from the posterior pituitary gland

      (1) Organic lesions of the hypothalamus, infundibular stem, or posterior pituitary gland can result from primary brain tumors, hypophysectomy, cerebral aneurysms, cerebral thrombosis, or closed head trauma

      (2) Organic brain lesions also may result from infections or immunologic disorders

    b. Nephrogenic diabetes insipidus usually is an acquired disorder that causes an inadequate kidney response to ADH; nephrogenic diabetes insipidus usually is caused by disorders and drugs that affect the kidneys

      (1) Disorders that may lead to nephrogenic diabetes insipidus include pyelonephritis, amyloidosis, sarcoidosis, destructive neuropathies, polycystic disease, intrinsic renal disease, multiple myeloma, and sickle cell disease

      (2) Nephrotoxic agents that can lead to nephrogenic diabetes insipidus include phenytoin, lithium carbonate, ethanol, demeclocycline, general anesthetics, and methoxyflurane

3. The impairment of ADH activity seen in diabetes insipidus causes immediate excretion of large amounts of dilute urine, thereby leading to increased plasma osmolality and decreased urine osmolality

4. In conscious patients, the hypothalamic thirst mechanism is stimulated and induces polydipsia

B. Clinical signs and symptoms

1. Polyuria with complaints of large, frequent, dilute voidings; urine output ranges from 165 to 500 ml/hour

2. Polydipsia

3. Tachycardia and hypotension

4. Hemoconcentration secondary to reduced circulating blood volume

5. Poor skin turgor and dry mucous membranes

C. Laboratory values

1. Elevated serum osmolality (greater than 295 mOsm/kg) and serum sodium level

2. Decreased urine osmolality (less than 500 mOsm/kg; may be as low as 50 mOsm/kg)

3. Low urine specific gravity (1.000 to 1.005)

4. Decreased urine sodium concentration (less than 20 mEq/L)

D. Diagnostic tests

1. In a patient with diabetes insipidus, a decreased urine output resulting from the vasopressin test confirms the diagnosis of neurogenic diabetes insipidus

   2. The water deprivation test differentiates psychogenic polydipsia from diabetes insipidus
E. Medical management
   1. Establish I.V. access for a dehydrated patient
   2. Administer oral or I.V. hypotonic fluids
   3. Restrict oral and I.V. fluid intake when administering the water deprivation test
      a. Explain the fluid restrictions to visitors and other health care providers
      b. Obtain frequent body weight measurements and vital sign readings during the test
      c. Consider discontinuing the test if the patient experiences a more than 3% weight loss
   4. Administer ADH replacement therapy
      a. Administer aqueous vasopressin (Pitressin) I.V. or S.C.
      b. Administer lypressin intranasally
      c. Administer desmopressin acetate (DDAVP) S.C. or intranasally
F. Nursing management
   1. Document the patient's medical history, noting risk factors that predispose the patient to diabetes insipidus, such as medications, recent exposure to general anesthesia, and impaired cognitive ability; identification of risk factors can help differentiate between diabetes insipidus and other polyuric states, including diabetes mellitus, HHNS, osmotic diuresis, and primary polydipsia
   2. Assess the patient's level of knowledge of the disease process; knowledge deficits must be addressed to increase awareness of early disease onset and to prevent a recurrence of diabetes insipidus
   3. Assess skin turgor and hydration of skin, mucous membranes, and eyeballs; these assessments are good indicators of hydration status, especially in patients who are unable to communicate
   4. Obtain an accurate baseline weight to help evaluate patient response to therapy
   5. Meticulously monitor input and output, noting frequent complaints of thirst and the color, amount, and specific gravity of urine; accurate input and output measurements, weight gain, and changes in plasma and urine values are the most accurate indicators of treatment efficacy and the most efficient methods by which to monitor and correct sustained dehydration or the development of water intoxication
   6. In neurosurgical patients, monitor input and output for 7 to 10 days postoperatively; neurogenic diabetes insipidus resulting from head trauma may appear to resolve and then reappear permanently if undetected and untreated
   7. Monitor serum electrolyte, glucose, and hemoglobin levels and hematocrit

     a. A normal glucose level eliminates DKA and HHNS as the cause of polyuria, polydipsia, and dehydration

     b. An elevated hemoglobin level and hematocrit may indicate hemoconcentration, a sign of dehydration

  8. Monitor pulse rate, ECG activity, and blood pressure; sinus tachycardia and hypotension may indicate hypovolemia, and the vasopressant effect of ADH replacement therapy may predispose patients (especially those with underlying coronary artery disease) to angina

  9. Monitor for the adverse effects of exogenous vasopressin administration: edema, low urine output, hyponatremia, headache, nasal congestion, nausea, slight increase in blood pressure, personality changes, and changes in the level of consciousness

  10. Water intoxication also is a possible adverse effect of high-dose exogenous vasopressin therapy and may occur with ADH therapy if excess fluids are ingested

  11. Administer chlorpropamide, as prescribed, to augment the renal response in patients with nephrogenic diabetes insipidus; this drug stimulates release of ADH from the posterior pituitary gland and augments renal tubular response to ADH

  12. Ensure adequate nutritional intake to prevent the hypoglycemia caused by increased pancreatic insulin production related to chlorpropamide administration

  13. Administer thiazide diuretics as prescribed; these medications induce mild sodium depletion and reduce the solute load, thus enhancing water reabsorption

  14. Restrict dietary sodium to induce sodium depletion; a 250-mg (11-mEq) daily sodium diet can effectively reduce urine output by 40% to 50%

  15. After the initial hypovolemia is resolved, educate the patient about risk factors, medication administration, adverse effects, and the potential for recurrence of symptoms to help prevent the severe complications associated with diabetes insipidus

VI. Diabetic ketoacidosis

  A. Description

    1. Diabetic ketoacidosis develops when there is an absolute or a relative deficiency of insulin and an increase in stress

     a. The lack of circulating insulin produces an accumulation of glucose in the blood that exceeds the renal threshold, thereby spilling glucose into the urine

     b. Excess serum glucose produces osmotic diuresis, extracting water from the vascular space and causing rapid dehydration

     c. The liver begins to break down fats and protein to provide energy to the glucose-deprived cells; this process is called gluconeogenesis

      d. The by-products of gluconeogenesis (keto acids, acetoacetic acid, and beta-hydroxybutyric acid) form acetone, which is responsible for the fruity odor noted on the patient's breath

      e. Ketones—the end products of fat metabolism (lipolysis)—form in the liver, accumulate in the bloodstream, and contribute to metabolic acidosis

      f. To compensate for metabolic acidosis, the lungs attempt to eliminate the excess carbonic acid by hyperventilating carbon dioxide (evidenced by Kussmaul's respirations)

      g. The body attempts to buffer excess hydrogen ions in the cell with proteins, phosphate, and bicarbonate, thus leading to the bicarbonate depletion noted in ABG values

      h. As hydrogen ions enter the cell, potassium ions are driven into the extracellular space (in ion exchange); elevated potassium levels in the range of 4.5 to 6.5 mEq/L commonly are seen in patients with DKA

  2. Patients with insulin-dependent diabetes and those newly diagnosed with diabetes are at greatest risk for DKA

  3. The mortality rate associated with DKA is 5% to 15%; in elderly patients and in patients with other chronic illnesses, the mortality rate ranges from 40% to 70%

      a. Death occurs not from hyperglycemia but from the complications of untreated hyperglycemia

      b. These complications include profound hypovolemic shock; inadequate organ and tissue perfusion with subsequent thrombus formation, infarction, or both; electrolyte imbalance with associated arrhythmias; and uncorrected, prolonged acidosis that may result from underlying, undetected sepsis

  4. The most common stressors that precipitate DKA are infections, trauma, surgery, myocardial infarction, and emotional stress

B. Laboratory values

  1. Serum glucose: 300 to 1,200 mg/dl

  2. Electrolytes: initially hyperkalemia and hypernatremia and then hypokalemia and hyponatremia

  3. Phosphate: decreased

  4. Magnesium: initially elevated and then decreased

  5. Blood urea nitrogen (BUN): elevated in severely dehydrated patients

  6. Serum osmolality: 295 to 330 mOsm/kg

  7. Hematocrit and white blood cell count: elevated

  8. Serum ketones: significantly elevated

  9. Anion gap: greater than 15 mEq/L

  10. ABG values: pH less than or equal to 7.20, HCO_3^- less than 10 mEq/L, decreased PCO_2 level

  11. Glycosuria, ketonuria, elevated acetone, proteinuria, decreased urine sodium level, and urine specific gravity greater than 1.025

C. Medical management
   1. Establish I.V. access
   2. Administer at least 2 L of normal saline solution; administer half-normal saline solution in place of normal saline solution or in alternation with normal saline solution after the initial 2 to 3 L have been infused
   3. Add potassium chloride to the maintenance I.V. infusion when the patient's potassium level is below 4 mEq/L; alternate potassium chloride with potassium phosphate after the vascular volume is stabilized
   4. Obtain serum electrolyte levels and ABG measurements at hourly intervals
   5. Administer sodium bicarbonate therapy, as prescribed, for patients with an arterial pH less than 7.10

D. Nursing management
   1. Assess for risk factors, including previously diagnosed diabetes, history of other endocrine disorders, recent reports of physical or emotional stress, and inadequate diabetic self-care practices; at least one-third of hospital admissions for DKA are associated with poor glucose control related to knowledge deficit and psychosocial distress
   2. Note blurred vision, abdominal pain, decreased level of consciousness, lethargy, fatigue, weakness, polyuria, nocturia, nausea, vomiting, abdominal bloating and cramping, polyphagia, polydipsia, and recent weight loss; cognitive and perceptual dysfunction as well as elimination and nutritional status are important indicators of the duration of illness and degree of dehydration
   3. Inspect for flushed and dry skin, dry mucous membranes, decreased skin turgor, sunken eyeballs, and medical identification information noting that the patient has diabetes; early detection of the physical signs and symptoms of diabetes can help in the rapid diagnosis of DKA, prompt treatment of dehydration and hyperglycemia, and prevention of multiple organ damage resulting from dehydration
   4. Check for tachycardia, hypotension, tachypnea, Kussmaul's respirations, and an acetone odor on the breath
   5. Assess intake and output, urine specific gravity, central venous pressure or pulmonary artery wedge pressure, skin turgor, and mucous membranes every hour; hourly assessments provide the most comprehensive information regarding hydration status and patient response to treatment
   6. Administer short-acting insulin I.V. to correct hyperglycemia; a bolus dose of 10 to 25 U (0.3 U/kg of body weight) of human regular insulin typically is administered
      a. I.V. insulin produces the stablest and most predictable reductions in serum glucose levels

b. Human insulin is preferred because some patients may develop antibodies to animal (beef or pork) insulin, especially those patients who have used animal insulin on an irregular basis

7. After the I.V. insulin bolus is administered, begin an insulin infusion by way of an infusion pump by mixing 100 U of regular insulin in 100 ml of normal saline solution; infuse at a rate of 5 to 10 U/hour

  a. The 1:1 ratio minimizes error in the delivery of the insulin infusion because the rate of delivery on the infusion pump (ml/hour) is the actual amount of insulin units the patient receives per hour

  b. This ratio also minimizes error because a 100-ml container of fluid is less likely to be mistaken as the maintenance I.V. fluid, thus preventing inadvertent increases or decreases in the insulin infusion

8. Use a diabetic flow sheet to monitor hourly glucose level, serum laboratory values (sodium, potassium, BUN, and creatinine), and ABG values; this form is helpful in identifying trends and changes in the patient's condition and in preventing the potential complications of hyperchloremic acidosis and hypoglycemia and the adverse effects of sodium bicarbonate therapy

9. Begin dextrose 5% in water (D_5W), D_5W in half-normal saline solution, or D_5W in 0.225% sodium chloride solution infusion at the decreased rate of 100 to 125 ml/hour when the patient's glucose level reaches approximately 250 mg/dl

  a. Adding dextrose to the infusion prevents hypoglycemia and accelerates the resolution of ketone bodies by decreasing lipolysis

  b. The decreased I.V. rate prevents fluid overload and rapid infusion of glucose

10. Maintain insulin infusion until ketones are absent from blood or urine

  a. Because the plasma glucose level generally falls before ketogenesis is reversed, the insulin infusion should be maintained at a low rate to prevent rebound hyperglycemia (the Somogyi effect) and acidosis

  b. The rationale is that if ketones still are present, then acidosis is not completely resolved

11. Administer regular and intermediate-acting insulin S.C. at least 2 hours (sometimes 4 to 6 hours) before discontinuing the I.V. insulin infusion; because the half-life of I.V. insulin is short, administering a longer-acting insulin helps prevent rebound hyperglycemia and acidosis

12. Provide the patient with information regarding procedures and the need for frequent laboratory specimens, ABG sampling, and vital sign readings; the neurologic changes and invasive procedures associated with DKA provoke fear and anxiety in the patient; information and reassurance can diminish the patient's anxiety and alleviate one source of stress

13. As the patient's condition improves, educate him or her about the precipitating factors of DKA and the need for more careful monitoring and control of diabetes

14. To decrease the risk of a recurrence of DKA, teach the patient correct insulin management, including measurement of doses, administration, rotation of injection sites, and glucose monitoring

VII. **Hyperosmolar hyperglycemic nonketotic syndrome**
   A. Description
      1. Hyperosmolar hyperglycemic nonketotic syndrome (HHNS), like DKA, is a condition of hyperglycemia and profound dehydration resulting from insulin deficiency
         a. Hyperosmolar hyperglycemic nonketotic syndrome is thought to result from the small amounts of circulating endogenous insulin that are sufficient to inhibit lipolysis but insufficient to prevent severe hyperglycemia and profound dehydration
         b. The resulting elevated blood glucose level produces osmotic diuresis, which leads to intracellular and extracellular dehydration
         c. As in DKA, sodium, potassium, and phosphorus are excreted through diuresis
         d. Severe dehydration results in hypoperfusion of the kidneys and altered glomerular filtration, leading to azotemia and acute tubular necrosis
         e. The impaired renal function exacerbates hyperglycemia
         f. If uncorrected, the high serum osmolality seen in HHNS leads to severe confusion, coma, and death
      2. Hyperosmolar hyperglycemic nonketotic syndrome is distinguished from DKA by the lack of ketosis and acidosis; however, the overall mortality rate for HHNS (15% to 20%) is higher than that for DKA
      3. Risk factors for HHNS include insulin-independent diabetes, obesity, advanced age, tube feedings and total parenteral nutrition, history of hypertension and coronary artery disease, pancreatitis, use of certain medications (thiazide diuretics, steroids, epinephrine, and phenytoin), and certain medical treatments (dialysis and burn therapy)
   B. Clinical signs and symptoms
      1. Severe confusion, generalized seizure disorder, positive Babinski's reflex, and nystagmus
      2. Rapid, shallow respirations
      3. Poor skin turgor and dry mucous membranes
      4. Tachycardia, hypotension, and arrhythmias
   C. Laboratory values
      1. Serum glucose: 400 to 4,000 mg/dl
      2. Sodium: high, normal, or low
      3. Potassium: high, normal, or low
      4. Serum osmolality: greater than or equal to 350 mOsm/kg

5. Blood urea nitrogen: greater than or equal to 20 mg/dl
6. Bicarbonate level: normal
7. Serum ketones: absent or minimal
8. pH: 7.30 to 7.50
9. Anion gap: less than 12 mEq/L

D. Medical management

1. Establish I.V. access and rapidly replace fluids, using crystalloid and colloid solutions; administer approximately 2 L of half-normal saline solution or normal saline solution during the first hour
2. Administer potassium and phosphorous replacement solutions
3. Administer insulin therapy by way of bolus and I.V. infusion; the dose of insulin administered to a patient with HHNS is lower than that administered to a patient with DKA
4. Add dextrose to the infusion when the glucose level reaches 250 mg/dl

E. Nursing management

1. Identify risk factors, such as insidious onset, advanced age, insulin-independent diabetes, and pancreatitis, that predispose the patient to HHNS; although DKA and HHNS are similar, HHNS usually is a more serious medical emergency
2. Assess for diminished skin turgor, dry mucous membranes, excessive thirst, frequent voidings of dark and concentrated urine, altered level of consciousness, and seizure activity; because dehydration typically is more severe in HHNS than in DKA, determination of the extent of dehydration is a priority assessment
3. Check for hypotension and tachycardia, signs of hypovolemia
4. Assess for shallow, rapid respirations; Kussmaul's respirations should not be present in a patient with HHNS and their absence can help make the differential diagnosis between DKA and HHNS
5. Monitor ECG for arrhythmias; hyperkalemia and hypovolemia can produce ECG changes that should resolve with medical treatment
6. Auscultate for breath sounds every 1 to 2 hours; the rapid administration of a saline solution to a debilitated, elderly patient significantly increases the risk of pulmonary edema
7. Monitor electrolyte levels, and expect a return to normal values after 1 week; keep in mind that an elderly patient may take longer to reach normal fluid and electrolyte levels because of the metabolic alterations associated with aging
8. Accurately record intake and output every hour; these measurements are the most efficient method of assessing the patient's response to fluid replacement and detecting the adverse effects of fluid overload
9. Use a diabetic flow sheet to monitor hourly blood glucose level, serum laboratory values, ABG values, and intake and output; hourly glucose checks help to prevent the development of hypoglycemia; other laboratory values are useful in assessing the patient's response to therapy

10. Maintain the patient on strict bed rest, and instruct the patient and family not to massage the lower extremities; these actions reduce the possibility of dislodging a thrombus formed by hemoconcentration and hyperviscosity of the blood

11. Educate the patient and family about the risk factors for HHNS as well as the signs and symptoms of hyperglycemia; early detection of blood glucose alterations and dehydration will ensure prompt treatment and prevent severe dehydration and hospital readmission

12. Teach the patient appropriate diabetic self-care management techniques, including the correct administration of oral and S.C. antidiabetic medications, signs and symptoms of hypoglycemia and hyperglycemia, and proper glucose monitoring techniques

13. Discuss dietary management of insulin-dependent diabetes and non-insulin-dependent diabetes, which is essential for good glucose control

VIII. Syndrome of inappropriate secretion of antidiuretic hormone

A. Description

1. Syndrome of inappropriate secretion of antidiuretic hormone is characterized by plasma hypotonicity and hyponatremia, which result from the aberrant or sustained secretion of ADH

   a. Syndrome of inappropriate secretion of antidiuretic hormone is caused by failure of the negative feedback system; ADH secretion continues despite low plasma osmolality and expanded volume

   b. The continuous release of ADH from the posterior pituitary gland causes the renal tubules and collecting ducts to increase their permeability to water and to promote water reabsorption

   c. Uninhibited ADH secretion ultimately leads to water retention and intoxication; symptoms usually resolve with the correction of hyponatremia

2. Several predisposing factors for SIADH exist

   a. Ectopic ADH production associated with leukemia and bronchogenic, prostatic, or pancreatic cancer

   b. Central nervous system disorders, such as brain trauma from injury, neoplasms, infections, or vascular lesions

   c. Antidiuretic hormone stimulation secondary to hypoxemia or decreased left atrial filling pressure; this may be caused by respiratory tract infections, heart failure, and the use of positive end-expiratory pressure (PEEP) during mechanical ventilation

   d. Use of medications that increase or potentiate ADH secretion, including chemotherapeutic drugs, exogenous vasopressin therapy, chlorpropamide, and thiazide diuretics

3. Syndrome of inappropriate secretion of antidiuretic hormone is confirmed by comparison of serum and urine osmolalities, with serum osmolality being considerably lower than urine osmolality

B. Clinical signs and symptoms

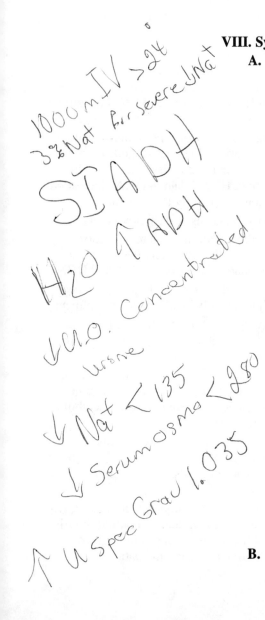

1. Symptoms of hyponatremia (serum sodium level less than 135 mEq/L): low urine output; dark, concentrated urine; thirst; impaired taste; dulled sensorium and fatigue; dyspnea on exertion; and weight gain without edema
2. Symptoms of severe hyponatremia (serum sodium level less than 115 mEq/L): confusion, lethargy, muscle twitching, and seizure activity

C. Laboratory values
1. Serum sodium level: less than 135 mEq/L
2. Serum osmolality: less than 280 mOsm/kg
3. Urine specific gravity and urine osmolality: increased; 1.035 and 800 mOsm/kg, respectively, after 12 hours with nothing by mouth
4. Serum ADH level: inappropriately elevated

D. Diagnostic tests
1. Normal kidney, adrenal, and thyroid function test results
2. Water-loading test demonstrating elimination of less than one-half of the fluid challenge

E. Medical management
1. Restrict combined I.V. and oral fluid intake to 1,000 ml or less every 24 hours; I.V. and oral intake usually are calculated based on urine output plus insensible losses
2. Administer hypertonic sodium chloride solution (such as 3% sodium chloride) to patients with severe hyponatremia
3. Monitor serial electrolyte levels for response to fluid and electrolyte interventions
4. Administer lithium or demeclocycline to increase urine output
5. Administer furosemide to increase urine output
6. Administer potassium supplements

F. Nursing management
1. Assess for precipitating factors: recent head trauma, medication use, known history of cancer or cancer treatment, and the use of PEEP; the onset of SIADH may be related to known precipitating events or previously undetected patient problems, such as ADH-secreting tumors
2. Observe the patient for CNS changes, such as headache, personality changes, confusion, irritability, dysarthria, lethargy, and impaired memory; assessment of the patient's neurologic status provides necessary information regarding the level of impairment caused by water intoxication and hyponatremia
3. Observe the patient for alterations in activity, such as restlessness, weakness, tremor, muscle twitching, seizure activity, excess fatigue, gait disturbances, and sleep pattern disturbances; changes in level of activity must be noted to address the patient's safety needs

SIADH

< 30 ml/hr

4. Assess for nutritional alterations, including nausea, anorexia, vomiting, and sudden weight gain without edema; changes in nutritional status are further evidence of electrolyte imbalance and onset of water intoxication

5. Monitor for alterations in elimination, such as a urine output less than 30 ml/hour and diarrhea; oliguria must be present to confirm a diagnosis of SIADH

6. Percuss for deep tendon reflexes, which are delayed in a patient who has severe hyponatremia

7. Assess kidney, adrenal, and thyroid function; normal function rules out other endocrine disorders as the cause of weight gain and low urine output

8. Monitor kidney function carefully, using BUN and creatinine values; assessment of kidney function is particularly important in patients who are receiving demeclocycline, a nephrotoxic drug

9. Meticulously record hourly intake and output, urine specific gravity, body weight, hydration status, and cardiovascular and neurologic status; hourly assessments provide the most accurate determination of treatment efficacy and the onset of adverse effects

10. Monitor the patient carefully for symptoms of hypernatremia, as evidenced by serum sodium level greater than 145 mEq/L, edema, and hypertension

    a. A sudden increase in the serum sodium level can cause brain damage and heart failure

    b. Osmotic demyelination syndrome can develop in patients with chronic hyponatremia who have had time to become adapted to the state

11. Maintain the patient on bed rest, and institute seizure precautions and safety measures to prevent self-injury; severe hyponatremia increases the risk of seizure activity, physical injury, and hypoxemia

12. To prevent injury, assist the patient with all activities

13. Frequently reorient the patient to the surroundings, and explain all procedures and treatments; reassure the patient that he or she is progressing well

    a. Diminished cognitive functioning is a frightening experience

    b. Frequent reorientation can help prevent injury and assist the patient in conserving energy for recovery

5 Hematologic and immunologic disorders

I. **Anatomy**
   A. Spleen
      1. The spleen is surrounded by a fibromuscular capsule that extends inward as trabeculae and forms partitions within the organ
      2. Smooth muscle in the surrounding capsule and trabeculae cause contractions that force additional blood cells into the circulation
      3. The internal structure of the spleen is composed of two types of tissue
         a. White pulp, which is randomly distributed throughout the spleen, contains lymph nodes and lymph strands
         b. Red pulp, which makes up the majority of tissue in the spleen, consists of reticular tissue and cells that make and store red blood cells (RBCs)
   B. Liver
      1. Divided into a larger right lobe and a smaller left lobe by the falciform ligament, the liver is attached to the diaphragm and moves with respirations
      2. The liver is protected by the lower right rib cage and is supplied with blood by the hepatic artery
      3. The lobules that form the functional units of the liver are interconnected by cords of hepatic cells; each lobule is surrounded by several portal triads that consist of a hepatic artery, a hepatic vein, and a branch of the biliary duct
   C. Bone marrow
      1. Productive bone marrow is located in the vertebrae, skull, rib cage, ilium, and proximal long bones
      2. The amount of productive bone marrow gradually decreases as a person ages
   D. Thymus gland
      1. The thymus gland is located behind the sternum in the upper part of the chest
      2. A large, two-lobed organ in infants and children, the thymus gland shrinks during adolescence; by adulthood, it is replaced by fibrous connective tissue and fat and is nonfunctional
      3. The thymus gland has a cortex and a medulla
         a. The cortex is composed of clusters of lymphocytes (thymocytes) but has no nodes
         b. The medulla contains loose thymocytes and Hassall's corpuscles

E. Lymph system
1. Lymph fluid is similar in composition to plasma and contains large quantities of leukocytes in the form of lymphocytes
2. Lymph capillaries are small, dead-end vessels that merge to form lymph vessels, including the right lymphatic duct and the thoracic duct; lymph capillaries are larger and have thinner walls and more valves than venous capillaries
3. Lymph vessels are more permeable than lymph veins and larger than lymph capillaries
4. Lymph nodes consist of oval bodies of lymph tissue encapsulated by fibrous tissue; internally, the nodes are a matrix of connective tissue forming small compartments that contain lymphocytes
   a. Lymph nodes are located along the lymph vessels and concentrated in the cervical, axillary, and inguinal areas
   b. Clusters of lymph nodes are found in the lungs, near the aorta, and in the intestinal mesentery

II. Physiology
A. Spleen
1. The white pulp in the spleen produces antibodies, lymphocytes, and monocytes and stimulates B-cell activity
2. The red pulp acts as a blood reservoir (holding 150 to 250 ml of blood); breaks down damaged RBCs; and produces, stores, and destroys platelets

B. Liver
1. The liver plays a significant role in the host defense against infection; Kupffer's cells located throughout the liver destroy bacteria in the blood
2. The liver also breaks down RBCs for bile production and destroys toxic substances that enter the circulatory system
3. The liver manufactures plasma clotting factors (factor VIII, vitamin K) and antithrombin
4. All blood from the GI tract passes through the liver before returning to the general circulation

C. Bone marrow
1. Bone marrow produces the precursors of RBCs and white blood cells (WBCs)
2. Erythrocytes, granulocytes, and thrombocytes are produced only in the bone marrow; bone marrow also is a site for the production of lymphocytes and monocytes
3. Bone marrow can remove very small protein toxins from the circulation

D. Thymus gland
1. The thymus gland produces thymic hormone, which stimulates the body's immune capabilities
2. It also regulates cellular immunity and T-cell activity

E. Lymph system

1. Lymph fluid contains glucose, amino acids, urea, and creatinine; this fluid does not circulate but flows toward the heart because of the increased interstitial pressure that forces fluid into the lymphatic system
2. Lymph capillaries carry lymph fluid to larger vessels
3. Lymph vessels filter the intercellular fluids, returning proteins to the blood
   a. The right lymphatic duct drains lymph from the right upper quadrant of the body and head to the right subclavian vein
   b. The thoracic duct drains lymph from the rest of the body to the left subclavian vein
4. Lymph nodes produce lymphocytes, monocytes, and plasma cells
   a. They also filter and remove foreign substances, dying cells, and microorganisms from the lymph fluid
   b. They produce globulins from the breakdown of cells and antibodies

F. Erythropoiesis
1. Erythropoietin stimulates the stem cells in the red bone marrow to produce mature RBCs; erythropoietin is secreted by the kidneys when the partial pressure of arterial oxygen level drops below normal
2. Red blood cells, or erythrocytes, are nonnucleated, round, biconcave cells with a life span of approximately 120 days
   a. The stroma, or inner part of an RBC, is the point of attachment for hemoglobin; the production of hemoglobin requires iron, vitamin B_{12}, and folic acid
   b. The stroma contains the antigens that determine blood type
3. Red blood cells are highly permeable to hydrogen ions, chloride ions, water, and bicarbonate ions
4. Aged or damaged RBCs are removed from the circulation by the liver and spleen

G. Leukopoiesis
1. Leukopoiesis refers to the formation and development of the various types of WBCs
2. White blood cells, or leukocytes, are the body's principal defense against foreign substances and infectious organisms
   a. White blood cells can move from one site of infection to another
   b. They are capable of reproducing rapidly and altering their structure according to the situation
3. Five types of leukocytes exist
   a. Neutrophils play a role in phagocytosis
   b. Eosinophils help in the detoxification of allergens, phagocytosis, antiparasitic action, and anaphylaxis
   c. Basophils play a role in allergies, hypersensitivity reactions, and chronic infections; basophils secrete heparin and histamine

Lymphocytes and their function

Although three types of lymphocytes exist, they are not produced in the same amounts in all bodies. The chart below provides approximate percentages of the three groups of lymphocytes, along with their function.

TYPE OF LYMPHOCYTE	NORMAL COUNT	FUNCTION
T cells	60% to 80%	Active in immune responses and immunoregulation
B cells	10% to 15%	Produce antibodies; destroy antigens
Null cells	5% to 15%	Attack and eliminate infected cells

Monocytes.
Lymphocytes.

    d. Monocytes, which are produced in the bone marrow, lymph nodes, and spleen, function in phagocytosis

    e. Lymphocytes are produced in the bone marrow and are divided into three groups (see *Lymphocytes and their function*)

      (1) T cells are produced in response to antigens and play a role in cellular immunity; there are four subtypes of T cells

        (a) Helper T cells (also known as T_H or T_4 cells) help B cells and begin the process of antigen destruction

        (b) Suppressor T cells (also known as T_S or T_8 cells) stop the immune response and destroy abnormal cells

        (c) Cytotoxic T cells (also known as T_C or killer cells) identify and directly or indirectly attack (lyse) infected cells

        (d) Memory T cells recall and respond to previously encountered antigens; they initiate a more rapid response

      (2) B cells produce antibodies and play a role in humoral immunity

      (3) Null cells are undifferentiated killer cells that help prevent cancer

H. Immunity

    1. Immunity is the body's ability to resist or combat invading organisms

    2. There are three types of immunity

      a. Innate immunity is derived from the body's inherent immune mechanisms; examples of innate immunity are the resistance of the skin, acidic secretions of the stomach, enzymes of the digestive tract, phagocytosis by blood cells, and the production of natural antibodies

      b. Passive immunity is a temporary form of acquired immunity produced by the injection of antibodies or sensitized lymphocytes; passive immunity can be acquired, for example, through injection of gamma globulin, tetanus toxoid, or antivenin (for snake bites)

     c. Active immunity is a type of acquired immunity in which the body creates its own antibodies in response to invasion by foreign organisms; humoral immunity and cellular immunity are the two types of active immunity

        (1) A humoral immune response produces immunoglobulins; in response to specific antigens, macrophages present antigens to the B lymphocytes, and in turn, the B cells differentiate into plasma cells, which produce antibodies

        (2) A cellular immune response results in the sensitization of T cells to specific antigens, such as viruses, fungi, cancer cells, and transplanted organs and tissues

I. Immunoglobulins

    1. Immunoglobulins are protein substances synthesized by lymphocytes and plasma cells

    2. Each of the five types of immunoglobulins function as antibodies

       a. Immunoglobulin G (IgG) comprises 80% of circulating antibodies and has primarily antibacterial and antiviral properties

       b. Immunoglobulin A comprises 10% to 15% of circulating antibodies and is found primarily in the mucous membranes, where it protects against antigen adherence and invasion

       c. Immunoglobulin M comprises 5% to 10% of circulating antibodies and is the first antibody to respond to bacterial and viral invasions

       d. Immunoglobulin D comprises less than 0.1% of circulating antibodies and activates B cells

       e. Immunoglobulin E comprises less than 0.01% of circulating antibodies and produces the symptoms of allergic reactions

III. Hematologic and immunologic assessment

  A. Noninvasive assessment techniques

    1. Inspect for enlarged lymph nodes, edema, erythema, red streaks on the skin, and skin lesions

    2. Palpate the superficial lymph nodes for enlargement, consistency, mobility, tenderness, and size, using the fingertips of the second, third, and fourth fingers

       a. A hard, discrete node may indicate a malignant tumor

       b. A tender node usually indicates inflammation

       c. A palpable supraclavicular node on the left side often indicates a malignant tumor in the chest or abdomen

  B. Key laboratory values

    1. White blood cell count (normal: 6,000 to 10,000 cells/mm^3)

    2. Differential WBC count: neutrophils (normal: 38 to 70 cells/mm^3), eosinophils (normal: 1 to 5 cells/mm^3), basophils (normal: 0 to 1 cell/mm^3), monocytes (normal: 1 to 8 cells/mm^3), and lymphocytes (normal: 15 to 45 cells/mm^3)

       a. Shift to the left indicates an infection and is seen in an increased number of immature neutrophils (bands)

[handwritten margin notes: Infection. 38 - 70 cell/mm³ Shift (Lt) immature neutrophils/bands.]

    b. Shift to the right usually indicates pernicious anemia or hepatic disease and is seen in an increased number of mature, hypersegmented neutrophils

    c. Degenerative shift indicates bone marrow depression and is indicated by an increased number of bands and a low WBC count

    d. Regenerative shift indicates stimulation of the bone marrow, as seen in pneumonia and appendicitis, and is indicated by an increased number of WBCs, bands, and myelocytes

3. Coombs' test, which is used to determine the presence of hemolyzing antibodies

    a. A direct Coombs' test is used to detect the presence of IgG in RBCs

    b. An indirect Coombs' test is used to detect the presence of IgG in plasma

IV. Acquired immunodeficiency syndrome

  A. Description

    1. Immunodeficiency disorders, such as acquired immunodeficiency syndrome (AIDS), result from defects in one or more immune system components

    2. The human immunodeficiency virus that causes AIDS attacks T cells and reduces their ability to destroy foreign organisms that enter the body

    3. Because most patients with AIDS, particularly those in the terminal stages of the disease, require extensive and specialized care, they typically are treated in the intensive care unit (ICU)

  B. Clinical signs and symptoms

    1. Recurrent high fevers

    2. Rapid, unplanned weight loss

    3. Swollen lymph nodes

    4. Constant fatigue

    5. Diarrhea and diminished appetite

    6. White spots and sores in the mouth

    7. Kaposi's sarcoma (a type of skin cancer that causes brown blotches on the skin and generally is fatal)

    8. *Pneumocystis carinii* pneumonia (a type of respiratory tract infection caused by a parasitic organism in the lungs; *P. carinii* pneumonia generally is fatal)

    9. Central nervous system (CNS) damage (infections of the CNS produce memory loss, an inability to make decisions, and loss of muscle control)

  C. Medical management

    1. Administer antibiotics and anticancer medications

    2. Administer zidovudine (Retrovir), interferon, and other medications approved for the treatment of AIDS

    3. Treat cancers that develop as a result of AIDS surgically or with radiation therapy

D. Nursing management

    1. Assess for risk factors for infection, such as altered immune response, malnutrition, chemotherapy, corticosteroid therapy, stress, and hospitalization, that reduce the body's ability to fight off infections and increase the patient's risk of acquiring a nosocomial infection

    2. Assess for signs and symptoms of infections, including chills, fever, tachycardia, generalized weakness, and open or draining wounds; in an immunosuppressed patient, the usual signs and symptoms of infection may not be present, and fever commonly is the only clinical sign

    3. Reduce the patient's exposure to infectious organisms by placing the patient in a private room, restricting the number of visitors, following proper hand-washing technique, and wearing a mask and gown for invasive procedures; to prevent the nurse's exposure to blood-borne pathogens, use universal precautions when working with blood or any body fluid that contains blood

    4. Monitor fluid and electrolyte status to prevent drying of the skin and mucous membranes, which can increase the risk of infection

    5. Assess skin condition and observe for irritation or breakdown; use measures to redistribute pressure on the skin, including turning, special mattresses, and heel and elbow protectors; immunosuppression and malnutrition increase the risk of skin breakdown and formation of pressure ulcers

    6. Check for the development of urinary tract infection (UTI), which is indicated by burning on urination and cloudy, strong-smelling urine; UTIs are a common complication of AIDS and can lead to sepsis

    7. Monitor for intravascular infection at the site of I.V. catheters and lines; these infections can lead to septicemia and frequently are fatal in immunosuppressed patients

    8. Monitor laboratory values, including blood urea nitrogen (BUN), creatinine, and electrolyte levels; complete blood count (CBC); and WBC count with differential; significant changes in the patient's condition can be determined by making comparisons with the baseline values

    9. Monitor nutritional intake, weight, and daily intake and output; GI functioning generally is impaired by the disease process, and the medications used to treat it, making adequate nutritional intake difficult; malnutrition can worsen the immunosuppression

    10. Assess the patient's elimination pattern; diarrhea is a common problem, and severe diarrhea may result in electrolyte imbalances and loss of potassium

    11. Implement measures to control diarrhea, including pharmacologic measures, special diets, and frequent, small, low-residue meals

12. Check for unusual or excessive bleeding; bone marrow depression and suppression of liver function can occur, leading to bleeding tendencies

13. Obtain culture specimens using appropriate techniques; successful antibiotic treatment depends on identification of the invasive microorganisms; keep in mind, however, that many pathogens found in hospitals are resistant to standard antibiotics

14. Help the patient maintain good oral hygiene; immunosuppressed patients are at increased risk of developing stomatitis from the disease and the medications used to treat it

15. Assess for signs of anxiety, which can lead to increased stress and further suppress the immune system; reduce anxiety by explaining all procedures, reassuring the patient, and encouraging the patient to participate in his or her care as much as possible

16. Assess the patient's knowledge of the disease process, and actively involve friends and family in the patient's care

17. Discuss the treatment regimen and discharge planning with the patient and family; accurate information about the disease can decrease anxiety and increase cooperation with treatment

18. Establish an atmosphere of mutual trust and caring by encouraging expression of feelings, identifying stressors, and developing strategies for dealing with stress

V. **Disseminated intravascular coagulation**

A. Description

1. A common complication of many severe illnesses, disseminated intravascular coagulation (DIC) is a pathophysiologic process resulting from the presence of thrombin in the systemic circulation, which causes microthrombi to form throughout the circulatory system

   a. The body responds to this diffuse coagulation with a massive release of fibrinolytic factors

   b. The result is the depletion of thrombin available for normal clotting and the circulation of an excessive amount of fibrinolytic enzymes, thus producing massive bleeding

2. Although any severe illness that induces a decrease in blood pressure can cause DIC, the condition most often is secondary to severe trauma, cancer, obstetric problems, sepsis, and autoimmune reactions

B. Clinical signs and symptoms

1. Excessive and unusual bleeding from the gums and mucous membranes and excess blood in stools and urine

2. Prolonged, severe headaches

3. Swollen joints and joint pain

4. Large ecchymotic areas resulting from minor trauma

5. Organ necrosis and tissue hypoxia

C. Medical management

        1. Transfuse whole blood and blood products, including platelets, plasma, and packed cells

        2. Administer heparin in the early stages of the disease

        3. Administer corticosteroids

D. Nursing management

        1. Assess mental status, orientation, and level of consciousness, and check for complaints of headache, dizziness, and behavioral changes; patients with DIC are at increased risk of intracranial bleeding, which can lead to cerebral hypoxemia and changes in neurologic status

        2. Assess cardiovascular status, including blood pressure, heart rate, central venous pressure, pulmonary artery wedge pressure, and cardiac output; ongoing assessments can help identify potential underlying bleeding and facilitate the evaluation of the patient's response to fluid and blood replacement

        3. Monitor peripheral circulation by checking skin color and temperature and quality of pulses; the presence of acrocyanosis indicates microthrombi within the peripheral circulation and blood vessels

        4. Check for transfusion reactions, which can result from the rapid administration of large quantities of blood and blood products

        5. Monitor blood loss and relevant laboratory test results, including CBC, partial thromboplastin time, prothrombin time, and fibrin degradation products; changes in these key laboratory values provide an indication of patient status and response to treatment

        6. Assess pulmonary status; the highly vascular pulmonary system, a prime area for increased bleeding, may cause decreased lung compliance and respiratory distress if bleeding occurs in this area

        7. Assess kidney status; urine output less than 30 ml/hour may indicate hypovolemia, kidney damage, or microemboli in the kidneys

        8. Assess the mobility of all extremities; thrombosis and bleeding into the joints and muscles may require that the patient limit movement to reduce the risk of injury

        9. Measure blood loss in urine, nasogastric and chest tube drainage, stools, and wound drainage; the multiple-organ effect of DIC requires a careful balance of fluids; both overhydration and underhydration are dangerous, and appropriate fluid replacement depends on accurate blood loss measurements

       10. Administer blood and fluid replacement therapy, using appropriate techniques; monitoring vital signs before, during, and after blood administration is necessary to detect transfusion reactions

       11. Prevent further bleeding by protecting the patient's skin from breakdown, using soft toothbrushes for oral care, suctioning only when necessary, avoiding the use of a blood pressure cuff, and avoiding I.M. and S.C. injections; damage to any tissues can result in massive bleeding

12. Administer medications, as prescribed and according to the dosing schedule, but avoid administering aspirin preparations because aspirin may trigger bleeding

13. Administer heparin as prescribed; sometimes heparin is used in the early stages of the disease but is of no value in the later stages; although heparin reduces the depletion of thrombin by preventing clot formation, its use in the treatment of DIC is controversial

14. Instruct the patient to avoid sneezing, vigorous coughing, and the Valsalva maneuver; any stress to blood vessels throughout the body can cause increased bleeding

15. Because the lungs generally are affected in DIC, maintain pulmonary status through proper oral hygiene, encouragement of deep breathing, and use of incentive spirometry; use nasal and endotracheal suctioning only as needed

16. Promote good skin care through frequent turning, use of air mattresses, and relief of pressure over bony prominences; in patients with DIC, even minor skin breakdown can cause significant blood loss

17. Assess the patient's and family's understanding of the disease; DIC usually is fatal, and the family should be prepared for this possibility

18. Allow the patient to express his or her fears and anxiety; this helps the patient reduce stress and conserve strength

VI. Organ transplantation

A. Description

1. Organ transplantation has become a fairly commonplace procedure

2. The kidneys, heart, lungs, pancreas, and liver as well as various tissues can be transplanted

3. Patients who undergo organ transplantation receive high dosages of immunosuppressant medications to prevent rejection of the transplanted organ; most patients spend a significant amount of time in the ICU during the postoperative period

4. In cases where a beating heart donor is required (as in heart, lung, and liver transplants), a donor's brain death may need to be determined (see *Determination of brain death*)

B. Medical management

1. Maintain the patient on mechanical ventilation as needed

2. Prescribe analgesic and sedative medications

3. Administer I.V. fluids

4. Prescribe antibiotics and immunosuppressant medications

C. Nursing management

1. Monitor cardiac output and vital signs (blood pressure, heart rate and rhythm, respiratory rate, and temperature) every 5 minutes while the patient is rewarmed, every 15 minutes until stable, and then every hour for 12 hours; frequent and thorough monitoring of vital signs allows early detection of complications and prompt treatment

Determination of brain death

These factors must be present to declare brain death:
• Generalized flaccidity
• No spontaneous muscle movement
• No posturing or shivering
• No spontaneous breathing or breathing movements for 3 minutes after disconnection from a ventilator
• Flat electroencephalogram (*Note:* This is not absolutely required when the patient is connected to life-support devices)
• No blood flow on brain scan or angiogram
• No cranial nerve reflexes
   –No pupil responses (fixed, may be dilated or constricted)
   –Absent corneal reflex
   –Absent response to upper and lower airway stimulation
   –Absent cold caloric response
• Negative responses not caused by induced hypothermia or central nervous system depressant medications.

2. Monitor hemodynamic parameters, including mean arterial pressure, pulmonary artery pressure, pulmonary artery wedge pressure, and central venous pressure; these parameters are critical indicators of cardiac function and are used to assess left ventricular function, fluid status, and arterial perfusion of vital organs

3. Monitor respiratory function and check endotracheal tube placement and patency; most patients are intubated after a heart transplant

4. Check the settings on the ventilator, and ensure that it is working properly; as a result of the administration of anesthesia and opioid analgesics, postoperative patients are dependent on the ventilator for adequate oxygenation and reduced workload of the heart

5. Monitor urine output every hour; urine output less than 30 ml/hour is a sign of possible heart failure, kidney failure, or hypovolemia

6. Monitor the amount and color of chest tube drainage; more than 100 ml of drainage per hour during the first 24 hours may indicate abnormal bleeding

7. Assess the patient's neurologic status every 1 to 2 hours for the first 24 hours; abnormal neurologic findings may indicate temporary or permanent disruption of CNS function related to anesthesia, use of the bypass machine, intraoperative cerebrovascular accident, or decreased cardiac output

8. Monitor laboratory blood values, including CBC, BUN and creatinine levels, WBC count with differential, and arterial blood gas analysis; significant changes in key blood values may indicate hemorrhage, bleeding disorders, kidney failure, decreased respiratory function, or infection

9. Check for signs and symptoms of infection, including fever, chills, tachycardia, weakness, fatigue, and localized pain; the use of immunosuppressant medications increases the patient's risk of infection and may mask the signs of infection

10. Assess for signs and symptoms of organ rejection, including decreased cardiac output, abnormal heart rhythms, chest pain, and enlargement of the heart; many patients experience some type of rejection episode approximately 1 week after transplantation; early detection allows for prompt treatment with increased doses of immunosuppressant medications

11. After extubation, encourage the patient to cough and deep breathe every hour to loosen and mobilize secretions and to prevent atelectasis and pneumonia

12. Reduce the patient's exposure to infectious organisms by placing the patient in a private room, restricting visitors to immediate family, following proper hand-washing technique, and wearing a mask and gloves for invasive procedures

13. Change dressings according to institutional protocol, and check the surgical site for signs of infection, such as redness, warmth, and purulent drainage

14. Obtain culture specimens from draining wounds or incisions; successful antibiotic treatment depends on identification of the invasive microorganisms

15. Provide adequate rest periods; sleep deprivation reduces the body's ability to cope with stress and may lead to disorientation and uncooperative behavior

16. Reorient the patient to surroundings frequently to reduce anxiety and stress

17. Allow family members to visit as much as possible based on the patient's condition; the family usually is the patient's primary support system and vital to his or her recovery

VII. Leukemias

A. Description

1. Leukemias are cancers that develop when immature WBCs grow without restraint, accumulating in the bone marrow and blood

2. This accumulation of abnormal leukemic WBCs interferes with the production of normal RBCs, WBCs, and platelets

3. Leukemias are classified according to the type of WBC that is most prevalent and whether the condition is acute or chronic

   a. Acute lymphocytic or lymphoblastic (ALL)

   b. Acute nonlymphocytic or myelogenous (ANLL) or (AML)

   c. Chronic lymphocytic (CLL)

   d. Chronic myelogenous (CML)

B. Clinical signs and symptoms

1. Anemia

2. Thrombocytopenia
3. Bone pain
4. Lymphadenopathy
5. Splenomegaly
6. Hepatomegaly
7. Headache
8. Cerebrovascular accident
9. Nausea, vomiting
10. Bleeding (joint swelling, ecchymosis, hemorrhage)
11. Weight loss
12. Complications
    a. Disseminated intravascular coagulation (DIC)
    b. Adult respiratory distress syndrome (ARDS)
    c. Increased intracranial pressure (ICP)
    d. Sepsis
    e. Leukostasis

C. Medical management
   1. Chemotherapy with a combination of drugs
   2. Admission to ICU with low WBC (less than 1,200), low platelet count (less than 20,000), indications of increased ICP, or active infections
   3. Transfusions of whole blood, packed cells, plasma, and other blood products
   4. Bone marrow transplantation (graft-versus-host rejection)
   5. Radiation therapy

D. Nursing management
   1. Monitor mental status (level of consciousness, orientation), hematologic status (joint pain and swelling; ecchymosis; active bleeding in stools, urine, gums), and infections
   2. Monitor fluid and electrolyte balance because the patient is being given large amounts of fluid and blood products
   3. Assess for tumor lysis syndrome
   4. Monitor and control adverse effects of chemotherapy and radiation therapy
   5. Maintain a strict aseptic environment (protective isolation) when the patient is in the acute stages of disease
   6. Administer medications as ordered, particularly antibiotics and blood products
   7. Monitor and control pain with pain medication, biofeedback, imaging, and other pain-control measures
   8. Increase fluid intake to 2 to 3 L/day (helps flush chemotherapeutic drugs from the system, preventing renal damage)

9. Perform active and passive range-of-motion exercises on all joints to maintain mobility and prevent contractures

10. Provide proper oral care; advise the patient to use a soft toothbrush and mouth rinses, and suction only when necessary

11. Promote the patient's appetite; allow a choice of meals as desired to ensure adequate intake of essential nutrients

12. Assess the patient's and family's understanding of the disease; provide education about treatments, complications, and prognosis

13. Reduce patient and family anxiety by allowing them to express feelings, fears, and concerns

6 Neurologic disorders

I. Anatomy and physiology

A. Skull

1. The brain is protected from superficial injury by the bony structure of the skull

2. A substantial blow to the skull can cause shifting of the brain itself, resulting in laceration or contusion of the brain tissues, or fracture of the bony segments, with the resultant fragments being propelled into the brain tissues

3. The skull is composed of eight flat, fused bones

   a. The frontal bone overlies the anterior aspect or frontal lobe of the brain

   b. The occipital bone overlies the posterior aspect or occipital lobe of the brain

   c. Two temporal bones overlie the inferolateral aspect or temporal lobe of the brain

   d. Two parietal bones overlie the superolateral aspect or parietal lobe of the brain

   e. The sphenoid bone is located at the base of the skull in front of the occipital and temporal bones and has at its center the sella turcica, in which the pituitary gland is located

   f. The ethmoid bone, or cribriform plate, fits into a notch in the frontal bone and forms the roof of the nasal fossa and the floor of the cranial cavity

4. At the base of the skull is a large opening, the foramen magnum, through which the brain stem extends and becomes continuous with the spinal cord

B. The meninges

1. The meninges, which comprise the dura mater, arachnoid mater, and pia mater, lie immediately below the skull and provide an additional layer of protection for the brain and spinal cord

2. The dura mater consists of two layers

   a. The outer layer forms a tough, fibrous periosteum that adheres to the cranial bones

   b. The inner layer, or meningeal dura, extends into the cranium and correlates with the division of hemispheres and lobes of the brain

   c. The outer dura separates from the meningeal dura to form sinuses that assist with venous drainage from the brain

   d. The meningeal dura has several extensions

      (1) The falx cerebri is located between the right and left hemi-spheres of the brain

      (2) The tentorium cerebelli supports the occipital lobe and covers the upper surface of the cerebellum

        (a) Structures above the tentorium cerebelli are called supra-tentorial

        (b) Structures below the tentorium cerebelli are called infratentorial or described as the posterior fossa

      (3) The falx cerebelli extends along the division of the lateral lobes of the cerebellum

      (4) The diaphragm sella canopies the sella turcica and thus encloses the pituitary gland

    e. The dura mater is separated from the next meningeal layer, the arachnoid, by a thin subdural space; this area is vulnerable to trauma because of the presence of a network of unsupported veins; if lacerated, these tiny veins form a subdural hematoma

  3. The arachnoid mater is a fragile membrane that surrounds the brain

    a. The arachnoid mater is separated from the pia mater by the relatively wide subarachnoid space, which contains cerebrospinal fluid (CSF), connective tissues, and cerebral arteries and veins

    b. The arachnoid villi connect the subarachnoid space to the sagittal and transverse sinuses

      (1) These structures facilitate the reabsorption of CSF from the subarachnoid space into the sinuses

      (2) Impedance of CSF reabsorption by the arachnoid villi is called communicating hydrocephalus; conditions that impede CSF reabsorption include hemorrhage in the subarachnoid space and bacterial or viral meningitis

  4. The pia mater is the innermost layer of the meninges

    a. It adheres to the entire surface of the brain, following its sulci and gyri, and to the surface of the spinal cord

    b. The pia mater contains the arterial blood supply for the tissues of the brain and is part of the choroid plexus (the structure that manufactures CSF)

C. Brain

  1. The *cerebrum* is the largest segment of the brain and constitutes up to 80% of its weight; it consists of two cerebral hemispheres, each of which is divided by anatomic demarcations into four paired lobes: the frontal, parietal, temporal, and occipital lobes

    a. The frontal lobes underlie the frontal bone and are separated from the parietal lobes by the central sulcus or fissure of Rolando and from the temporal lobes by the lateral cerebral sulcus or fissure of Sylvius; the frontal lobes have several functions

      (1) They control voluntary motor functions

      (2) They control some autonomic nervous system functions

[handwritten margin notes: "2 hemispheres", "Cerebrum", "4 paired lobes."]

(3) They play a role in cognition, memory, language, personality, and higher intellectual functions

b. The parietal lobe, which is posterior to the frontal lobe and separated by the central sulcus, also has several functions

(1) It integrates sensations

(2) It controls sensory functions of the contralateral side of the body (referred to as the postcentral gyrus)

(3) It translates sensory information that pertains to shape, texture, and size

(4) It interprets sensory information related to kinesthesia and spatial relationships

c. A portion of the parietal lobe and the temporal lobe combine to form Wernicke's area, an area associated with the sensory aspects of speech and interpretation of written language; damage in this area results in receptive aphasia

d. The temporal lobe underlies the temporal bone; it interprets auditory stimuli, translates written language, and forms memory

e. The limbic area is anatomically integrated with the temporal lobe to form the borders of the lateral ventricles; the limbic lobe contains the uncus, hippocampus, primary olfactory cortex, and amygdaloid nucleus; the limbic lobe has several functions

(1) It initiates actions of self-preservation

(2) It stimulates emotions

(3) It stores short-term memory

(4) It interprets smell

f. The occipital lobe is the most posterior of the cerebral lobes; the occipital lobe plays a role in vision by translating visual stimuli into integrated meaning

2. The *cerebral cortex* forms the outer layer of the cerebrum

a. It is composed of unmyelinated cells (gray matter)

b. The myelinated tracts (white matter) below the cerebral cortex function in the transmission of impulses from the cerebral cortex to the rest of the brain

(1) The commissural fibers create a tract of communication between the cerebral cortex of one hemisphere and the corresponding parts in the other hemisphere; the largest of these tracts is the corpus callosum

(2) Projection fibers create a tract of communication between the cerebral cortex and the lower brain and the spinal cord; these tracts consist of ascending or afferent tracts, which are located primarily in the thalamus, and descending or efferent tracts, which are found in the motor area of the cortex

      (3) Association fibers communicate within the different areas of the same hemisphere and serve to bring all parts of that hemisphere into a functional relationship; they are classified as short fibers or long fibers

  c. The prefrontal sections of the cerebral cortex are associated with thought, feeling, and emotions

  d. The premotor sections are associated with common body movements

      (1) They are linked with cranial nerves III (oculomotor), IV (trochlear), VI (abducens), IX (glossopharyngeal), X (vagus), and XII (hypoglossal)

      (2) They coordinate movement of the eyes with the head, and the head with the shoulders and torso

      (3) The premotor section known as Broca's area is associated with the motor aspects of speech; damage to this area results in expressive aphasia

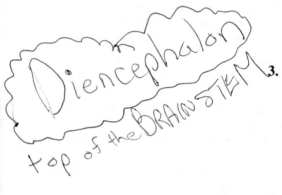

Diencephalon
top of the BRAIN STEM

3. The *diencephalon* is positioned at the top of the brain stem, where the olfactory nerve (cranial nerve I) and the optic nerve (cranial nerve II) begin; it consists of the thalamus, hypothalamus, subthalamus, and epithalamus

  a. The thalamus, which forms the lateral walls of the third ventricle, has several functions

      (1) It relays motor and sensory information

      (2) It conveys all sensory information (except olfactory) to the appropriate area of the cerebral cortex

      (3) It coordinates the functions of the parietal lobe of the cerebrum and cerebral cortex for both sensory and motor stimuli

      (4) It processes basic brain functions and more complex behavior

  b. The hypothalamus, located below the thalamus, forms the floor and anterior wall of the third ventricle; it is responsible for regulating temperature, autonomic responses, water and food intake, behavioral responses, and hormonal secretions

4. The *autonomic nervous system* consists of parasympathetic and sympathetic responses

  a. Parasympathetic responses stimulate the body to slow down activities and conserve energy

  b. Sympathetic responses, also known as fight-or-flight responses, stimulate the body to increase activities and consume energy

5. The *pituitary gland* is located below the hypothalamus in the sella turcica; connected to the hypothalamus by the pituitary stalk, the pituitary gland secretes several hormones: corticotropin (also known as adrenocorticotropic hormone), thyroid-stimulating hormone, growth hormone, prolactin, follicle-stimulating hormone, luteinizing hormone, melanocyte-stimulating hormone, antidiuretic hormone, and oxytocin

6. The *internal capsule* is composed of fiber tracts that lie between the cerebrum and the spinal cord

   a. Afferent (sensory) fibers travel from the spinal cord through the brain stem, thalamus, and internal capsule to the cerebral cortex

   b. Efferent (motor) fibers travel from the cerebral cortex through the internal capsule to the spinal cord

7. The *basal ganglia* make up the central gray matter of the cerebrum and lie between the white matter of the cerebrum and the thalamus

   a. These fibers are primarily motor tracts and influence the ability to produce smooth, coordinated, voluntary movements and to maintain balance

   b. Damage to the basal ganglia results in several clinical syndromes related to motor dysfunction

   (1) Chorea manifests as random, uncontrolled contractions of different muscle groups that occur in place of the normal progression of voluntary movement

   (2) Athetosis causes continuous writhing movements of the upper extremities

   (3) Hemiballismus is an uncontrollable succession of violent jerking motions on one side of the body that results from injury to the contralateral area of the basal ganglia

   (4) Parkinsonism is characterized by tremor at rest, muscle rigidity, loss of involuntary movements (akinesia), shuffling gait, poor posture, and increased salivation

8. The *brain stem* is continuous with the spinal cord and extends through the foramen magnum of the skull; the brain stem consists of the medulla oblongata, pons, midbrain, and reticular formation

   a. The medulla oblongata is the site where decussation (crossing) of motor tracts occurs; at this level, stimulation from one side of the brain affects movement on the contralateral side of the body

   (1) Involuntary swallowing, hiccuping, coughing, vomiting, and vasoconstriction are wholly or partly controlled by the medulla

   (2) The respiratory center, which is located in the medulla, acts in concert with the apneustic and pneumotaxic centers of the pons to control respiratory rhythm

   (3) Also arising in the medulla are the beginnings of the reticular formation and cranial nerves IX (glossopharyngeal), X (vagus), XI (spinal accessory), and XII (hypoglossal)

   b. The pons is located immediately superior to the medulla

   (1) It is a major relay station for the transmission of impulses from the cerebellum to the cerebral cortex; this contributes to smooth body movements

   (2) The apneustic respiratory center, which is located in the pons, controls the length of inspiration and expiration

Midbrain

Reticular formation

Cerebellum

(3) Cranial nerves V (trigeminal), VI (abducens), and VII (facial and acoustic) originate in the pons

c. The midbrain forms the connection between the pons and the diencephalon

  (1) It relays voluntary motor activity

  (2) It is the site of origin of cranial nerves III (oculomotor) and IV (trochlear)

  (3) It also is the location of the extrapyramidal tracts that control the involuntary tone of flexor muscles (rubrospinal) and the involuntary reflex motor movements resulting from auditory or visual stimuli (tectospinal)

  (4) The aqueduct of Sylvius also is located in the midbrain

d. The reticular formation is located in the central core of the brain stem and projects into the cerebral cortex

  (1) All sensory input to the brain stem is relayed through the reticular formation on its way to the cerebral cortex

  (2) Composed of motor and sensory tracts, the reticular formation has both excitatory and inhibitory capacities

  (3) The primary function of the reticular formation is to maintain normal muscle tone through inhibition or excitation of nerve impulses

  (4) Injury to the cerebral cortex, cerebellum, or basal ganglia—all of which lie above the reticular formation—results in continuous stimulation of motor neurons, causing distinctive posturing known as decerebrate (unnatural extension) or decorticate (unnatural flexion)

  (5) Within the reticular formation lie the centers for control of blood pressure and heart and respiratory rates

  (6) Through the reticular activating system, the reticular formation is responsible for wakefulness, consciousness, and sleep

9. The *cerebellum* is located at the posteroinferior aspect of the cerebrum

a. Equilibrium, spatial orientation, coordination of movement, and proprioception are integrated functions of the cerebellum

b. Dysfunction of or injury to the cerebellum can result in ataxia and dysarthria

  (1) Incoordination of movements, which affects both large skeletal muscle movement and the muscles associated with speech, may occur

  (2) Past-pointing, the inability to inhibit movement after it has begun, results from a loss of the ability to predict spatial orientation

  (3) Intentional tremor results from the inability to dampen stimuli that produce motor responses

D. Ventricular system of the brain

1. The ventricles of the brain consist of four connected compartments filled with CSF
2. The largest ventricles, called the lateral ventricles, are paired, with one ventricle located within each of the cerebral hemispheres; the lateral ventricles connect with the third ventricle through the foramen of Monro

    a. Each lateral ventricle consists of a body, frontal horn, temporal horn, and occipital horn

    b. The frontal horn of the lateral ventricle most frequently is selected as the site used for intracranial pressure (ICP) monitoring.

3. The third ventricle is centrally located immediately above the midbrain and between the thalamic structures of the diencephalon; it is linked to the fourth ventricle by the aqueduct of Sylvius
4. The fourth ventricle is situated behind the pons and medulla and in front of the cerebellum; within the fourth ventricle are two openings (known as the foramen of Luschka and the foramen of Magendie) that allow CSF to flow into the subarachnoid space for reabsorption by the arachnoid villi
5. Cerebrospinal fluid is formed almost wholly by the choroid plexus located in the four ventricles; a scant amount is secreted by the ependymal cells that line the ventricles and the spinal cord and by the capillaries of the pia mater

    a. Cerebrospinal fluid is an odorless, colorless, clear substance that contains a small amount of protein (5 to 25 mg/dl) and glucose (50 to 75 mg/dl, which is approximately two-thirds of the amount of glucose found in serum)

    b. Cerebrospinal fluid provides support for the central nervous system (CNS), cushions the CNS against trauma, and assists in the removal of waste products and the delivery of nutrients

    c. Approximately 25 ml of CSF are produced every hour, for a total of 500 ml every day; no feedback mechanism regulates the production of CSF

    (1) With an average circulating volume of 135 to 150 ml, approximately 350 ml of CSF must be reabsorbed every day or hydrocephalus will result

    (2) An obstruction of the cerebral aqueducts within the ventricular system, such as from a tumor or blood clot, blocks the flow of CSF and causes noncommunicating hydrocephalus

    d. Cerebrospinal fluid is thought to be a filtrate of blood resulting from active transport and osmotic pressure; thus, blood pressure is a key element in the production of CSF, as is serum osmolality and cerebral metabolism

    e. Normal CSF pressure at the level of the lumbar cistern, when the patient is in a recumbent position, is 70 to 200 mm H_2O; in the cerebral ventricle, the normal pressure of CSF is 3 to 15 mm Hg

Cerebrospinal Fluid

f. Cerebrospinal fluid flows through a closed system from secretion in the lateral cerebral ventricles through the foramen of Monro to the third ventricle, which secretes more CSF; the CSF then travels through the aqueduct of Sylvius to the fourth ventricle, where more CSF is added; it continues through the foramina of Magendie and Luschka to the subarachnoid space

    (1) From the subarachnoid space, CSF travels down the spinal cord and up over the surface of the brain to be reabsorbed by the arachnoid villi

    (2) The arachnoid villi empty into the intracerebral and meningeal veins, which drain into the venous sinuses

    (3) The venous sinuses drain into the internal jugular vein and back into the central venous circulation

E. Blood-brain barrier

  1. The existence of the blood-brain barrier is based on the theory of "tight junctions" among the capillary endothelium cells of the brain

  2. The blood-brain barrier protects delicate neurons by keeping out toxins and harmful elements by means of selective permeability

    a. The blood-brain barrier is easily permeable to oxygen, water, glucose, and carbon dioxide; most lipid-soluble substances that are stable at body pH cross the blood-brain barrier without difficulty

    b. Chemotherapeutic agents, which are toxins, do not cross the blood-brain barrier; this not only allows these drugs to be administered systemically without harm to the sensitive neurons but also renders them ineffective against most neoplasms in the CNS

    c. Antibiotics, although permeable to the blood-brain barrier, cross more slowly and thus are found in smaller concentrations

  3. The blood-brain barrier exists throughout the brain, except in the hypothalamus, pineal region, and floor of the fourth ventricle; the hypothalamus, because of its involvement in water regulation, requires contact with a greater amount of solutes to sense changes in serum osmolality, glucose, and carbon dioxide levels

  4. The blood-brain barrier can be altered by trauma, induction of some toxic elements, intracranial tumor, and brain irradiation

F. Circulatory system of the CNS

  1. Approximately 80% of the blood flow to the CNS is supplied by the carotid arteries, and 20%, by the vertebral arteries; blood is returned by way of the venous system

  2. The external carotid artery supplies blood to the scalp, face, skull, and middle meningeal artery; laceration of the middle meningeal artery, which lies between the dura and the skull, causes an epidural hematoma

  3. The internal carotid artery proceeds up through the base of the skull, where it connects to the anterior aspect of the circle of Willis, a ring of anastomotic vessels

    a. Immediately before connecting to the circle of Willis, the internal carotid artery branches into the ophthalmic artery

    b. The ophthalmic artery supplies blood to the optic nerve and the eye

4. The two vertebral arteries travel posteriorly after branching from the subclavian arteries and proceed upward through the cervical spine, where they enter the skull through the foramen magnum

    a. The vertebral arteries come together at the level of the posterior rim of the pons to form the basilar artery

    b. The basilar artery supplies blood to the brain stem and the cerebellum before branching into paired posterior cerebral arteries that form the posterior portion of the circle of Willis

    c. The circle of Willis consists of an anterior communicating artery, paired posterior communicating arteries, and paired anterior, posterior, and middle cerebral arteries

        (1) The anterior cerebral arteries supply blood to the medial surfaces of the frontal and parietal lobes

        (2) The middle cerebral arteries supply blood to the surface of the frontal, parietal, and temporal lobes; basal ganglia; internal capsule; and thalamic nuclei

        (3) The posterior communicating arteries supply blood to the medial and inferior aspects of the occipital lobes and the medial and lateral aspects of the temporal lobe

5. The venules move venous blood from the capillaries to the paired cerebral veins

    a. The venous sinuses, established through the cranium, drain venous blood from the cerebral veins

    b. The venous blood then is returned to the heart by way of the internal jugular veins

6. The resistance of the cerebral arterioles is regulated by the vascular system to produce a constant flow, regardless of the systemic arterial pressure

    a. The mechanism that produces this constant flow is called autoregulation

    b. When the systemic mean arterial pressure (MAP) falls below 50 mm Hg or rises above 150 mm Hg, autoregulation fails and the cerebral blood flow mirrors systemic pressures; thus, hypotension may cause cerebral ischemia

7. The gases found in arterial blood have strong vasoactive properties

    a. Hypercapnia (high carbon dioxide content) causes vasodilation, which increases circulating cerebral blood volume and in turn increases ICP

    b. Hypocapnia (low carbon dioxide content) causes vasoconstriction, which decreases circulating blood volume

        (1) Induced hypocapnia, such as that resulting from hyperventilation, causes cerebral vasoconstriction and is an effective method of decreasing ICP

(2) Prolonged hypocapnia (characterized by partial pressure of arterial carbon dioxide [$PaCO_2$] less than 20 mm Hg) produces cerebral ischemia

c. Hypoxemia (characterized by low partial pressure of arterial oxygen [PaO_2]) causes vasodilation, which increases cerebral blood flow and thus increases ICP; PaO_2 less than 50 mm Hg exposes the brain to ischemia as a result of low circulating PaO_2 and increased ICP

G. Spinal cord

1. The spinal cord extends from the brain stem at the level of the foramen magnum to the level of the first or second lumbar vertebra, where it tapers and forms the conus medullaris

2. At the level of the conus medullaris, 31 pairs of nerve roots—known as the cauda equina (horse's tail)—exit from the spinal cord and travel down the intervertebral foramen

3. Bony support for the vertebral column is provided by 33 vertebrae: 7 cervical (C1 through C7), 12 thoracic (T1 through T12), 5 lumbar (L1 through L5), 5 sacral (S1 through S5), and 4 coccygeal

4. Twenty-four intervertebral disks provide flexible support for the spinal cord

5. The spinal cord contains 31 pairs of spinal nerves: 8 cervical, 12 thoracic, 5 lumbar, 5 sacral, and 1 coccygeal

   a. The first 7 pairs of cervical nerves exit above the similarly numbered cervical vertebrae

   b. The eighth cervical nerve pair exits below the seventh cervical vertebra and above the first thoracic vertebra (there is no eighth cervical vertebra)

   c. Each vertebral nerve pair after the eighth one exits below the similarly numbered vertebra

6. A horizontal cross section of the spinal cord shows a central core of gray matter in the shape of an H surrounded by myelinated white matter

   a. The white matter of the spinal cord contains ascending and descending tracts that conduct impulses to and from the brain; these tracts are labeled with names that identify their origin and destination

      (1) The prefix identifies the tract's origin in the spinal tract and the suffix identifies its destination

      (2) The prefix *spino* denotes an ascending sensory tract; for example, the spinothalamic tracts are ascending sensory tracts that conduct impulses upward to the thalamus

      (3) The suffix *spinal* denotes a descending motor tract; for example, the corticospinal tracts are descending motor tracts that originate in the cortex

   b. Each projection of the gray matter (the "H") forms an anterior (ventral) or posterior (dorsal) horn for the left and right sides of the spinal cord

(1) The anterior horns contain motor cells

(2) The posterior horns contain axons from the peripheral sensory neurons

(3) Lateral horns arising at the level of T1 through L2 contain sympathetic fibers, and those of S2 through S4 contain parasympathetic fibers of the autonomic nervous system

H. Nervous system cellular functions

1. The neuron is the basic structural unit of the nervous system

2. Neurons consist of a cell body, dendrites, and an axon

   a. The cell bodies form the gray matter of the brain, brain stem, and spinal cord; ganglia are cell bodies in the peripheral nervous system that lie close to the CNS

      (1) The cell body contains the nucleus, which stores deoxyribonucleic acid (DNA) and ribonucleic acid (RNA) and synthesizes RNA

      (2) The cell body also contains the Golgi apparatus, which stores protein, lysosome-intracellular scavengers, and structures that synthesize cell membrane

      (3) Nissl bodies within the cell body store RNA and synthesize protein

   b. Dendrites are short fibers that branch outward from the cell body

      (1) Dendrites receive stimuli moving toward the cell body

      (2) Each cell body may contain several dendrites

   c. Axons are fibers that branch outward from the cell body in varying lengths; some are several feet long

      (1) Axons transmit stimuli away from the cell body

      (2) Each cell body contains only one axon

      (3) Some axons are covered by a protein-lipid complex known as a myelin sheath

         (a) The myelin sheath is produced by Schwann cells in the peripheral nervous system and by oligodendroglia in the CNS

         (b) The sheath is not a continuous covering but is broken at intervals by nodes of Ranvier

         (c) The sheath acts as an insulator for the conduction of nerve impulses and allows for the efficient conduction of nerve impulses from one node of Ranvier to the next

         (d) Demyelinization of the sheath disrupts conduction of nerve impulses away from the neuron and is seen in degenerative diseases, such as multiple sclerosis

3. Neuroglial cells protect, structurally support, and nourish neurons

   a. Unlike neurons, neuroglial cells retain mitotic function; this may cause CNS neoplasms

   b. Four types of neuroglial cells exist

      (1) Astroglial cells help form the blood-brain barrier

        (2) Ependymal cells are found in the choroid plexus of the ventricular system

        (3) Microglial cells are phagocytic cells found in white matter

        (4) Oligodendroglial cells make up the myelin sheath for axons in the CNS

  4. A nerve impulse can be defined as a physiochemical change in the nerve fibers that is self-propagating once it is initiated

      a. Transmission of nerve impulses in neurons begins with the depolarization of the cell membrane

      b. Depolarization begins with an impulse from another cell in the form of a chemical stimulus

      c. The chemical stimulus triggers the release of neurotransmitters from the bouton terminal or presynaptic terminal at the end of the axon; the impulse then crosses the synaptic cleft to reach the postsynaptic membrane of another nerve cell's dendrite or cell body

      d. The speed of nerve impulse transmission depends on the degree of myelinization (or lack thereof) of the nerve

        (1) In unmyelinated nerve cells, the impulse must travel the length of the nerve fiber

        (2) In myelinated nerve cells, the impulse travels faster by jumping from one node of Ranvier to the next

          (a) The velocity of transmission of the nerve impulse in myelinated nerves increases because less energy is expended

          (b) The conduction of nerve impulse from node to node is known as saltatory conduction

  5. Neurotransmitters are classified as excitatory or inhibitory

      a. Excitatory neurotransmitters foster the transmission of a nerve impulse across the synaptic cleft

      b. Inhibitory neurotransmitters chemically block or slow the transmission of a nerve impulse by increasing the negativity of the cell, thus increasing the cell's resistance to depolarization

  6. Impairment of the synaptic pathway causes increased transmission of some impulses and faulty or no transmission of others

      a. Myasthenia gravis, a disease characterized by weakness and rapid exhaustion of skeletal muscles after exertion, is caused by diminished receptors for the neurotransmitter acetylcholine on the postsynaptic membrane

      b. Parkinsonism, a disease characterized by tremors, rigidity, and fragmentary or incomplete voluntary movements, is caused by a deficiency of dopamine in the basal ganglia, which results in unsuppressed activity of excitatory neurotransmitters

II. Neurologic assessment

  A. Description

1. A neurologic assessment consists of five key components that are meaningful only if evaluated together
   a. Level of consciousness
   b. Motor function
   c. Pupil and eye signs
   d. Respiratory pattern
   e. Vital signs
2. A sixth component, often of clinical significance, is the medical history of the patient and family
B. Level of consciousness
   1. The two principal elements in the assessment of level of consciousness are alertness and awareness
      a. Assessment of alertness is an evaluation of the reticular activating system and its link to the thalamus and cerebral cortex
      b. Assessment of awareness is an evaluation of the patient's orientation to person, place, and time; awareness requires a higher level of brain function than alertness
   2. Changes in the level of consciousness generally are subtle but frequently are the first signs of neurologic deterioration
   3. The Glasgow Coma Scale is the tool most commonly used to assess level of consciousness
      a. On this scale, a score of 15 is best, 3 is the lowest, and 7 or below denotes coma; however, more important than a particular score, the assessment of level of consciousness depends on recognition of subtle changes from a baseline level of consciousness
      b. The Glasgow Coma Scale can be used to assess the level of consciousness only; it cannot be used to rate motor deficits of one side of the body compared with the other, pupillary changes and comparisons, or aphasia
      c. The scale does not clearly differentiate between extremities and thus does not take into account lateralizing signs that may be of primary and emergent importance
      d. The scale also does not reflect the quality of the commands given by the rater
         (1) Commands should be simple and clear and given in the absence of other verbal or tactile stimuli to avoid misinterpreting reflex responses as following the command
         (2) A command that frequently is used but may be misinterpreted is requesting that the patient clasp and release the hands; to avoid random reflex responses to commands, a more appropriate command is to ask the patient to show a particular finger or thumb or to turn the palm up or down
         (3) In patients who are unable to follow commands, the rater often must use noxious stimuli to assess motor function

Cranial nerves and their functions

Each cranial nerve has one or more specific functions. These functions can be described as motor or sensory; some cranial nerves have both. The chart below details the location of each cranial nerve as well as its function.

CRANIAL NERVE	LOCATION	FUNCTION
I. Olfactory	Diencephalon (olfactory tract), with interpretation in temporal lobe	Smell
II. Optic	Diencephalon (optic chiasm), with interpretation in occipital lobe	Sight
III. Oculomotor	Midbrain	Movement of eyes and eyelids and pupillary constriction
IV. Trochlear	Midbrain	Movement of eyes
V. Trigeminal	Pons	Facial sensations and mastication
VI. Abducens	Pons	Movement of eyes
VII. Facial	Medulla and caudal pons	Taste, facial expression, and secretion of saliva and tears
VIII. Acoustic	Medulla, with interpretation in temporal lobe	Hearing and balance
IX. Glossopharyngeal	Medulla, with interpretation of taste in temporal lobe	Taste, swallowing, gag reflex, secretion of saliva, and phonation
X. Vagus	Medulla	Pain and temperature sensations near the ears, gag reflex, coughing, swallowing, and visceral sensations from the abdomen and thorax
XI. Accessory	Medulla and C1 through C5	Movement of head and shoulders
XII. Hypoglossal	Medulla	Movement of tongue

     (a) Examples of acceptable noxious stimuli are pressure applied to the patient's nail bed with a hard, dull object (such as a pen), pinching the trapezius muscle, firmly patting the sternal area, and pinching the sensitive inner aspect of the thigh or arm

     (b) Examples of unacceptable noxious stimuli are pressure applied to the supraorbital area, rubbing the sternal area with the knuckles, and pinching the nipples, breasts, groin, or testicles

C. Motor function

    1. The assessment of motor function includes evaluation of motor tone, motor strength, posturing, and the ability to follow commands appropriately

Remembering cranial nerve functions

Use the two mnemonic phrases below to recall the cranial nerves and their motor, sensory, or mixed functions. Read each phrase vertically: the first letter of each word in the phrase corresponds to the name of the cranial nerve or its function.

CRANIAL NERVE	MNEMONIC FOR NAME	MNEMONIC FOR FUNCTION
I. Olfactory	On	Some (sensory)
II. Optic	Old	Say (sensory)
III. Oculomotor	Olympus'	Marry (motor)
IV. Trochlear	Towering	Money (motor)
V. Trigeminal	Tops	But (both)
VI. Abducens	A	My (motor)
VII. Facial	Finn	Brother (both)
VIII. Acoustic	And	Says (sensory)
IX. Glossopharyngeal	German	Bad (both)
X. Vagus	Viewed	Business (both)
XI. Spinal accessory	Some	Marry (motor)
XII. Hypoglossal	Hops	Money (motor)

2. Coordinated motor function requires an intact motor cortex, basal ganglia, and descending motor pathways (including the corticospinal tract, extrapyramidal tract, cerebellum, lower motor neurons, neuromuscular junctions, and skeletal muscle)

3. Because the bulk of corticospinal neurons decussate in the medulla, motor impairment of one side of the body reflects deficits in the ipsilateral side of the brain

4. Assessment of the 12 pairs of cranial nerves can help in the identification of the area of injury in a neurologically impaired patient (see *Cranial nerves and their functions*); the cranial nerves have motor (III, IV, VI, XI, and XII), sensory (I, II, and VIII), or mixed (V, VII, IX, X) functions (see *Remembering cranial nerve functions*)

5. The Romberg test can be used to evaluate cerebellar intactness, balance, and proprioception; in this test, a patient stands with feet together and closes the eyes and normally would be able to remain erect

6. Assessment of Babinski's reflex is used to determine corticospinal tract intactness

   a. This test involves stroking the lateral part of the sole and the ball of the foot

   b. An abnormal response is dorsiflexion of the big toe, while a normal response is plantar flexion

7. Meningeal irritation can cause muscle spasm or abnormal posturing
   a. Nuchal rigidity describes the involuntary muscle spasm that prevents a patient from putting chin to chest
   b. Opisthotonos is an extreme spasm of the spinal muscles and causes drastic extension of the spine; it also is seen in tetanus and decerebrate posturing
   c. A positive Kernig's sign results when resistance to extension and pain occurs when the leg is flexed at a 90-degree angle and the thigh already is flexed at a 90-degree angle to the hip; this sign may be seen in tumors of the cauda equina, herniated disks, and meningeal irritation
   d. Brudzinski's sign is an involuntary flexion of the hip and knees produced by flexion of the neck; it is indicative of meningeal irritation
   e. Abnormal posturing includes flexor spasm and extensor spasm
      (1) Decorticate posturing manifests as abnormal flexion in the upper extremities with accompanying extension of the lower extremities; it indicates an interruption in a corticospinal pathway by a lesion in the cerebral hemisphere, basal ganglia, or diencephalon
      (2) Decerebrate posturing manifests as abnormal extension of the upper extremities and the lower extremities; it indicates injury to the brain stem

D. Pupil and eye signs
   1. Assessment of pupil size, shape, equality, and degree of response to light stimuli is valuable primarily because it may delineate the path of innervation from the autonomic nervous system
      a. Sympathetic innervation of the pupil starts in the hypothalamus and runs the length of the brain stem
         (1) Intact sympathetic stimulation causes pupillary dilation
         (2) Disrupted sympathetic control—resulting from conditions involving pathologic brain stem involvement or lesions of the pons that interrupt sympathetic pathways before they enter the brain stem—results in pinpoint, nonreactive pupils
      b. The parasympathetic response is controlled by the oculomotor nerve (cranial nerve III), which exits the brain stem at the level of the midbrain and tentorial notch
         (1) Intact parasympathetic stimulation causes pupillary constriction
         (2) Disrupted parasympathetic control, which occurs when increased ICP compresses the oculomotor nerve against the tentorial notch, results in dilated, nonreactive pupils that are absent of consensual response
            (a) A unilaterally dilated pupil absent of light response in a patient at risk for increasing ICP signifies possible brain herniation

(b) Patients who have undergone cardiopulmonary resuscitation (CPR) may show anoxic pupillary dilation, which carries a grave prognosis if it lasts more than a few minutes; however, patients who receive mydriatic agents (for example, atropine) during CPR may have dilated pupils from the medication and do not necessarily have a poor prognosis

2. Pupil reactivity may be the most important clinical sign in the differentiation of metabolic coma from structural injury coma; in the presence of metabolic disturbances, pupil reactivity remains relatively intact

   a. Pupils should always be assessed relative to baseline or previous assessments and relative to each other

   b. Pupil reactivity and size can be affected by medications and previous injuries or surgery to the eye; the patient's medication and medical history should be considered before inferences are made from pupillary signs

3. The function of three cranial nerves—the oculomotor (III), trochlear (IV), and abducens (VI)—can be assessed by evaluating the ability of the eye to move through the six points of the cardinal fields of gaze

   a. This assessment can be performed only if the patient is alert and cooperative

   b. Unconscious patients can be assessed for intactness of cranial nerve function by evaluating the oculocephalic (doll's eyes) reflex and the oculovestibular reflex; these reflexes are used to assess the intactness of cranial nerves III through VIII and reflect brain stem integrity; tests of these reflexes should not be performed on a conscious patient

      (1) In the oculocephalic reflex, the nurse holds the patient's eyelids open while briskly turning the head to one side; this test should not be performed if a cervical injury is suspected

         (a) If the reflex is intact, the eyes move in the direction away from which the head is turned (doll's eyes are present); this normal reflex indicates intact brain stem function

         (b) If the eyes drift in an irregular manner or move in opposite directions when the head is turned (doll's eyes are abnormal), the patient has some degree of brain stem impairment

         (c) If the eyes move with the head as it is turned and maintain the same position as though fixed in place (doll's eyes are absent), significant brain stem impairment has occurred

      (2) In the oculovestibular reflex, 20 to 50 ml of cold water is instilled into the external auditory canal with a large-bore syringe

         (a) The normal response is nystagmus with movement toward the ear into which the water was instilled, indicating intact brain stem function

         (b) Movement away from the stimulated ear is an abnormal response, indicating some brain stem impairment

         (c) No movement in any direction is an absent reflex, indicating significant brain stem injury

  E. Respiratory pattern

     1. Respiratory patterns are closely associated with and should be assessed in conjunction with clinical assessment of vital signs and level of consciousness

     2. Cheyne-Stokes respirations are characterized by periodic waxing and waning of respiratory excursion with alternating periods of apnea and hyperpnea; they usually result from upper brain stem lesions

     3. Central neurogenic hyperventilation may be caused by middle brain stem lesions; this respiratory pattern is characterized by sustained, deep, rapid hyperpnea with resultant hypocapnia; arterial blood gas (ABG) values show elevated PaO_2 level, elevated pH, and decreased $PaCO_2$ level

     4. A protracted peak inspiration pattern is characteristic of apneustic breathing; in the absence of unopposing stimuli from the pneumotaxic center (which normally limits the rate of inspiration), the apneustic center continues unchecked, thus resulting in this respiratory pattern

     5. Cluster breathing, characterized by irregular clusters of breaths followed by irregular pauses, indicates lower brain stem herniation

     6. Ataxic breathing, or Biot's respirations, may result from medullary lesions or rapid cerebellar or pontine hemorrhage; this respiratory pattern is characterized by an irregular rate and depth of respirations accompanied by irregular periods of apnea

     7. Kussmaul's respirations, characterized by slow, deep, and labored breathing, are a sign of metabolic acidosis—not neurologic dysfunction

  F. Vital signs

     1. Changes in vital signs, like changes in pupillary response, are late signs of neurologic deterioration compared with changes in the level of consciousness

     2. In a neurologically injured patient, vital signs may reflect changes in autoregulation; for example, intracranial injury often results in loss of cerebral autoregulation

     3. Autoregulation is a compensatory mechanism whereby the cerebral vessels constrict or enlarge in response to increasing or decreasing arterial pressure

        a. Autoregulation remains functional within the following parameters: MAP of 50 to 150 mm Hg, ICP less than 33 mm Hg, and normal PaO_2 (80 to 100 mm Hg) and $PaCO_2$ (35 to 45 mm Hg)

    b. When autoregulation fails, the cerebral vessels relax and allow the volume in the cerebral tissues to mirror the systemic arterial pressure

      (1) In the face of failed autoregulation, increased systemic arterial pressure increases blood flow to the brain

      (2) Increased blood flow to the brain increases volume in the cranial vault, resulting in increased ICP

    c. In the brain stem, the center for regulation of blood pressure loses its ability for autoregulation when injury to the brain increases ICP and causes medullary hypoxia

      (1) As a result, arterial pressure increases in an attempt to raise oxygenation by means of increased perfusion

      (2) Increased perfusion results in increased ICP, which produces parasympathetic stimulation of the lower brain stem with ensuing bradycardia

      (3) If left unchecked, this results in destruction of the medullary centers and causes signs of decompensation, hypotension, tachycardia, and respiratory arrest

  4. Cushing's triad consists of three clinically significant signs of decreased cerebral perfusion pressure and cerebral ischemia

    a. These signs are increased blood pressure with widening pulse pressure, bradycardia, and abnormal respiratory function

    b. In an attempt to increase cerebral perfusion, heart rate slows; this in turn increases the stroke volume and raises systolic blood pressure

  5. Temperature dysfunctions can arise from disruption of the sympathetic pathways between the hypothalamus and the peripheral vessels; such disruptions can result from spinal cord injury or infection and cause a chain of deleterious effects

    a. Elevated temperature increases the metabolic rate

    b. An elevated metabolic rate causes increased levels of carbon dioxide

    c. Increased levels of carbon dioxide cause dilation of the cerebral vasculature

    d. Increased dilation leads to cerebral edema and elevated intracerebral pressure

III. Diagnostic tests

  A. Noninvasive diagnostic tests

    1. X-rays of the skull or spine are the most frequently used noninvasive diagnostic test in a patient with suspected neurologic injury; X-rays also are helpful in diagnosing skull fractures, tumors, vascular calcification, and vertebral fractures or dislocations

    2. Computed tomography (CT) scans can be used to assess hydrocephalus, infarction, tumors, atrophy, abscess, and cerebral swelling; when used with contrast media (making the scan an invasive test), CT scans provide greater visualization of cerebral vasculature and thus can help identify congenital malformations and aneurysms

3. Magnetic resonance imaging (MRI) is used to evaluate cerebral edema, infection, bone lesions, infarction, and blood vessels

4. An EEG monitors brain wave activity by means of electrodes placed on the scalp

   a. The EEG is useful for determining the focus of seizure activity or the cause of coma and can indicate an area of lesions

   b. The EEG is of particular importance in determining brain death

5. Evoked potentials are another diagnostic tool involving surface electrodes; in this test, the patient's response to visual, auditory, and tactile stimulation is measured along a specific neuronal pathway and graphically depicted using computer analysis

   a. Visual responses aid in the evaluation of posttraumatic injury

   b. Auditory responses help in the evaluation of brain stem function, multiple sclerosis, auditory lesions, and coma

   c. Tactile responses are useful in the evaluation of peripheral nerve disease and lesions of the brain and spinal cord involving demyelinated neurons

6. Electromyography (EMG) is a useful diagnostic tool for muscular dystrophies, myasthenia gravis, amyotrophic lateral sclerosis, and peripheral nerve dysfunctions; through electrical stimulation of specific muscle groups, EMG can help differentiate neuromuscular junction disease from lower motor neuron disease

B. Invasive diagnostic tests

   1. Digital subtraction angiography uses computerized fluoroscopy to visualize cerebral vessels and carotid blood flow

      a. After a baseline scan is made, contrast dye is injected and a second scan is done; the computer then "subtracts" the first scan from the second, providing greater definition of the targeted vasculature

      b. As with CT scans that require contrast media, the contrast dye is hypertonic and may temporarily reduce cerebral edema; however, in the absence of actions to correct the cause of the condition, cerebral edema will return

   2. Cerebral angiography is used to diagnose malformations of the cerebral vasculature and requires the injection of radiopaque dye into the cerebral circulation

      a. Cerebral angiography may indicate tumors if vessel displacement is observed or may identify arteriovenous malformations (AVMs) and aneurysms

      b. It also is used to diagnose vessel thrombosis, arterial spasm, cerebral edema, and herniation

   3. Positron emission tomography measures tissue uptake of a radionuclide that is inhaled or administered I.V.

      a. Positron emission tomography assesses tissue metabolism and cerebral blood flow

      b. Uptake of the isotope by different regions of the brain may reveal hemorrhage, infarction, abscess, or tumor

4. Brain scans involve the use of an I.V. radionuclide and measurement of its uptake by the brain; areas of greater uptake indicate disturbances in the blood-brain barrier, such as in contusions, tumors, hemorrhage, infarction, and abscess

5. Lumbar puncture requires the insertion of a hollow needle into the subarachnoid space of the spine, generally at the L3 or L4 level; this test usually is performed when meningitis or subarachnoid bleeding is suspected

   a. During the lumbar puncture, CSF pressure is measured (normal pressure is 50 to 200 cm H_2O) and samples of CSF are taken and evaluated for the presence of blood cells, protein, glucose, electrolytes, and microorganisms

   (1) The presence of more than 5 white blood cells (WBCs) per millimeter of CSF indicates inflammation within the ventricular system or meninges

   (2) The presence of red blood cells (RBCs) in the CSF suggests subarachnoid hemorrhage or cerebral laceration

   (3) Protein levels greater than 40 mg/dl may indicate Guillain-Barré syndrome, tumor, or infection

   (4) The CSF glucose level should be two-thirds of the level found in serum; low CSF glucose levels signify infection

   (5) Low chloride levels in the CSF suggest meningitis

   b. Medication may be injected during the lumbar puncture to bypass the blood-brain barrier

   c. Contrast media (myelogram) may be injected to diagnose ventricular or subarachnoid space abnormalities

   d. Testing for Queckenstedt's sign, which detects obstruction in the subarachnoid space resulting from tumor or vertebral fracture, may be performed during the lumbar puncture; in this test, the jugular veins are compressed for approximately 10 seconds to test for a normally rapid rise in lumbar pressure with a rapid fall to normal levels when the veins are no longer compressed

   e. Lumbar puncture is contraindicated in patients with increased ICP resulting from space-occupying lesions of the brain or acute head trauma

   (1) In these patients, the release of pressure in the subarachnoid space below the brain may force the brain to herniate through the foramen magnum

   (2) Cisternal puncture is an alternate method of obtaining access to the subarachnoid space in patients in whom total spinal blockage is apparent or lumbar access is not feasible

6. ICP monitoring assesses the static and dynamic pressures exerted by the volume of intracranial contents

   a. The Monro-Kellie doctrine describes the volume-pressure relationship within the brain and the pathologic condition associated with increased ICP

   (1) This doctrine asserts that the skull is a rigid compartment of limited space

(2) This space is filled to capacity by three components—brain tissue, blood, and CSF—all of which have a fairly constant volume

(3) An increase in any one component necessitates a concomitant decrease in one of the other components or cerebral edema and increased ICP will result

b. Herniation of cerebral tissues is caused by compression and displacement of areas of the brain against the bony cranial compartment or its structures; increased ICP caused by tumors, hemorrhage, or cerebral edema produces this displacement

(1) Supratentorial herniation involves the structures located above the tentorial notch: the cerebral hemispheres, basal ganglia, and diencephalon

(a) Cingulate or transflex herniation develops when one cerebral hemisphere is shifted laterally, forcing the cingulate gyrus under the falx cerebri; the lateral shifting compresses and displaces the large cerebral veins of that hemisphere

(b) Central or transtentorial herniation occurs when increased, diffuse pressure is exerted downward, forcing the cerebral structures down through the tentorial opening and resulting in rostral-caudal herniation

(c) Early rostral-caudal herniation is characterized by a decreased level of consciousness, normal respiratory control but an atypical respiratory pattern with frequent sighs or yawns, and small but equally reactive pupils; as the herniation continues and more structures become compressed, deep coma, pathologic respiratory patterns, and pupillary and reflex changes associated with brain stem involvement occur

(d) Uncal herniation is the lateral compression of cerebral tissues downward through the tentorial opening; the lateralizing signs present with uncal herniation differentiate it from central herniation; in uncal herniation, the typically decreased level of consciousness is accompanied by a unilaterally dilated pupil, which signifies the beginning of brain stem involvement and rapid deterioration to coma and brain death

(2) Infratentorial herniation involves the structures located below the tentorial notch: the cerebellum and lower brain stem

(a) Infratentorial herniation develops when a tumor, an abscess, or hemorrhage forces the cerebellum and brain stem to shift laterally, upward through the tentorial opening, or downward through the foramen magnum

(b) Lumbar puncture in a patient with high ICP may cause a rapid downward shift of cerebral tissues that leads to infratentorial herniation; signs of compression usually are unilateral and deterioration is rapid

(3) Transcranial herniation involves the cerebral tissues throughout the cranial vault; it is caused by cerebral extrusion through a skull fracture, craniotomy site, or opening in the skull caused by a bullet wound

c. Cerebral edema causes increased ICP

   (1) Vasogenic cerebral edema results from disruption of the blood-brain barrier, causing extracellular edema; this in turn causes osmotic pressure gradients in the cerebral vessels that move water from the intravascular space to the cerebral interstitium, thus increasing the edema; vasogenic edema may be caused by trauma, infection, abscess, hypoxia, or tumor

   (2) Cytotoxic cerebral edema results from failure of the sodium-potassium pump, which allows potassium to leave the cell while sodium, chloride, and water enter the cell and cause it to swell; this intracellular edema can be caused by hypoxic states, administration of hypotonic fluids (such as dextrose 5% in water, other hypo-osmotic conditions, and certain diseases (such as Reye's syndrome)

   (3) Interstitial (hydrocephalic) cerebral edema is extracellular edema that results from a buildup of CSF pressure within the ventricular system; this produces transudation of CSF into the periventricular areas; hydrocephalus can be acute or chronic and may be communicating (nonobstructive) or noncommunicating (obstructive)

     (a) Communicating hydrocephalus is caused by increased production or decreased absorption of CSF; meningeal tumors, congenital malformations, and infection can result in communicating hydrocephalus

     (b) Noncommunicating hydrocephalus is caused by adhesions or mechanical obstructions; subarachnoid hemorrhage and infection may cause noncommunicating hydrocephalus

d. Venous outflow has a role in determining ICP

   (1) The two major outflow vessels for venous cerebral blood are the internal jugular veins and the basal cerebral veins

   (2) ICP can be increased if these outflow tracts are impeded, which can result from the following actions

     (a) Placing the head of the bed in a flat position

     (b) Rotating the head to one side or neck flexion

     (c) Taping the endotracheal tube too tightly

     (d) Engaging in any activity that increases intra-abdominal or intrathoracic pressure, such as the Valsalva maneuver, coughing, suctioning, use of positive end-expiratory pressure, during mechanical ventilation, and positioning the patient in the prone position or with hips flexed more than 90 degrees

e. Compliance is the term used to describe the mechanisms that maintain fairly constant ICP (normal range is 0 to 15 mm Hg, with 10 mm Hg being ideal) in the face of increased volume

  (1) Compliance mechanisms include the following

    (a) Relocation of CSF from the intracranial cavity to the spinal space

    (b) Constriction of cerebral blood vessels that decreases circulating blood volume

    (c) Decreased production or increased reabsorption of CSF

    (d) Expansion of the skull to accommodate increased volume in children whose cranial sutures have not yet fused

  (2) Compliance is effective only to a certain degree; compliance is most effective when volume increases slowly, allowing compensatory mechanisms to work

  (3) Once compliance mechanisms reach their limit of effectiveness, small increases in volume result in significant increases in ICP

f. Cerebral perfusion pressure (CPP) is a measure of the pressure gradient between the systemic MAP and the opposing ICP

  (1) Cerebral perfusion pressure is a measure of the ability to sufficiently perfuse the cerebral tissues; it is calculated as follows: CPP = MAP – ICP

  (2) Normal CPP is 80 to 100 mm Hg; a CPP of at least 60 mm Hg is necessary to sustain cerebral tissues

  (3) Autoregulation fails with a CPP of 40 mm Hg or less, and irreversible hypoxic states occur when the CPP is 30 mm Hg or less

g. Decompensation occurs when a patient can no longer compensate for changes in MAP or ICP; there are four stages of compensation-decompensation

  (1) Stage I: intracranial volume increases without a concomitant increase in ICP as a result of active compliance mechanisms; no changes are evident in vital signs or level of consciousness; compensation is present

  (2) Stage II: intracranial volume increases with a concomitant increase in ICP; compliance mechanisms are reaching end-stage effectiveness, and slight changes in vital signs, level of consciousness, and motor functions may be evident; compensation is beginning to fail

  (3) Stage III: ICP approaches arterial blood pressure, and compliance methods are no longer effective; Cushing's triad and decreased level of consciousness are present; decompensation begins

  (4) Stage IV: autoregulation fails; cerebral blood flow is greatly decreased or absent; decompensation is present and death results if the condition is not immediately reversed

h. Intracranial pressure can be monitored using one of several methods

  (1) In the intraventricular method, a catheter is inserted into the anterior or occipital horns of the lateral ventricle; a three-way stopcock attached to the catheter permits monitoring of ICP through a pressure transducer and permits drainage of CSF

    (a) Advantages of this method are that it allows direct measurement of ICP and instillation of medication or contrast media to visualize the size and patency of the ventricular system

    (b) Disadvantages include risk of infection, hemorrhage, loss of CSF, and difficulty inserting the catheter in the presence of collapsed ventricles, midline shifting, and marked cerebral edema

  (2) A subarachnoid screw—a screw with a hollow core—is inserted into the subarachnoid space by means of a burr hole, usually over the frontal lobe area; a three-way stopcock attached to the screw allows monitoring of ICP through a pressure transducer and allows drainage of CSF

    (a) Advantages of this method are that it permits direct measurement of ICP, the screw is easy to insert, and the infection rate is lower than in ventricular monitoring

    (b) Disadvantages include risk of infection, possibility of inaccurate measurements if the screw lumen becomes occluded, and need for a firm skull (this method usually cannot be used on patients under age 6); the screw also is more easily dislodged than a catheter

  (3) In the epidural sensor method, a fiber-optic sensing device is inserted by means of a burr hole into the space between the skull and the dura, with the sensor membrane placed against the dura

    (a) Advantages of this method are that it is less invasive than other methods and the device is easy to insert

    (b) Disadvantages include the lack of a route for CSF drainage and the questionable accuracy of this method (readings are higher than those obtained by other methods; inaccurate readings may result if the dura is compressed or thickened or if increased surface tension exists)

  (4) In the lumbar subarachnoid method, an epidural catheter is inserted into the subarachnoid space below the L2 level of the spinal cord

    (a) Advantages of this method are that it is less invasive and allows for drainage of CSF and instillation of intrathecal medications

    (b) Disadvantages include a greater likelihood of contamination and a catheter that can be easily dislodged

7. A normal ICP waveform has some similarity to an arterial hemodynamic waveform
   a. A normal ICP waveform has a sharp upward slope followed by a more gradual downward slope with a dicrotic notch
   b. An abnormal ICP waveform may be one of three types
      (1) A waves, also known as plateau waves, are the most clinically significant
         (a) A waves are tall, flat-topped waves lasting 5 to 20 minutes with ICP readings between 50 and 100 mm Hg
         (b) A waves signify a reduction in CPP with ensuing hypoxia and decompensation
         (c) A waves are an ominous sign and require emergency treatment
      (2) B waves are peaked, saw-toothed, rhythmic oscillations lasting 0.5 to 2 minutes with ICP readings of 50 mm Hg; although the clinical significance of B waves has not been established, they are thought to denote a decrease in compliance and may be precursors to A waves
      (3) C waves are rapid, rhythmic waves lasting 1 to 2 minutes that appear every 4 to 8 minutes with ICP readings between 20 and 50 mm Hg; C waves are thought to be related to respiratory and hemodynamic parameters
C. Key laboratory values
   1. The laboratory tests with the most clinical significance in a patient with neurologic problems are ABG analysis, CSF analysis, and drug screens
   2. Other laboratory tests, such as for blood glucose, calcium, and sodium levels, are used to rule out other diseases that may produce neurologic symptoms

IV. **Nursing care common to all neurologic disorders**
   A. Assessment of changes in neurologic status
      1. Check pupillary and eye signs
      2. Monitor vital signs, including quality of respirations and heart rhythm
      3. Assess motor and sensory abilities
      4. Check for alterations in level of consciousness
   B. Maintenance of adequate ventilatory status
      1. Maintain airway
      2. Prevent aspiration
      3. Treat hypoxemia
   C. Prevention of complications associated with decreased mobility
      1. Turn the patient frequently and use special mattresses to prevent pressure ulcers from developing over bony prominences
      2. Maintain adequate nutrition and hydration
      3. Assess for phlebitis

      4. Position the patient to prevent aspiration

      5. Maintain good pulmonary toilet

   D. Maintenance of normal temperature

      1. Use thermic blankets and tepid soaks

      2. Investigate the cause of temperature elevations

   E. Education of patient and family members

      1. Communicate calmly and clearly

      2. Explain procedures before they are implemented

      3. Explain the reasons for interventions

      4. Orient the patient to the environment

V. Acute spinal cord injuries

   A. Description

      1. Injuries to the spinal cord are classified by the area and mechanism of injury

      2. The area of injury refers to the level of the spine (cervical, thoracic, or lumbar) injured; the higher the level of injury, the greater the degree of injury

      3. Mechanisms of injury include hyperflexion, hyperextension, rotation, axial loading or compression, and penetration by a knife or bullet

         a. Hyperflexion most commonly is seen in cervical injuries (C5 to C6); it is caused most often by sudden deceleration, with the resulting dislocated or subluxated intervertebral disk or bone fragments compressing the spinal cord nerve roots

         b. Hyperextension commonly is seen in whiplash injuries; it results from backward and downward movement, which stretches the spinal cord, disrupts disks, and tears ligaments

         c. Rotation occurs in combination with flexion or extension injuries; rotational forces tear spinal ligaments, resulting in displacement of disks and compression of nerve roots

         d. Axial loading or compression results from an impact great enough to cause the intervertebral disks to burst; this mechanism of injury is seen in falls from heights and generally results in complete neurologic damage below the level of injury

         e. A penetrating injury, such as a knife or bullet wound, usually causes complete transection of the spinal cord

   B. Clinical signs and symptoms

      1. The signs and symptoms associated with acute spinal cord injuries depend on the level of vertebral damage (see *Consequences of spinal cord injuries,* page 158)

      2. Although the level of vertebral and spinal nerve damage can be used as a guidepost, anatomic and functional levels of injury also bear consideration

Consequences of spinal cord injuries

The signs and symptoms that accompany spinal cord injury can help diagnose the extent of the injury. Likewise, knowing the level of injury and the body areas affected can help the critical care nurse plan appropriate interventions. The chart below details the motor function, sensation, and outcome for certain levels of spinal cord injury. Keep in mind that the motor function and sensation of a particular level of spinal cord injury also include features noted in the levels above.

LEVEL OF INJURY	MOTOR FUNCTION	SENSATION	OUTCOME
C4 or above	Movement of head and upper neck; respiratory paralysis	Full sensation to head and upper neck	Quadriplegia; patient may require mechanical ventilation
C4 to C5	Control of head, neck, shoulders, trapezius, and elbow flexion	Shoulders, back, anterior chest, and lateral upper arms	Quadriplegia; patient requires assistive devices for limited participation in activities of daily living
C5 to C6	Index finger and thumb, some extension of wrist, phrenic nerve intact	Index finger and thumb	Quadriplegia; patient has increased ability to help with some activities of daily living
C6 to C7	Elbow extension	Middle and ring fingers	Patient is capable of some finger commands as well as performing some activities of daily living, feeding, and dressing
C7 to T1	Hand movement	Complete hand and medial arm	Patient has greater independence
T1 to T2	Upper extremity control	Some upper trunk sensation above the nipple line	Paraplegia; patient has full use of hands and arms with no trunk control
T3 through T8	Back and chest to nipple line	Some trunk sensation below the nipple line, increasing as the injury occurs lower in the spinal cord (autonomic dysreflexia may occur with injuries at the level of T4 through T6 and above)	Patient has some trunk control
T9 to T10	Muscles of the trunk and upper thigh	Intact to below the waist	Bowel and bladder reflex
T11 to L1	Most leg and some foot movement	Lower leg and dorsal foot	Leg brace, ambulation
L1 to L2	Reflex centers for lower legs, feet, and perineum	Bowel, bladder, and sexual function	Continued dysfunction of bowel, bladder, and sexual reflexes if S2 through S4 spinal nerves are involved

3. The anatomic level of injury refers to damage of the upper or lower motor neurons; the upper motor neurons descend from the brain to the spinal cord and begin and end with the CNS; the lower motor neurons originate in the anterior horns of the spinal cord and end in the muscle tissues

   a. Damage to a specific motor neuron results in pathologic signs, such as a positive Babinski's reflex, muscle spasticity, or muscle flaccidity

   b. If damage to an upper motor neuron occurs above the level of decussation at the medulla, contralateral dysfunction is seen; if damage occurs below the level of decussation for upper or lower motor neurons, ipsilateral dysfunction occurs

4. The functional level of injury refers to the extent of disruption of normal spinal cord functions; functional injuries are classified as complete or incomplete

   a. A complete injury generally involves permanent loss of motor and sensory function in the nerve fibers distal to the injury; complete injuries at the level of the cervical spine result in quadriplegia, and those at the level of the thoracic or lumbar spine result in paraplegia

      (1) Complete transection of the spinal cord can result in spinal or neurogenic shock, with immediate loss of all neurologic function below the level of injury

         (a) Complete transection causes loss of motor neuron function, as evidenced by the absence of reflex activity and flaccid paralysis below the level of injury

         (b) All sensation of temperature, vibration, touch, proprioception, and pain are lost below the level of injury

         (c) Loss of autonomic function results in lowered and unsteady arterial blood pressure and an inability to perspire

         (d) Loss of vascular tone causes venous pooling and warm, dry skin that is prone to heat loss and thus lowers the body temperature

         (e) Bradycardia is present because of the lack of parasympathetic opposition; if hypotension accompanies bradycardia in a patient with spinal cord injury, spinal shock is likely; if hypotension accompanies tachycardia, hemorrhagic shock should be suspected

      (2) Spinal shock lasts between 1 and 6 weeks, at which point 50% of patients regain some degree of spinal cord function; as reflexes return, a hyperactive state is seen with spastic paralysis of the upper motor neurons and continued flaccidity of the lower motor neurons

   b. In an incomplete injury, function of a portion of the spinal cord remains intact; a patient may suffer from one of several types of incomplete injuries

(1) Damage to the anterior horns of the spinal cord involves the motor tracts, spinothalamic (pain perception) tracts, and corticospinal (temperature perception) tracts

   (a) Anterior cord damage generally is seen in flexion and dislocation injuries of the cervical cord

   (b) Pain and temperature sensations and motor function are lost at the level below the injury

   (c) Touch, proprioception, pressure, and vibration senses remain intact

   (d) Babinski's reflex is pathologically positive, and spastic paralysis is seen

(2) Damage to the posterior horns of the spinal cord results in loss of proprioception and the sensation of light touch

   (a) Pain and temperature sensations and motor function remain intact

   (b) Posterior cord injuries, which are rare, generally are associated with hyperextension of the cervical spine

(3) Damage to the central gray matter of the spinal cord results in significant loss of upper-extremity motor function with an accompanying, but less significant, loss of lower-extremity motor function

   (a) Some patients do not experience loss of lower-extremity motor function; this results from the central placement of the upper motor neurons in the cord and the peripheral placement of the lower motor neurons

   (b) Central cord injuries typically are seen in hyperextension of the cervical spine and in older patients in whom degenerative changes of the vertebrae and disks allow central cord compression to occur

(4) Damage to one side of the cord, called Brown-Séquard syndrome or transverse hemisection, results in ipsilateral loss of motor function

   (a) It also causes ipsilateral loss of touch, proprioception, pressure, and vibration sensations and contralateral loss of pain and temperature sensations

   (b) Brown-Séquard syndrome is caused by penetrating wounds, such as bullet or knife wounds that transect one side of the cord; this syndrome also is seen in surfers who suffer traumatic injury caused by the surfboard hitting them in the neck and rupturing the intervertebral disk

(5) Damage to spinal nerve roots in the sacral area from trauma resulting in a fracture dislocation causes neurologic deficits specific to the nerve roots involved; damage can be unilateral or bilateral, and both motor and sensory loss may be apparent

    (6) Damage to the spinal cord at the level of T4 through T6 or above can lead to autonomic dysreflexia, an emergency clinical condition characterized by an exaggerated autonomic response (life-threatening hypertension) to a stimulus; the triggering stimulus can be bladder distention, bowel distention, a hot or cold stimulus, or a skin stimulus (such as from tight clothing, a pressure ulcer, or an ingrown toenail)

        (a) Impulses from a full bladder or other stimuli are sent by way of the spinothalamic tracts and posterior columns toward the brain but are blocked at the level of injury

        (b) As these impulses travel up the spinal cord, they stimulate a sympathetic reflex in the gray horns of the thoracolumbar spinal cord; normally, these reflexes are inhibited by impulses from the brain

        (c) Because the initial impulses to the brain are blocked at the level of injury, no inhibitory signals are sent to counter the sympathetic reflexes, thereby resulting in a tremendous sympathetic response

        (d) Symptoms of this sympathetic response include diaphoresis and flushing above the level of injury, with chills and severe vasoconstriction below the level of injury; paroxysmal hypertension, bradycardia, headache, and nausea also are present

        (e) Autonomic dysreflexia is treated by removing the cause (for example, emptying the bladder or bowel) and administering antihypertensive drugs; the best treatment involves identifying the patient as susceptible to autonomic dysreflexia and preventing the syndrome through elimination of drafts, good skin and nail care, and regular bowel and bladder regimens

C. Diagnostic tests

  1. A series of spinal X-rays is done to check for fractures, dislocations, and degenerative changes of the vertebral column

  2. Axial tomography may be used to check for bony lesions

  3. A myelogram also may be performed

D. Medical management

  1. Treat the acute symptoms and stabilize the injury

  2. Use surgical interventions, if indicated, to repair fractures or decrease pressure on the spinal cord

E. Nursing management

  1. Assess motor function and sensory abilities to detect changes from baseline values

  2. Prevent further damage by immobilizing the area, using special equipment as needed

3. Keep in mind that immobilization places the patient at risk for hypoventilation, pneumonia, and pulmonary embolism; encourage coughing and deep breathing and use suctioning to prevent these complications

4. Prevent skin breakdown by using proper positioning, frequent turning, and therapeutic range-of-motion exercises

5. Provide supportive care and treat complications resulting from the injury

   a. Arrhythmias, especially tachycardia and bradycardia, are common in patients with spinal cord injuries

   b. Respiratory disturbances also are common and are associated with the level of injury

VI. Aneurysms

A. Description

   1. An aneurysm is a dilated area in an artery wall that weakens the vessel wall

   2. Aneurysms are classified as *saccular* or *berry* (bulging or ballooning of the vessel wall with a stemlike attachment to the vessel), *fusiform* (a usually large atherosclerotic outpouching), *dissecting* (blood leaking from a tear in the intima of the vessel wall into the layers of the arterial wall), or *mycotic* (an infected lesion or embolism of the arterial wall)

   3. Eighty-five percent of cerebral aneurysms are formed at the bifurcation of the arteries and are of the saccular type

   4. Traumatic injury to a vessel also can cause an aneurysm to form

   5. Some aneurysms are congenital defects; of these, a small percentage are caused by AVM

      a. Arteriovenous malformations occur when a miscommunication develops between arteries, veins, and capillaries, resulting in shunting of arterial blood directly into the venous system, thus bypassing the capillaries

      b. This "stealing" of blood causes ischemia and atrophy in the tissues from which the arterial blood is shunted

      c. The higher-than-normal pressures exerted on the venous side by the arterial flow create engorgement of the veins into which the arterial blood is shunted

B. Clinical signs and symptoms

   1. Sometimes asymptomatic

   2. Severe headaches, vomiting, photophobia, and nuchal rigidity (caused by leakage of small amounts of blood into the subarachnoid space) followed by loss of consciousness (as a result of aneurysm rupture)

   3. Signs and symptoms associated with meningeal irritation

   4. Headaches or seizures resulting from enlargement of the vessels and ischemic changes in patients with AVM

Grades of subarachnoid hemorrhage

The five grades of subarachnoid hemorrhage are based on the severity of the neurologic symptoms.

Grade I: Slight headache, slight nuchal rigidity, or asymptomatic
Grade II: Moderate headache, nuchal rigidity, and slight neurologic deficits
Grade III: Confusion, drowsiness, and mild neurologic deficits
Grade IV: Stupor, moderate hemiparesis, and beginning of decerebrate posturing
Grade V: Comatose, decerebrate or decorticate posturing, and clinical deterioration

    a. Hemorrhage caused by AVM is more common in patients ages 15 to 35; other types of aneurysms are more common in middle-aged patients

    b. Arteriovenous malformation has a 20% mortality rate; rupture of the aneurysm causes hemorrhage into the subarachnoid space (see *Grades of subarachnoid hemorrhage*)

C. Diagnostic tests

    1. Cerebral aneurysm most often is diagnosed with a CT scan, followed by a cerebral angiogram

    2. Lumbar puncture is attempted only if there are no signs of increased ICP; if performed, the lumbar puncture will show bloody or xanthochromic (yellow) CSF with elevated CSF protein and cell counts and, usually, elevated CSF pressure

D. Medical management

    1. Resect the affected vessel or surgically reinforce the walls of the vessel

    2. In patients with AVM, consider surgical intervention to clamp the diverting arteries if the area of AVM is not so deep into the brain as to make it inaccessible; nonsurgical intervention (embolization of the AVM with injection of Silastic beads) may be used alone or in conjunction with surgical intervention

    3. Treat complications; rebleeding is the most common cause of death in a patient with cerebral aneurysm; vasospasm also is associated with rupture of a cerebral aneurysm and is likely to occur 7 to 10 days after the initial event

        a. Rebleeding occurs in 30% of all patients, and of those 30%, two-thirds die because of rebleeding

        (1) Rebleeding is related to the body's natural fibrinolytic process; as the clot that sealed the initial bleeding undergoes fibrinolysis, the risk of rebleeding increases

        (2) Rebleeding most often occurs 7 days after the original event

        (3) Aminocaproic acid (Amicar), a drug that inhibits fibrinolysis, is used at some institutions to decrease the incidence of rebleeding; however, the effectiveness of the drug has not been clearly established, and some clinicians believe that it increases the incidence of vasospasm

    b. The chief consequence of cerebral vasospasm is ischemia in large areas of the cerebral hemispheres, thereby leading to cerebral infarction and death

        (1) Cerebral vasospasm can be treated by vasodilation through the use of the spasmolytic agent papaverine, which produces vasodilation by causing the smooth muscles to relax

        (2) Another treatment option is the use of calcium channel blockers (nimodipine), serotonin antagonists (reserpine), and beta-adrenergic agents (isoproterenol [Isuprel]) in tandem with a smooth-muscle relaxant (aminophylline)

        (3) Hypervolemic hypertension also can be used to treat vasospasm

           (a) During this treatment, the patient is given fluid and volume expanders to increase the systolic blood pressure to between 150 and 160 mm Hg

           (b) Two potential complications of this therapy are rebleeding of an unstable aneurysm and the development of pulmonary edema associated with fluid overload

           (c) This therapy should be used only after surgical clipping has secured the initial bleed site and hemodynamic monitoring is being used to track fluid status

E. Nursing management

    1. Prevent and control conditions that contribute to increased ICP

    2. Assess neurologic status (compare with baseline values) and determine the grade of subdural hemorrhage

    3. Maintain a patent airway; hypoxia may cause brain cell death, and hypercapnia may cause increased ICP and decreased cerebral perfusion

    4. Maintain the patient on bed rest with the head of the bed elevated 15 to 30 degrees to facilitate venous drainage; position the patient with neck midline, avoid crossing the patient's legs, and use pillows under the patient's knees to allow for free flow of blood and to decrease the possibility of thrombus formation

    5. Ensure that the patient has adequate rest periods; activity increases metabolic demands as well as ICP

VII. Cerebral embolism

    A. Description

        1. Cerebrovascular accidents (CVAs) are obstructive strokes, not hemorrhagic events

        2. Cerebrovascular accidents generally are caused by thrombotic or embolic events that block cerebral blood flow enough to cause cerebral ischemia or infarction

           a. These embolic events may be transient, with resolution of symptoms within 24 hours; such events are called transient ischemic attacks

              b. These events may be reversible, with resolution of symptoms after 24 hours and subsequent complete resolution; such events are called reversible ischemic neurologic deficit

              c. If the symptoms do not resolve, a completed stroke has occurred

       3. The clinical signs and symptoms of patients experiencing a hemorrhagic or embolic stroke depend on the cerebral area involved

B. Clinical signs and symptoms

       1. Absent or diminished proprioception, indicating cerebellar or posterior ascending spinothalamic tract dysfunction; to detect this dysfunction, the Romberg test (the ability to stand steady with eyes closed) is performed

       2. Absent or diminished tactile sensation, indicating damaged sensory pathways or parietal lobe dysfunction; to detect this dysfunction, the patient is asked to identify an object by touch with the eyes closed

       3. Aphasia (impairment of speech or communication)

              a. In expressive, or Broca's, aphasia, speech and writing are impaired, but verbal comprehension and reading ability usually remain intact; this type of aphasia results from damage to the posteroinferior frontal lobe

              b. In receptive, or Wernicke's, aphasia, verbal comprehension and reading are impaired, but speech usually is intact; this type of aphasia results from damage to the posterosuperior temporal lobe

              c. In global aphasia, both expressive and receptive abilities are impaired; global aphasia results from damage to the frontotemporal lobe

       4. Dysarthria (impairment of speech muscles)

       5. Dysphagia (impairment of swallowing muscles)

       6. Diplopia (double vision)

       7. Hemiparesis (loss of contralateral sensation)

       8. Hemiplegia (loss of contralateral movement)

       9. Homonymous hemianopia (contralateral loss of vision in the same side of each eye)

C. Diagnostic tests

       1. A brain scan or CT scan may be performed to pinpoint the area of injury

       2. An MRI scan or EEG also may be used to determine the location of the embolism

D. Medical management

       1. Treat acute symptoms through supportive care

       2. Prescribe physical and occupational therapy to help the patient regain lost abilities

       3. Prevent recurring embolic events with anticoagulant therapy

E. Nursing management

       1. Assess for worsening neurologic impairment

2. Use communication techniques appropriate for the patient's deficits
3. Use caution when moving the patient to avoid dislocation of flaccid extremities
4. Position the patient carefully to prevent pressure on affected areas; this helps prevent skin breakdown
5. Provide emotional support to the patient and family

VIII. Encephalitis

A. Description
   1. Encephalitis is an inflammation of the brain tissues that usually is caused by a virus, fungus, bacterium, parasite, or *Rickettsia*
   2. Acute encephalitis typically is caused by a virus
      a. Known infective viruses are herpes simplex virus, equine virus, and arbovirus
      b. Equine virus and arbovirus are transmitted by ticks and mosquitoes

B. Clinical signs and symptoms
   1. Headache, fever, nausea, and vomiting
   2. Nuchal rigidity, positive Kernig's sign, positive Brudzinski's sign, photophobia, altered level of consciousness, and seizures

C. Diagnostic tests
   1. Diagnosis generally is determined by lumbar puncture
   2. In viral encephalitis, the CSF sample is cloudy and shows elevated protein level, normal glucose level, and the presence of WBCs

D. Medical management
   1. Control the symptoms, using steroids (except in cases of herpesvirus) and antiviral medications
   2. Administer antibiotic and antifungal medications after the causative organism has been identified
   3. Control increased ICP with osmotic diuretics (such as mannitol)

E. Nursing management
   1. Continuously assess for changes in level of consciousness and temperature
   2. Monitor for causes of increasing ICP
   3. Maintain an environment of subdued stimulation to decrease the risk of seizures
   4. Suppress elevated temperatures, which can cause increased ICP, through the use of antipyretics and hypothermia blankets or tepid soaks
      a. The measures used to decrease temperature should not induce shivering
      b. Shivering raises the metabolic rate and may increase ICP

IX. Head trauma

A. Description

1. Head trauma is caused by acceleration-deceleration, rotation, or missile injuries
   a. Acceleration-deceleration injuries occur when the skull strikes or is struck by an object
      (1) The brain is carried by force of movement until it strikes the inside of the skull (coup injury)
      (2) If the impact is strong enough, the force that has not yet dissipated pitches the brain in the reverse direction, where it strikes the opposite side of the skull (contrecoup injury)
   b. Rotation injuries, which occur in conjunction with acceleration-deceleration injuries, result in tearing or shearing of tissues
   c. Missile injuries are direct penetrating injuries, such as those that occur from a bullet wound
2. Whatever the cause of injury, traumatic head injuries are classified according to the ensuing loss of function
   a. Concussions are the mildest form of brain injury and are characterized by brief loss of consciousness, no structural break in the skull or dura, no visible damage to the brain, and lack of residual deficits; the patient experiences headache, dizziness, and possibly nausea and vomiting
   b. Contusions are closed head injuries that cause small, diffuse, venous hemorrhage (bruising); they usually occur in the frontal lobe; unconsciousness usually is prolonged with evident neurologic deficits
   c. Cerebral lacerations are tears in the brain tissue caused by shearing forces
      (1) Lacerations generally cause a greater amount of hemorrhage than contusions and may affect both arterial and venous vessels
      (2) Lacerations tend to cause a deteriorating state unless the bleeding and increased ICP are treated
3. Trauma to the head can fracture the skull
   a. In a linear skull fracture, the skull is broken but the bone is not displaced; this type of fracture generally requires no treatment unless a concomitant injury to the cerebral vasculature has occurred
   b. In a depressed skull fracture, the skull is broken and the bone is displaced downward toward the brain; this type of fracture usually requires surgical intervention to raise the bony fragments and repair any cerebral injury
   c. In a compound skull fracture, the break in the skull exposes the brain; if the dura has been lacerated, CSF may leak out
      (1) This type of fracture is associated with a high risk of infection and meningitis
      (2) Treatment involves the use of antibiotics, debridement of the wound, and subsequent closure of the skull

      d. In a basilar skull fracture, the skull is fractured at the base of the brain and injury to the cervical spine is likely; the fracture is repaired surgically and the neck is immobilized to prevent further damage to the area; Battle's sign (bruising behind the ears at the mastoid process), raccoon eyes (bruising around the eyes), otorrhea (CSF leaking from the ears), and rhinorrhea (CSF leaking from the nose) may be present

      e. In a comminuted skull fracture, the skull is splintered, and the bony fragments must be removed surgically

B. Diagnostic tests

    1. A brain scan or CT scan may be performed to pinpoint the area of injury

    2. An MRI scan may also be used to determine the location and extent of the head injury

C. Medical management

    1. Expect surgical intervention for injury repair, ventriculostomy placement, or ICP monitor insertion

    2. Control ICP with osmotic diuretics, hyperventilation, and CSF drainage   *MANNITOL.*

    3. Reduce <u>cerebral metabolic rate</u> with sedatives, antipyretics, and paralytic agents

    4. Maintain blood pressure to ensure adequate cerebral perfusion

D. Nursing management

    1. Have any drainage tested for halo (presence of a yellow ring, which indicates that the fluid is CSF) and glucose (CSF contains glucose; mucus does not)

    2. Position the patient according to the location of the injury

    3. Do not use suctioning unless the patient is intubated and ICP is controlled

    4. Do not insert a nasogastric tube, which may introduce infectious organisms into the cranial vault

    5. If the patient is alert, instruct him or her not to blow the nose

X. Infections of the nervous system

A. Meningitis

    1. Description

      a. Meningitis is an infection of the membranes of the pia mater and arachnoid mater

      b. The infective agent can be introduced by way of the sinuses, ear canal, or bloodstream or through a penetrating head wound

        (1) In 80% to 90% of cases, meningitis is caused by streptococcal pneumonia, *Haemophilus influenzae,* or *Neisseria*

        (2) Mumps virus, tuberculosis, and fungal agents also may cause meningitis

    2. Clinical signs and symptoms

      a. Headache, fever, nausea, and vomiting

Meningitis (handwritten in margin)

      b. Nuchal rigidity, positive Kernig's sign, positive Brudzinski's sign, photophobia, altered level of consciousness, and seizures

  3. Diagnostic tests

      a. Diagnosis generally is determined by lumbar puncture

      b. The CSF is cloudy or xanthochromic (yellow) and shows elevated pressure, elevated protein level, decreased glucose level, and the presence of WBCs

  4. Medical management

      a. Control symptoms; patients with meningococcal meningitis must be isolated

      b. Administer antibiotics specific to the bacterial or fungal causative agent; antibiotics are not given for viral or aseptic meningitis

  5. Nursing management

      a. Continuously assess for changes in level of consciousness and temperature

      b. Monitor for causes of increasing ICP

      c. Maintain an environment of subdued stimulation to decrease the risk of seizures

      d. Suppress elevated temperatures, which can cause increased ICP, through the use of antipyretics and hypothermic blankets or tepid soaks

         (1) The measures used to decrease temperature should not induce shivering

         (2) Shivering raises the metabolic rate and may increase ICP

B. Brain abscesses

  1. Description

      a. Abscesses are pockets of infection in the tissues of the brain

      b. They most commonly are caused by an infectious agent that has originated from an infected site elsewhere in the body and is carried in the bloodstream to the brain; examples of infections that can lead to brain abscesses include bacterial endocarditis, lung or skin abscesses, and ear, sinus, or tooth abscesses

      c. The most common sites for abscesses to settle in the brain are the epidural and subdural spaces or the cerebrum

  2. Clinical signs and symptoms

      a. Fever and lethargy

      b. Focal neurologic deficits, speech and motor deficits, and seizures

  3. Diagnostic tests

      a. The diagnosis is made by using a CT scan and lumbar puncture

      b. Aspiration of the abscess, with culture and sensitivity testing, identifies the organism and the appropriate medications

  4. Medical management

      a. Administer I.V. and intrathecal antibiotics

        b. Use surgical excision and drainage of the abscess to drain as much purulent fluid as possible

    5. Nursing management

        a. Use the same interventions as for a patient with meningitis (see A page 168.)

        b. If the patient undergoes surgery, ensure that the head of the bed is elevated postoperatively to facilitate venous drainage

C. Reye's syndrome

    1. Description

        a. Reye's syndrome is a viral inflammation of the brain

        b. This syndrome is triggered by the use of aspirin in children under age 12; it is followed by severe metabolic, hepatic, and neurologic dysfunctions and has a 40% to 50% mortality rate

    2. Clinical signs and symptoms

        a. Fever, nausea, and vomiting

        b. Increased ICP, seizures, and enlarged liver

    3. Diagnostic tests

        a. Diagnosis primarily is determined through patient history, clinical presentation, and laboratory values

        b. Laboratory values show an ammonia level above 300 µg/ml, serum osmolality level greater than 350 mOsm/L, partial thromboplastin time less than 30% of control, respiratory alkalosis in the presence of metabolic acidosis, and hypoglycemia

    4. Medical management

        a. Correct fluid and electrolyte imbalances, hypoxia, acidosis, hypoglycemia, and increased ICP

           (1) Induce barbiturate coma, if necessary, to decrease cerebral metabolic demands and the incidence of seizures

           (2) Suppress the absorption of ammonia with neomycin

        b. Treat bleeding with fresh frozen plasma and vitamin K supplements

    5. Nursing management

        a. Continuously assess for changes in level of consciousness and temperature

        b. Monitor for causes of increasing ICP

        c. Maintain an environment of subdued stimulation to decrease the risk of seizures

        d. Suppress elevated temperatures, which may cause increased ICP, through the use of antipyretics and hypothermic blankets or tepid soaks

           (1) The measures used to decrease temperature should not induce shivering

           (2) Shivering raises the metabolic rate and may increase ICP

D. Guillain-Barré syndrome

    1. Description

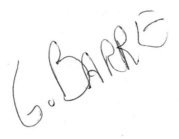

    a. Guillain-Barré syndrome is an inflammatory process of the nervous system characterized by demyelination of peripheral nerves; it results in progressive, symmetrical, ascending paralysis

    b. The exact cause is unknown, but the syndrome usually is preceded by a suspected viral infection accompanied by fever 1 to 3 weeks before the onset of acute bilateral muscle weakness in the lower extremities; autodigestion of the myelin sheath continues to ascend with development of flaccid paralysis within 48 to 72 hours

  2. Clinical signs and symptoms

    a. Cranial nerve (IX, X, and XII) impairment, as evidenced by difficulties in speech, swallowing, and mastication

    b. Inability to wrinkle the forehead or close the eyelids

    c. Impaired facial expressions and disconjugate eye movements, indicating impairment of cranial nerves II, IV, V, VI, and VII

    d. Impairment of the muscles of respiration as the paralysis continues to ascend and the cervical nerve roots are affected; respiratory failure occurs and supportive treatment is required to prevent death

    e. Ascending bilateral flaccid paralysis with pain but no decrease in level of consciousness

  3. Diagnostic tests

    a. The hallmark of Guillain-Barré syndrome is the presence of albuminocytological dissociation (high protein count in the CSF)

    b. Sometimes lumbar puncture, MRI scan, and CT scan are used to diagnose this syndrome

  4. Medical management

    a. Provide supportive care while myelin is regenerated; symptoms usually begin to subside within 2 weeks, with recovery in 2 years

    b. Consider using plasmapheresis to eliminate the protein causing the autoimmune demyelination

  5. Nursing management

    a. Implement appropriate airway management techniques

    b. Observe for signs of phlebitis; passive range-of-motion exercises, antiembolism stockings, and anticoagulant therapy may be indicated

    c. Maintain adequate hydration and nutrition

E. Myasthenia gravis

  1. Description

    a. Myasthenia gravis is an autoimmune disorder characterized by muscle fatigue that improves with rest but is exacerbated by activity

Myasthenia gravis

M. GRAVIS

b. The disorder is caused by an autoimmune response that destroys the acetylcholine receptor sites at the neuromuscular junction

2. Clinical signs and symptoms

a. Skeletal muscle weakness that increases with repetitive exercise and is accompanied by cranial nerve VII deficits

b. Respiratory muscle impairment, which usually is the reason patients are treated in the intensive care unit

3. Diagnostic tests

a. Antibodies to acetylcholine receptors are found in the serum of 90% of patients with myasthenia gravis

b. Electromyography is used to measure the electrical activity of muscle cells

c. The Tensilon test is used to determine whether the patient is experiencing myasthenic or cholinergic crisis

  (1) Tensilon (edrophonium chloride) is an anticholinesterase agent that, when given I.V. or I.M., dramatically revitalizes skeletal muscle function in a patient in myasthenic crisis; this recuperation lasts for only a few minutes

  (2) When Tensilon is given to a patient in cholinergic crisis, symptoms are exacerbated; although the exacerbation of symptoms lasts for only a minute, respiratory support must be available

4. Medical management

a. Administer anticholinesterase agents (such as pyridostigmine bromide [Mestinon]) to block the hydrolysis of acetylcholine at the neuromuscular junction

b. Consider surgical excision of the thymus or plasmapheresis to decrease the autoimmune response

c. Administer corticosteroids and other immunosuppressant drugs, if indicated

d. Keep in mind that a patient in myasthenic crisis (inadequate anticholinesterase) presents a clinical picture much like that of a patient in cholinergic crisis (overdose of anticholinesterase); a patient in myasthenic crisis experiences increased blood pressure and tachycardia, whereas a patient in cholinergic crisis experiences GI symptoms (for example, nausea, vomiting, salivation, and abdominal cramps), decreased blood pressure, bradycardia, and blurred vision

  (1) Treatments for these crises are diametric opposites; therefore, it is of utmost importance to distinguish between the two types of crisis

  (2) Neostigmine bromide (Prostigmin Bromide) usually is the drug of choice for myasthenic crisis; atropine, a cholinergic blocker, is the drug of choice for cholinergic crisis

5. Nursing management

a. Administer medications as prescribed and according to the dosing schedule

thymus
Plasmapheresis to ↓ autoimmune response

Myasthenic crisis
↑ BP ↑ HR

Cholinergic crisis
GI symptoms.
↓ BP ↓ HR
BLURRED Vision.

b. Observe the patient closely for evidence of respiratory failure

c. Continuously assess muscle strength

XI. Intracranial hemorrhage

  A. Description

   1. Cerebral hematomas are classified by the space into which the bleeding occurs

    a. Epidural hematomas are formed by bleeding into the space between the skull and the dura

    b. Subdural hematomas are formed by bleeding into the space below the dura

    c. Intracerebral hematomas are formed by bleeding into the tissues of the brain

   2. Epidural hematomas usually are caused by arterial bleeding

    a. They most often are caused by a blow to the temporal area, which results in a skull fracture and shearing of the middle meningeal artery

    b. Because the bleeding is coming from an artery, not a vein, deterioration is rapid; this accounts for the high mortality rate (approximately 30%)

   3. Subdural hematomas usually are caused by shearing of the cortical veins that bridge the dura and arachnoid membrane

    a. They typically result from acceleration-deceleration and rotational forces impinging the surface of the skull, causing cerebral contusion

    b. The skull may remain intact

   4. Hematoma formation caused by subdural hematomas may be classified as acute, subacute, or chronic

    a. Acute subdural hematomas cause clinical symptoms immediately or within the first 24 to 48 hours after the trauma

    b. Subacute subdural hematomas develop 3 to 20 days after the trauma

    c. Chronic subdural hematomas are seen more than 20 days after the trauma

     (1) In chronic subdural hematomas, fibroblasts accumulate around and encapsulate the hematoma

     (2) As the RBCs of the clot hemolyze, blood proteins disintegrate and the encapsulated area has a higher osmotic concentration than the surrounding tissues

     (3) The osmotic gradient induces an influx of water into the capsule, causing it to swell

   5. Intracerebral hematomas may be caused by trauma, tumors, blood dyscrasias, anticoagulant therapy, or hypertension; 90% of cases result from congenital aneurysm, and 10% result from infection, trauma, or idiopathic causes; whatever the cause, the result is a pooling of blood within the cerebral tissues

    a. If the hematoma results from trauma, the usual cause is a missile injury or severe acceleration-deceleration force that causes laceration of deep cerebral tissues

    b. When caused by hypertension, the hematoma is called a hemorrhagic stroke

    c. The vessels usually involved are those of the circle of Willis, located at the base of the brain

B. Clinical signs and symptoms

  1. Epidural hematoma: brief loss of consciousness at the time of injury; the patient awakens and is lucid for several hours and then lapses into unconsciousness with rapid deterioration in neurologic status

  2. Subdural hematoma: decreased level of consciousness and lateralizing signs

    a. Patients with acute and subacute subdural hematoma may exhibit a decreased sensorium that progresses to unconsciousness

      (1) In acute subdural hematoma, the patient commonly becomes unconscious immediately after the traumatic event and never regains consciousness

      (2) In subacute subdural hematoma, hematoma formation occurs at a slower rate; thus, symptoms appear more slowly but are nonetheless acute when they develop

    b. Chronic subdural hematoma: decreased level of consciousness with a history of changes in behavior but not necessarily a history of a recent trauma

      (1) Patients with chronic subdural hematoma usually are elderly or alcoholics and have decreased cerebral volume as a result of atrophy

      (2) The initial hemorrhage is not enough to cause significant clinical symptoms; it is the resultant swelling, which applies pressure to the surrounding cerebral tissues, that causes symptoms

      (3) Symptoms generally are insidious (for example, headache, absentmindedness, and lethargy) and may be misdiagnosed as Alzheimer's disease or ascribed to the aging process or cerebral atrophy

  3. Intracerebral hematoma: possibly signs of increased ICP; symptoms vary according to the area of the brain in which the bleeding occurs and the rate of bleeding

C. Diagnostic tests

  1. The diagnosis for epidural, subdural, and intracerebral hematomas generally is based on the patient's clinical presentation and medical history and on the results of a CT scan

  2. Skull and cervical spine X-rays may help identify associated fracture

  3. Lumbar puncture is contraindicated by the presence of increased ICP

D. Medical management

    1. Intervene accordingly, based on the location and extent of the bleeding ,

    2. Take immediate action for acute symptoms

        a. Acute intervention generally entails immediate surgical intervention to remove the clot and cauterize the vessels and to prevent rapid neurologic deterioration

        b. Osmotic diuretics should not be administered before surgery because the bleeding initially is stopped by the tamponade effect of the clot's expansion against the skull; decreasing the swelling by administering osmotic diuretics would allow bleeding from the vessel to continue

        c. Surgery may be deferred when there is a very small amount of bleeding, the patient remains neurologically stable, and there is no midline shifting of the cerebral structures

E. Nursing management

    1. Continuously assess for changes in neurologic status

    2. Maintain the patient's airway if inadequate oxygenation and ventilation are present

    3. Keep the cervical spine immobilized until injury has been ruled out

    4. If the patient undergoes surgery, ensure that the head of the bed is elevated postoperatively to facilitate venous drainage

XII. Seizures

A. Description

    1. Seizures are sudden paroxysmal discharges of a group of neurons that interfere with normal mental and behavioral activities

    2. Seizures may be triggered by toxic states, electrolyte imbalances, tumors, anoxia, inflammation of CNS tissue, increased ICP, trauma, hyperpyrexia, multiple sclerosis, Huntington's disease, Alzheimer's disease, or idiopathic causes

    3. Seizure activity is thought to be associated with an imbalance between the excitatory and inhibitory synaptic influences on the postsynaptic neurons; when this imbalance occurs, an area of excessive depolarization results, causing an abnormal pattern of electrical activity or a paroxysmal depolarization shift

    4. There are three theories of the causation of this imbalance: alteration in the cellular sodium pump, acetylcholine-cholinesterase imbalance, and alteration in the conversion of glutamic acid to gamma-aminobutyric acid (GABA)

        a. The cellular sodium pump preserves the normal resting membrane potential by moving potassium out of the cell and sodium into the cell during depolarization; this active transport mechanism relies on sufficient amounts of oxygen and glucose

            (1) When deprived of sufficient oxygen and glucose, the transport mechanism fails and sodium is allowed to diffuse into the cell abnormally

(2) The resting membrane potential of the cell is lowered, making it more vulnerable to paroxysms of electrical activity

b. Synaptic impulse transmission relies on the excitatory transmitter acetylcholine; the resting membrane potential is decreased in the presence of increased levels of acetylcholine

(1) Decreased levels of cholinesterase, an inhibitory neurotransmitter, decrease postsynaptic inhibition

(2) Increased levels of acetylcholine and decreased levels of cholinesterase make neuronal synaptic membranes more susceptible to repetitive electrical discharges

c. The coenzyme pyridoxine is essential for the conversion of glutamic acid to the synaptic inhibitor GABA; inadequate amounts of pyridoxine result in decreased levels of GABA and loss of inhibition

5. Seizures are classified as partial (focal) or generalized

   a. Partial seizures involve a localized or focal area of the brain

   b. Generalized seizures involve the entire brain and are associated with bilateral neuronal discharges

B. Clinical signs and symptoms

1. Partial seizures usually do not impair consciousness and involve either motor or sensory symptoms

a. For example, a jacksonian seizure involves the clonic activity of a muscle that progresses to adjoining muscles

b. The successive progression of the seizure reflects the wave of neuronal discharge activity in the brain

c. Clinically, the patient experiences decreased level of consciousness, impaired mentation and sensation, and amnesia

2. Generalized seizures affect consciousness and concurrently affect motor and sensory functions

a. Absence (petit mal) seizures cause transient loss of consciousness without tumultuous muscle motion and last for a few seconds

(1) Absence seizures may be accompanied by a vacant, blinking stare during the state of decreased consciousness

(2) Absence seizures are seen most frequently in children

b. Generalized tonic-clonic (grand mal) seizures manifest initially as a preictal or aura phase consisting of vision disturbances or irritability

(1) Loss of consciousness is followed by stiffening of skeletal muscles (tonic phase) with progression to jerking movements (clonic phase)

(2) Breathing is halted during the tonic phase; the clonic phase is characterized by hyperventilation

(3) Autonomic dysfunction is demonstrated by the loss of bowel and bladder control

           (4) The postictal phase is characterized by flaccidity with progressive return to consciousness and subsequent amnesia

  c. Myoclonic seizures cause brief, sudden contractions that generally involve the upper extremities

  d. Akinetic seizures cause brief, sudden episodes of loss of muscle control

  e. Status epilepticus is a clinical emergency distinguished by continually recurring generalized tonic-clonic seizures that do not allow for recovery at the end of the postictal phase; the principal concerns with status epilepticus are anoxia, arrhythmias, and acidosis

C. Diagnostic tests

  1. The use of radiologic tests depends on the causative pathology

  2. An EEG is used to identify the area of seizure focus

  3. Laboratory tests are performed to look for abnormalities in sodium and potassium levels

D. Medical management

  1. Correct the causative pathology if the patient is not in status epilepticus

  2. For status epilepticus, administer diazepam (Valium) to interrupt the seizure activity and maintain the airway; intubation may be necessary

    a. Because diazepam cannot prevent a recurrence of seizures, phenytoin (Dilantin), phenobarbital, pentobarbital, or general anesthetic agents may be administered

    b. Once the seizure activity has been stemmed, correction of the primary cause can be addressed

E. Nursing management

  1. Assess the seizure, noting the part of the body involved, the duration of the seizure, the type and quality of movement, changes in neurologic status, and any precipitating events

  2. Provide supportive care and institute measures to prevent injury during the seizure

7

Gastrointestinal disorders

I. Anatomy

  A. Mouth
  1. The mouth comprises the lips, cheeks, teeth, gums, tongue, palate, and salivary glands; the tongue is a mass of striated and skeletal muscles covered by mucous membranes
  2. The mouth is connected to the esophagus by the pharynx; the walls of the pharynx are composed of fibrous tissues surrounded by muscle fibers

  B. Esophagus
  1. Located behind the trachea, the esophagus is 10″ to 12″ (25.4 to 30.5 cm) long and passes through the thoracic cavity and the abdominal cavity
  2. The top one-third of the esophagus consists of striated muscle; the bottom two-thirds consists of smooth muscle
  3. The superior end of the esophagus is opened and closed by the hypopharyngeal sphincter; the distal end is opened and closed by the gastroesophageal sphincter
  4. Peristaltic waves move food through the esophagus to the stomach

  C. Stomach
  1. The stomach is located in the epigastric umbilical and left hypochondriac areas of the abdomen
  2. It is divided into the fundus, or upper part; the greater curvature, which lies below the fundus; the body, which makes up the largest portion of the stomach; the pyloric part, near the outlet to the intestines; and the lesser curvature, which lies between the pyloric sphincter and the esophagus
  3. The stomach consists of an outer layer of longitudinal muscle fibers, a middle layer of circular fibers, and an inner layer of transverse fibers
  4. Gastric mucosa, which contains large numbers of gastric glands, lines the interior of the stomach
  5. The submucosal layer of the stomach is composed of blood vessels, lymph vessels, and connective and fibrous tissues
  6. Rugae (folds) on the interior of the stomach allow for distention

  D. Small intestine
  1. The small intestine is a tubular structure that extends from the pyloric sphincter to the cecum

2. It is divided into three sections: the duodenum, which makes up the first several inches; the jejunum, which is about 8′ (2.4 m) long and extends from the ileocecal valve; and the ileum, which is about 12′ (3.6 m) long

3. The lumen contains small, fingerlike projections called villi that vastly increase the surface area of the small intestine

4. The small intestine also contains several glands, including the crypts of Lieberkühn, which are found between the villi and produce mucus; absorptive and secreting cells; Brunner's glands; and Peyer's patches, which play a role in the immune system

E. Large intestine

  1. Also called the colon, the large intestine extends from the ileum to the anus

  2. Approximately 5′ to 6′ (1.5 to 1.8 m) long and 2.5″ (6.3 cm) in diameter, the large intestine is divided into three segments: the cecum, the colon (ascending, transverse, and descending), and the rectum

  3. The large intestine contains no villi

F. Innervation of the GI system

  1. The GI tract has its own intrinsic nervous system, which is under the control of the autonomic nervous system; the autonomic nervous system can change the effects of the GI system at any point

  2. Cranial nerve X (vagus nerve) is the primary nerve for the parasympathetic nervous system; sympathetic nervous fibers parallel the major blood vessels of the entire GI tract

    a. Parasympathetic stimulation increases the activity of the GI tract

    b. Sympathetic stimulation decreases, or may even halt, the activity of the GI tract

G. Accessory organs of the GI system

  1. Salivary glands

    a. There are three salivary glands: the parotid gland, submandibular gland, and sublingual gland

    b. Each salivary gland occurs in pairs

  2. Pancreas

    a. The pancreas is both an endocrine and a digestive system organ

    b. This fish-shaped, lobulated gland lies behind the stomach

      (1) The head and neck of the pancreas lie in the C-shaped curve of the duodenum

      (2) The body lies behind the duodenum

      (3) The tail is a thin, narrow segment that is below the spleen

    c. The duct of Wirsung is the main pancreatic duct and runs the entire length of the organ

    d. Small pancreatic sacs called acinar cells manufacture the juices used in digestion

    e. The ampulla of Vater is the short segment of the pancreas, located just before the common bile duct

      f. Pancreatic function is controlled by the phases of digestion and the vagus nerve of the parasympathetic system

  3. Gallbladder

      a. The gallbladder can store up to 50 ml of bile, which is released when fatty food is present in the small intestine

      b. There are four parts to the gallbladder

        (1) The fundus is the distal portion of the body and forms a blind sac

        (2) The body connects the fundus to the infundibulum

        (3) The infundibulum connects the body to the neck of the gallbladder

        (4) The cystic duct merges with the duct system of the liver to form the common bile duct

  4. Liver

      a. The largest single organ in the body, the liver weighs 3 to 4 lb (1.4 to 1.8 kg)

      b. The liver is located in the right upper quadrant of the abdomen, lying against the right inferior diaphragm

      c. It is divided into a right and left lobe by the falciform ligament

        (1) The right lobe is larger than the left

        (2) The falciform ligament attaches the liver to the abdominal wall

      d. The hepatic lobule is the functioning unit of the liver

        (1) Each lobule has its own hepatic artery, a portal vein, and a bile duct; these structures constitute the portal triad

        (2) Sinusoids are intralobular cavities between columns of epithelial cells and are lined with Kupffer's cells

II. Physiology

  A. Mouth

    1. Food that enters the mouth is altered mechanically by mastication

    2. To help break down starch, the food is mixed with saliva

  B. Esophagus

    1. When a bolus of food enters the esophagus, the hypopharyngeal sphincter opens

    2. Gravity and peristaltic wave motion advance the bolus of food down the esophagus

    3. When the gastroesophageal sphincter opens, the food passes into the stomach

  C. Stomach

    1. When the upper portion of the stomach receives the bolus of food, the gastric glands are stimulated to secrete lipase, pepsin, intrinsic factor, mucus, hydrochloric acid, and gastrin

    2. The food bolus is churned until it becomes a semiliquid mass called chyme

Where nutrients are absorbed in the GI tract

LOCATION	NUTRIENT
Duodenum-jejunum	Triglycerides, fatty acids, amino acids, simple sugars (glucose, fructose, galactose), fat-soluble vitamins (A, D, E, and K), water-soluble vitamins (C, B complex, niacin), folic acid, calcium, electrolytes, and water
Ileum	Bile salts, vitamin B_{12}, chloride, and water
Colon	Potassium and water

   3. Gastric motility—the ability of the stomach to churn the food—is affected by the quantity and pH of the contents, the degree of mixing, peristalsis, and the ability of the duodenum to accept the food mass
   4. The stomach empties at a rate proportional to the volume of its contents and can distend to hold a large quantity of food
  D. Small intestine
   1. The principal function of the small intestine is to absorb nutrients from the chyme (see *Where nutrients are absorbed in the GI tract*)
      a. The chyme leaving the stomach is not sufficiently broken down to be absorbed
      b. The pancreas, liver, and gallbladder contribute to the additional breakdown of the chyme
   2. Food is absorbed in the small intestine through hydrolysis, nonionic movement, passive diffusion, facilitated diffusion, and active transport
   3. The small intestine uses mixing contractions to mix the food with digestive juices and propulsive contractions to move the food through the system
      a. The myenteric reflex occurs when distention of the small intestine activates the nerves to continue the contraction sequence
      b. The gastroileal reflex regulates the movement of chyme from the small intestine to the large intestine
   4. The bacteria found in the small intestine (primarily *Escherichia coli*) help break down and digest protein and, to some degree, fat
   5. The ileocecal valve at the terminal ileum prevents the chyme from returning to the ileum from the large intestine
  E. Large intestine
   1. The large intestine absorbs water and some electrolytes and retains the chyme for elimination of waste products
      a. The chyme moves slowly through the large intestine to allow for water reabsorption
      b. Normally, the large intestine removes 80% to 90% of the water from the chyme

2. Haustral contractions are weak peristaltic contractions that move the chyme through the large intestine

F. Pancreas
1. The acinar glands secrete water, salt, amylase, and lipolytic and proteolytic enzymes as well as nuclease and deoxyribonuclease
   a. Amylase digests starches
   b. The lipolytic enzymes lipase and phospholipase break down fats of all types
   c. The proteolytic enzyme trypsin breaks down protein
   d. The enzymes nuclease and deoxyribonuclease break down the nucleotides in deoxyribonucleic acid and ribonucleic acid
2. The cells lining the acinar glands contain large amounts of carbonic anhydrase and make the pancreatic secretions strong bases
3. Pancreatic secretion is triggered by the presence of undigested food in the small intestine

G. Liver
1. The liver synthesizes and transports bile and bile salts for fat digestion
2. The hepatic cells synthesize bile, which flows through a series of ducts to the common hepatic duct and the gallbladder

H. Gallbladder
1. The gallbladder stores and concentrates bile
   a. Bile salts react with water, leaving a fat-soluble end product to mix with cholesterol and lecithin
   b. Bile pigments and bilirubin result from the breakdown of hemoglobin
   c. Vagal stimulation increases bile secretions through the sphincter of Oddi
2. During normal digestion, the gallbladder contracts in response to the hormone cholecystokinin when food is present in the small intestine

III. **Gastrointestinal assessment**
A. Noninvasive assessment techniques
1. Inspect the abdomen from above and from the side
   a. Note any distention of the abdomen and check for symmetry, skin texture, color, scarring, lesions, rashes, and moles
   b. Note the location and condition of the umbilicus, and assess abdominal movements, breathing, and pulses
   c. Normally, the abdomen should be flat with no scars and the umbilicus in midline
2. Lift the head and observe the abdominal muscles
3. Auscultate all four quadrants, noting normal and abnormal sounds
4. Percuss all four quadrants, noting the presence of fluid, air, or masses; tympany is the normal sound in the abdomen

5. Percuss the liver
   a. To percuss the liver, first percuss from the umbilicus up the right abdomen for a change in sound from tympany to dullness and mark this site; then, percuss downward from above the nipple on the right midclavicular line for a change in sound from resonance to dullness and mark this site
   b. The space between the two sites indicates where the liver is situated; measure this space (the normal size of the liver is 2.4″ to 3.9″ [6 to 10 cm])
6. Percuss for the spleen in the left lateral area between the sixth and tenth ribs
7. Lightly palpate (indent the skin $1/2''$ [1.3 cm]) all four quadrants to assess for tenderness, guarding, and masses
8. Deeply palpate the abdomen (indent the skin 2″ to 3″ [5 to 7.6 cm]) to identify tenderness and masses in deeper tissues and rebound tenderness
9. Palpate the liver, spleen, and kidneys; normally, most abdominal organs are *not* palpable
10. Assess for inguinal lymph nodes

B. Invasive assessment techniques
   1. Esophagoscopy is the direct visualization of the esophageal mucosa through the use of a flexible fiber-optic endoscope
   2. Gastroscopy is the direct visualization of the gastric mucosa through the use of a flexible fiber-optic endoscope
   3. Esophagogastroduodenoscopy (EGD) is the direct visualization of the esophageal and gastric mucosa plus the pylorus and duodenum using a flexible fiber-optic endoscope; EGD can be extended to include the pancreas and gallbladder
   4. Proctoscopy and sigmoidoscopy is the direct visualization of the mucosa of the distal segment of the colon and rectum using a rigid or flexible fiber-optic sigmoidoscope
   5. Colonoscopy is the direct visualization of colonic mucosa up to the ileocecal valve using a flexible fiber-optic colonoscope
   6. Barium enema (lower GI series) involves the introduction of liquid barium by enema into the colon to visualize the movement, position, and filling of the various segments of the colon
   7. Barium swallow (upper GI series) involves the swallowing of liquid barium to visualize the position, shape, and activity of the esophagus, stomach, duodenum, and jejunum
   8. Cholecystography involves the ingestion of a contrast medium and consumption of a fatty meal, after which X-rays of the dye-filled gallbladder are taken to assess gallbladder function and presence of gallstones
   9. Cholangiography visualizes the hepatic, cystic, and common bile ducts for patency, using an I.V. contrast medium

C. Diagnostic tests

1. Gastric analysis with histamine or Histalog is conducted by obtaining a sample of gastric contents and analyzing it for the presence of hydrochloric acid after histamine has been administered I.M. or S.C.

2. Insulin gastric analysis (Hollander test) is conducted by obtaining and analyzing gastric contents for hydrochloric acid after I.V. administration of insulin; this test is used to assess the effectiveness of a vagotomy

3. Fecal occult blood test is used to detect the presence of blood in the stool after a specimen has been removed from the rectum

4. Bromsulphalein test (normal value: 5% retention in 45 minutes)
   a. Elevated values occur in acute hepatic disease
   b. Decreased values are not seen

D. Key laboratory values

1. Amylase (normal value: 80 to 150 U/ml)
   a. Elevated amylase level is caused by acute pancreatitis, duodenal ulcer, cancer of the head of the pancreas, and pancreatic pseudocysts
   b. Decreased amylase level is seen in chronic pancreatitis, pancreatic fibrosis and atrophy, cirrhosis of the liver, and acute alcoholism

2. Ascorbic acid (normal value: 0.4 to 1.5 mg/dl)
   a. Elevated level is uncommon
   b. Decreased level results from collagen disease, decreased intake of vitamin C, or hepatic disease

3. Bilirubin (normal value: total, 0.1 to 1.0 mg/dl; direct, 0.1 to 0.2 mg/dl; indirect, 0.1 to 0.8 mg/dl)
   a. Elevated bilirubin level is caused by biliary obstruction, hepatocellular damage, pernicious anemia, hemolytic anemia, and hemolytic disease of newborn
   b. Decreased bilirubin level is seen in certain malnutrition states

4. Cholesterol (normal value: 120 to 200 mg/dl)
   a. Elevated level results from hyperlipidemia, obstructive jaundice, diabetes, and hypothyroidism
   b. Decreased level is seen in pernicious anemia, hemolytic jaundice, hyperthyroidism, severe infections, and terminal diseases

5. Fibrinogen (normal value: 0.10 to 0.4 g/dl)
   a. Elevated level occurs in pneumonia, acute infections, nephrosis, and carcinoma
   b. Decreased level results from cirrhosis, acute toxic necrosis of the liver, and anemia

6. Iron (normal value: 65 to 150 μg/dl)
   a. Elevated level is seen in pernicious anemia, aplastic anemia, hemolytic anemia, hepatitis, and hemochromatosis
   b. Decreased level results from iron deficiency anemia

7. Leucine aminopeptidase (normal value: 1 to 3 μmoles/hour/ml)

  a. Elevated value is seen in liver and biliary tract disease, pancreatic disease, metastatic cancer of the liver or pancreas, and biliary obstruction

  b. Decreased value is not associated with any disease states

 8. Lipase (normal value: 0.2 to 1.5 U/ml)

  a. Elevated level occurs in acute or chronic pancreatitis, biliary obstruction, cirrhosis, hepatitis, and peptic ulcer

  b. Decreased level results from fibrotic disease of the pancreas

 9. Pepsinogen (normal value: 200 to 425 U/ml)

  a. Elevated level is not associated with any disease states

  b. Decreased level results from decreased gastric acidity conditions, pernicious anemia, and achlorhydria

 10. Protein (total) (normal value: 6 to 8 g/dl)

  a. Elevated level is seen in hemoconcentration and shock states

  b. Decreased level results from malnutrition or hemorrhage

 11. Aspartate aminotransferase (AST) (normal value: 15 to 45 U/ml)

  a. Increased level is seen in liver disease, myocardial infarction, and skeletal muscle disease

  b. Decreased level is not associated with any disease states

 12. Alanine aminotransferase (ALT) (normal value: 5 to 36 U/ml)

  a. Highly elevated level is seen in liver disease

  b. Decreased level is not associated with any disease states

 13. Gastric analysis

  a. The normal value for free hydrochloric acid is 0 to 30 mEq/L; for total acidity, 15 to 45 mEq/L; and for combined acid, 10 to 15 mEq/L

  b. All values are increased in peptic ulcer disease; all values are decreased in pernicious anemia, gastric carcinoma, gastritis, and aging

IV. Acute abdominal trauma

 A. Description

  1. Abdominal trauma is defined as any injury that occurs from the nipple line to midthigh; it is seldom limited to a single organ

  2. Abdominal trauma is classified as blunt or penetrating

   a. Blunt trauma commonly results from motor vehicle accidents, assaults, falls, and sports injuries

   b. Penetrating trauma may be caused by motor vehicle accidents, assaults, and knife or gunshot wounds

  3. Because a patient with bowel trauma may have other abdominal injuries, the focus should be on the risk of hemorrhage and peritonitis associated with abdominal trauma rather than on the pathological changes in a specific organ

 B. Clinical signs and symptoms

  1. Slightly distended abdomen with multiple ecchymotic areas

  2. Acute upper thoracic and abdominal pain

3. Tenderness on palpation

4. Hypotension and tachycardia

5. Cold, clammy skin

6. Laboratory tests showing decreased hemoglobin level and hematocrit as well as abnormal liver enzyme, blood urea nitrogen (BUN), and creatinine values; the abnormal values depend on the organs affected by the injury

C. Medical management

1. Insert a central I.V. line and begin fluid replacement

2. Insert a nasogastric (NG) lavage tube

3. Administer supplemental oxygen

4. Review abdominal X-rays, computed tomography (CT) scans, and magnetic resonance imaging (MRI) scans to assess the extent of the injury

5. Recommend surgery, if indicated

D. Nursing management

1. Continuously monitor vital signs (blood pressure, heart rate and rhythm, respiratory rate, and temperature); in patients with multisystemic trauma, close monitoring of vital signs permits identification of overt or covert changes in the patient's status

2. Continuously assess arterial oxygen saturation (SaO_2) level, which reflects oxygen perfusion of tissues, using pulse oximetry

3. Frequently assess breath sounds and respiratory effort; patients who have experienced blunt abdominal trauma must be observed closely for complications

4. Perform adequate inspection while maintaining spinal immobilization

   a. Although the initial examination may rule out neurologic involvement, this determination is not absolute in the immediate postinjury phase

   b. Further diagnostic tests, such as X-rays and, possibly, CT or MRI scans, may be necessary to determine the extent of the injury

   c. Extreme care must be taken when moving the patient to prevent spinal injury

5. Check the abdomen for ecchymoses and assess for Cullen's sign (ecchymosis around the umbilicus) and Turner's sign (ecchymosis in either flank)

   a. Ecchymosis may indicate internal bleeding

   b. Cullen's sign may indicate retroperitoneal bleeding into the abdominal wall

   c. Turner's sign indicates retroperitoneal bleeding

6. Assess for Kehr's sign (left shoulder pain); this sign—a classic finding in patients with splenic rupture—is caused by the presence of blood below the diaphragm that irritates the phrenic nerve

7. Auscultate the abdomen for bowel sounds; absent or diminished bowel sounds may result from the presence of blood, bacteria, or a chemical irritant in the abdominal cavity

8. Auscultate the abdomen for bruits, which indicate renal artery injury

9. Percuss the abdomen, noting any resonance over the right flank with the patient lying on the left side (Ballance's sign); percuss for resonance over the liver and for areas of dullness over hollow organs, such as the stomach, large intestine, and small intestine, that normally contain gas

   a. Ballance's sign indicates a ruptured spleen

   b. Normal percussion over the liver elicits a dull sound; resonance, which is caused by free air, is pathological

   c. Dullness over hollow organs may indicate the presence of blood or fluid

10. Lightly palpate the abdomen to identify areas of tenderness, rebound tenderness, guarding, rigidity, and spasm

11. Check for rectal bleeding; assess urine output every hour and monitor for protein or blood in the urine; and check the amount of gastric drainage from an NG tube every hour and monitor for bleeding

    a. Close observation of the patient is necessary in the initial postinjury phase to identify overt or covert signs of bleeding

    b. Signs of bleeding may necessitate an exploratory laparotomy to repair abdominal injuries

12. Assess verbal complaints of pain, including the severity, location, and intensity of the pain; a complete and continuing assessment of the patient's pain permits planning of the most effective interventions to relieve the pain and provides information about the extent of tissue, nerve, or vessel damage caused by blunt trauma

13. Perform a patient assessment (including ABC [airway-breathing-circulation] with cervical spine precautions and hemorrhage control), and monitor the patient every 15 minutes until stable and then every hour; frequent monitoring permits identification of overt or covert changes in patient status

14. Perform an abbreviated neurologic examination, using the Glasgow Coma Scale and assessing pupillary responses, every 15 minutes until the patient is stable and then every hour; changes in neurologic status may indicate cerebral ischemic conditions

15. Perform capillary refill checks when vital signs are assessed, and continue to monitor urine output, noting the color, amount, consistency, and specific gravity of the urine; these assessments reflect the adequacy of tissue perfusion

16. Establish a patent airway, using a chin-lift or jaw-thrust maneuver without hyperextending the neck; a patent airway provides the initial route for adequate intake of oxygen

17. Provide high-flow oxygen at 6 to 10 L/minute, using a mask, cannula, or oral or nasal adjuncts; oxygen delivery in the proper amount using the appropriate method helps maintain adequate tissue oxygenation

18. Use mechanical ventilation as needed to maintain forced inspiratory oxygen at 100%; patients with an obstructed airway may require ventilatory support by means of endotracheal or nasotracheal intubation, cricothyrotomy, or tracheotomy

19. Monitor serial arterial blood gas (ABG) values as prescribed; ABG measurements accurately reflect gas exchange requirements in injured patients with decreased tissue perfusion

20. Monitor breath sounds every 15 minutes until the patient is stable and then every hour, and observe for tracheal shifting to the contralateral side; although the initial respiratory assessment may be negative, tension pneumothorax may develop as a result of blunt trauma to the chest

21. Position the patient supine with legs elevated, unless contraindicated because of hypertension; the best position for a hypotensive patient is supine with legs elevated because this prevents blood from pooling in the lower extremities and allows maximum perfusion of vital organs
    a. A modified Trendelenburg's position initially facilitates venous return and augments blood pressure
    b. Continued use of the Trendelenburg position causes overstimulation of the baroceptors in the carotid arteries and aortic arch, decreasing blood pressure and producing rebound hypotension

22. Continue to assess for signs of occult bleeding, such as a rigid abdomen, and review the results of guaiac stool tests; continued assessment for occult bleeding is necessary to prevent missed injuries and to note the changing patient status

23. To replace lost fluid volume, maintain large-bore I.V. infusions with crystalloids, colloids, and blood, as prescribed
    a. Crystalloids are replaced at a rate of 3 ml for each milliliter of blood loss
    b. Blood is replaced in a 1:1 ratio, that is, at a rate of 1 ml for each milliliter of blood loss

24. Assist the doctor with insertion of peripheral or central I.V. lines, which provide quick fluid access to central circulation

25. Consider using a pneumatic antishock garment, and if used, monitor the patient's response; a pneumatic antishock garment enhances peripheral resistance, achieves arterial tamponade, promotes shunting of blood to vital organs, and splints fractures to decrease blood loss

26. Monitor serial hematocrit and white blood cell (WBC) counts as well as chemistry and enzyme laboratory test results

   a. The initial hemoglobin level and hematocrit do not reflect true blood loss—the values appear higher than they actually are because of hemoconcentration resulting from volume loss; serial hemoglobin and hematocrit measurements can identify true blood loss

   b. An elevated WBC count may indicate a ruptured spleen

   c. Elevated serum amylase concentrations may signal injury to the pancreas or the bowel

27. Obtain a baseline 12-lead electrocardiogram (ECG) and perform continuous ECG monitoring

28. Consider implementing hemodynamic monitoring to detect the status of cardiopulmonary function and measure cardiac output

29. Position the patient to alleviate pain or reduce discomfort; medication for pain may not be administered in the immediate posttraumatic phase because it may mask the physical symptoms of injury

30. Administer pain medication, as prescribed, and monitor the patient's response

31. Communicate frequently with the patient and family to establish a trusting relationship; encourage the patient and family to verbalize feelings and involve them in the treatment plan

32. Explain all procedures before implementing them to help decrease the patient's anxiety

33. Refer the patient to support services, as needed, including social services, pastoral care, and psychological counseling; these services can be of value during the acute and rehabilitative treatment phases

V. Acute GI hemorrhage

A. Description

1. Gastrointestinal bleeding is responsible for only a small percentage of all medical and surgical hospital admissions in the United States

2. Common causes of GI hemorrhage include duodenal ulcer, gastric ulcer, erosive gastritis, varices, esophagitis, Mallory-Weiss syndrome, and bowel infarction

B. Medical management

1. Administer colloids, crystalloids, and whole blood or packed cells to maintain blood pressure

2. Administer vitamin K, calcium, or platelets to reduce bleeding

3. Initiate vasopressin therapy to reduce bleeding

4. Administer histamine$_2$-receptor antagonists to reduce stomach acidity

5. Administer antacids to maintain a pH of 5 or greater

6. Administer lactulose to reduce stomach acidity

7. Administer sorbitol or magnesium citrate to facilitate passage of blood from GI tract

8. Insert a Sengstaken-Blakemore tube with proper balloon inflation to control bleeding from esophageal varices

C. Nursing management

1. Monitor vital signs (blood pressure, heart rate and rhythm, respiratory rate, and temperature) every 5 minutes until the patient is stable; frequent monitoring of vital signs allows early detection of abnormalities and prompt initiation of treatment to prevent further complications

2. Monitor cardiac output and hemodynamic pressures, including central venous pressure (CVP), right arterial pressure, pulmonary artery wedge pressure (PAWP), and pulmonary artery pressure (PAP); these parameters are critical indicators of cardiac function and reflect left ventricular function, fluid status, and arterial perfusion of vital organs

3. Monitor hemoglobin level and hematocrit; these measurements serve as indicators of further hemorrhage, with decreased levels seen 4 to 6 hours after a bleeding episode; these measurements also are decreased by hemodilution and crystalloid fluid replacement

4. Monitor BUN and serum electrolyte, creatinine, and ammonia levels

a. Sodium and potassium levels are transiently decreased after volume restoration and are increased after a bleeding episode; the body responds to bleeding by conserving sodium and water to maintain volume

b. The potassium level increases over time as transfusions free potassium and it goes into serum; the breakdown of red blood cells in the intestines frees additional potassium

c. The calcium level decreases after massive transfusions of stored blood; citrate in the stored blood binds circulating calcium

d. Blood urea nitrogen and creatinine levels increase after a bleeding episode as the breakdown of blood into intestinal products overwhelms the ability of the kidneys to excrete these products; hypovolemia and shock lead to decreased glomerular filtration

e. The ammonia level increases because liver dysfunction impairs clearance of the intestinal products of blood breakdown, with resulting encephalopathy

5. Monitor ABG values and keep in mind that respiratory alkalosis can develop early; decreased perfusion of the lungs during shock stimulates hyperventilation, and lactic acid buildup leads to metabolic acidosis

6. Frequently assess for chest congestion, as evidenced by crackles and wheezes, dyspnea, shortness of breath, orthopnea, and cough with pink, frothy sputum; patients with GI hemorrhage are at high risk for impaired gas exchange related to hemoglobin deficit and for pulmonary edema resulting from fluid overload

7. Assess urine output and specific gravity hourly; a high urine specific gravity and urine output less than 30 ml/hour indicates kidney failure secondary to decreased circulating volume or compensatory vasoconstriction

8. Monitor for signs of respiratory distress or back pain, which may indicate esophageal rupture or tracheal occlusion caused by the balloon of the Sengstaken-Blakemore tube

9. Monitor for hypertension, chest pain, abdominal pain, and oliguria; they are possible adverse effects of vasopressin or nitroglycerin therapy

10. Monitor for signs of continued bleeding by checking gastric aspirate and stools, which may appear black, sticky, or dark red if they contain blood; prompt recognition of further bleeding episodes allows early intervention to stem the bleeding and prevent hypovolemic shock

11. Assess the patient's level of consciousness and neuromuscular function and response; these signs and symptoms may result from elevated serum ammonia level secondary to increased protein load caused by GI bleeding

12. Maintain traction on the Sengstaken-Blakemore tube and keep the gastric and esophageal balloons at the correct pressures, with periodic deflation and inflation as prescribed; traction of inflated balloons against varices maintains tamponade of bleeding mucosal surfaces; periodic deflation and inflation of the balloons prevents tissue necrosis

13. Maintain patent gastric aspiration and oropharyngeal ports; because these tubes are not vented, intermittent suction must be applied to maintain patency

14. Keep the head of the bed elevated to maximize ventilation of the lungs

15. Administer supplemental oxygen, as prescribed, to maintain or reestablish normal oxygenation status

16. If symptoms of encephalopathy develop, orient the patient to person, place, and time as necessary to decrease anxiety and fear; increased anxiety level and fear could directly affect the central nervous system (CNS) and influence hemodynamic stability

17. Explain all procedures before implementing them to help decrease the patient's anxiety

18. Encourage the patient to verbalize his or her feelings; this allows the patient to develop adaptive coping skills

VI. Acute pancreatitis

A. Description

1. Acute pancreatitis is an inflammation of the tissues of the pancreas

2. It is caused by the premature activation and release of proteolytic enzymes, which autodigest the organ itself

3. The inflammatory response within the pancreas can be hemorrhagic (with tissue necrosis extending to the vascular compartment) or nonhemorrhagic (acute interstitial or acute edematous inflammation caused by the escape of digestive enzymes into the surrounding tissue)

4. The inflammatory and autodigestive process leads to tissue necrosis, precipitation of calcium with resultant hypocalcemia, release of necrotic toxins (which serve as precursors to sepsis), leakage of large volumes of albumin-rich pancreatic exudates into the peritoneum and, ultimately, shock and death

B. Clinical signs and symptoms
1. Severe epigastric pain
2. Nausea and vomiting
3. Hypotension and tachycardia
4. Distended abdomen with distant bowel sounds and guarding on palpation
5. Laboratory tests showing increased amylase and lipase levels, increased WBC count, and decreased potassium level

C. Medical management
1. Withhold food and fluids and keep the environment free of food odors to reduce pancreatic secretions
2. Insert an NG tube for drainage or suction
3. Administer I.V. meperidine and assess its effectiveness in relieving pain
4. Administer antacids to decrease inflammation
5. Keep the patient on nothing-by-mouth status and maintain NG tube drainage until bowel sounds return and abdominal pain subsides
6. While the patient is on nothing-by-mouth status, administer I.V. fluid solutions; add potassium chloride, multivitamin supplements, thiamine, and folic acid to these solutions to maintain nutritional status
7. Consult with a nutritional support team or a dietitian regarding the patient's nutritional status and a nutrition repletion program
8. Institute alternate feeding methods if nothing-by-mouth status must be prolonged

D. Nursing management
1. Monitor vital signs (blood pressure, heart rate and rhythm, respiratory rate, and temperature) every 5 to 15 minutes until the patient is stable and then every 30 to 60 minutes; frequent monitoring of vital signs permits early recognition of abnormalities and prompt initiation of treatment to prevent further complications
2. Monitor hemodynamic parameters (CVP, PAP, PAWP, and cardiac output) as ordered; the patient's hemodynamic status provides an indication of the effectiveness of interventions

3. Monitor for signs and symptoms of hypovolemia and shock: increased pulse rate; normal or slightly decreased blood pressure; urine output less than 30 ml/hour; restlessness, agitation, and change in mentation; increasing respiratory rate; diminished peripheral pulses; cool, pale, or cyanotic skin; increased thirst; and decreased hemoglobin level and hematocrit

   a. Hypovolemia secondary to pancreatitis may have several origins, including decreased oral intake, nothing-by-mouth status, and excess fluid loss through NG tube drainage or vomiting

   b. In addition, pancreatic enzymes destroy vessel walls, resulting in bleeding; plasma shifts (secondary to increased vascular permeability resulting from the inflammatory response) also contribute to hypovolemia

   c. The compensatory response to decreased circulatory volume is to increase blood oxygen by increasing heart and respiratory rates and decreasing circulation to the extremities, causing decreased pulse rate and cool skin

   d. Diminished oxygen to the brain causes changes in mentation

   e. Decreased circulation to the kidneys leads to decreased urine output

4. Monitor fluid status by assessing parenteral and oral intake, urine output, and fluid loss resulting from NG tube drainage or vomiting

   a. Fluid shifts, NG suctioning, and nothing-by-mouth status can disrupt fluid balance in a patient with acute pancreatitis; stress may cause sodium and water retention

   b. Early detection of a fluid deficit allows prompt intervention to prevent hypovolemic shock

5. Collaborate with the doctor to replace fluid losses at a rate sufficient to maintain urine output greater than 0.5 ml/kg/hour; this measure promotes optimal tissue perfusion

6. Monitor for signs and symptoms of hypocalcemia, which include changes in mental status, numbness and tingling of fingers and toes, muscle cramps, seizures, and ECG changes

   a. Hypocalcemia may result from the inability of the kidneys to metabolize vitamin D, which is needed for calcium absorption

   b. Retention of phosphorus causes a reciprocal drop in the serum calcium level

   c. Low serum calcium level produces increased neural excitability, which leads to muscle spasms and CNS irritability (manifested as seizures); it also causes cardiac muscle hyperactivity, as evidenced by ECG changes

   d. Calcium binds with free fats, which are excreted because of a lack of lipase and phospholipase—enzymes needed for digestion

7. If hypocalcemia occurs, administer calcium by way of a bolus infusion as prescribed, consult with a dietitian regarding the need for a high-calcium, low-phosphorus diet, monitor for hyperphosphatemia and hypomagnesemia, and observe for ECG changes

8. Monitor glucose levels in blood and urine; injury to pancreatic beta cells decreases insulin production, whereas injury to pancreatic alpha cells increases glucagon production

9. Continue to monitor serum glucose level every 30 minutes until the patient is stable; careful monitoring enables early detection of medication-induced hypoglycemia or continued hyperglycemia

10. Monitor for signs and symptoms of hyperglycemia, including polyuria and polydipsia

   a. Without insulin, cells cannot utilize glucose

   b. As a result, protein and fats are metabolized, leading to the production of ketones

11. Monitor for later manifestations of ketoacidosis, such as serum glucose level greater than 300 mg/dl, positive serum and urine ketones, acetone breath, headache, Kussmaul's respirations, anorexia, nausea, vomiting, tachycardia, decreased blood pressure, polyuria, polydipsia, and decreased serum sodium, potassium, and phosphate levels

   a. Excessive ketone bodies cause headaches, nausea, vomiting, and abdominal pain

   b. The respiratory rate and depth increase in an attempt to increase carbon dioxide excretion and reduce acidosis

   c. Glucose inhibits water reabsorption in the renal glomerulus, leading to osmotic diuresis with severe loss of water, sodium, potassium, and phosphate

12. If ketoacidosis occurs, initiate appropriate treatment protocols: administer normal or half-normal saline solution I.V., begin an I.V. infusion of dextrose 5% when the serum glucose level is between 250 and 300 mg/dl, add insulin (approximately 6 to 10 U/hour) to I.V. fluids, administer I.V. potassium and phosphate supplements, and administer bicarbonate I.V. as prescribed; these interventions restore the insulin-glucagon ratio and treat circulatory collapse, ketoacidosis, and electrolyte imbalance in a patient with severe acidosis

13. Monitor serum potassium, sodium, and phosphate levels

   a. Acidosis causes hyperkalemia and hyponatremia

   b. Insulin therapy promotes the return of potassium and phosphate to the cells, causing serum hypokalemia and hypophosphatemia

14. Monitor BUN and serum albumin, protein, and cholesterol levels as well as hemoglobin level and hematocrit

   a. The presence of insufficient pancreatic enzymes in the GI tract results in insufficient protein catabolism and decreased protein absorption, producing decreased levels of BUN and serum albumin, cholesterol, and transferrin

   b. Decreased transferrin level causes inadequate iron absorption and transport, resulting in decreased hemoglobin level and hematocrit

15. Monitor serum amylase, lipase, calcium, bilirubin, and alkaline phosphatase levels; urine amylase level; and WBC count

    a. Elevated levels of serum amylase, serum lipase, and urine amylase are signs of pancreatic cell injury

    b. Serum calcium level decreases as fatty acids combine with calcium during fat necrosis

    c. The serum bilirubin and alkaline phosphatase levels and WBC count are increased by hepatobiliary involvement, obstructive processes, and the inflammatory response

16. Monitor for signs and symptoms of alcohol withdrawal: tremors, diaphoresis, anorexia, nausea, vomiting, increased heart and respiratory rates, agitation, visual or auditory hallucinations, and alcohol withdrawal delirium

    a. Chronic alcohol abuse may cause pancreatitis, and the signs and symptoms of alcohol withdrawal may be apparent even when the patient denies alcoholism

    b. Signs of alcohol withdrawal begin 24 hours after the last drink and can continue for 1 to 2 weeks

17. Monitor SaO$_2$ to detect hypoxia and hypoxemia

18. Monitor for signs and symptoms of hypovolemic shock; if hypovolemic shock occurs, place the patient in the supine position with legs elevated (unless contraindicated)

19. Monitor neurologic status every hour; fluctuating glucose level, acidosis, and fluid shifts can affect neurologic functioning

20. Monitor cardiac function and circulatory status by assessing skin color, capillary refill time, peripheral pulses, and serum potassium level

    a. Severe dehydration can reduce cardiac output and cause compensatory vasoconstriction

    b. Arrhythmias can be caused by potassium imbalances

21. Monitor for signs of paralytic ileus, which may manifest as localized, sharp, or intermittent pain

    a. Paralytic ileus results from impaired peristaltic activity of the bowel, caused by ischemia from hypovolemia

    b. It also can be related to the use of opioid analgesics, which affect peristaltic action

22. Assess the location of pain (epigastric area, back, or chest) and whether it is caused by flatus or the presence of an NG tube; determining the source and nature of the pain helps guide interventions

23. Assess pain severity after each pain-relief measure by having the patient rate the pain on a scale of 1 to 10, with 1 indicating no pain and 10 indicating the greatest pain possible; because a patient in chronic pain may exhibit no outward signs, a rating scale provides a good method of measuring the subjective experience of pain

24. Assess for physical signs of acute pain, such as increased heart and respiratory rates, elevated blood pressure, restlessness, facial grimacing, and guarding; some patients are reluctant to admit that they are in pain, and the assessment of these signs and symptoms may be the only method of detecting pain

25. Assess verbal complaints of abdominal pain, and determine the specific location and intensity of the pain; acute pancreatitis can cause severe and diffuse pain

26. Work with the patient to determine the most effective methods of decreasing the pain

27. Do not ignore a patient's complaints of pain; a patient who must convince health care providers that he or she is in pain experiences an increased level of anxiety, which can further increase the perception of pain

28. Implement appropriate interventions to decrease anxiety and pain; these interventions may have a direct, positive effect on respiratory rate and pattern because they help prevent the release of catecholamines in response to pain and anxiety

29. Intervene to reduce accumulated gas, which may be painful; encourage frequent position changes, administer nonnarcotic analgesics, advance the diet slowly and avoid large meals, and restrict dietary fat intake

30. Ensure that the NG tube is properly secured, apply a water-soluble lubricant around the nares, and turn the patient every 2 hours; these interventions help reduce the discomfort associated with NG tube placement

31. Monitor the frequency, consistency, odor, and amount of stools
    a. Decreased secretion of pancreatic enzymes impairs protein and fat digestion; these undigested fats are excreted in the stool
    b. Steatorrhea (large amounts of fat in the stool) indicates impaired digestion

32. Assess the patient's nutritional status by weighing the patient on admission and daily thereafter, checking intake hourly, and inspecting for signs of malnutrition, such as fragile and lackluster hair, sunken eyes with pale conjunctivae, dry and swollen oral mucous membranes, and smooth or coated tongue
    a. Pancreatitis can negatively affect nutrition because of decreased intake and impaired digestion
    b. Changes in weight provide an indication of nitrogen balance; weight loss reflects a negative nitrogen balance and breakdown of muscle mass (catabolism), whereas weight gain reflects a positive nitrogen balance and buildup of muscle mass (anabolism)

33. Evaluate the adequacy of the patient's diet in meeting nutritional requirements

34. Assess the patient's complaints of nausea, vomiting, stomatitis, gastritis, and flatus; these symptoms can adversely affect eating patterns

35. Position the patient on the side with the knees flexed to reduce pressure and tension on the abdominal muscles

36. Place the patient in semi-Fowler's position to allow for maximum expansion of the diaphragm; this helps decrease ventilatory effort and increase ventilation

37. Restrict the patient to bed rest, and provide a quiet environment; keeping the patient rested and in bed decreases the metabolic rate, GI stimulation, and GI secretion, thereby reducing abdominal pain

38. Restrict the patient's movement and level of activity to help decrease tissue demand for oxygen

39. Provide reassurance, simple explanations, and emotional support to help reduce the patient's anxiety; a high level of anxiety increases the metabolic demand for oxygen

40. Explain all procedures before implementing them to decrease the patient's anxiety

VII. Bowel infarction, obstruction, and perforation
  A. Description
  1. Bowel infarction results from decreased blood flow to the bowel, which causes vasoconstriction and vasospasm
    a. Vasoconstriction and vasospasm can lead to ischemic bowel, tissue necrosis, gangrenous changes, peritonitis, and local abscess
    b. Bowel infarction is associated with mural thrombosis during the postmyocardial infarction period, decreased cardiac output, arteriosclerosis, cirrhosis, emboli, dislodged plaques, and hypercoagulability
  2. Bowel obstruction occurs when the normal flow of intestinal contents is impeded by a disturbance in the neural stimulation of bowel peristalsis or by other factors (such as inflammation, edema, Crohn's disease, and tumors)
  3. Chronic inflammation and thinning of the bowel mucosa can predispose the bowel to perforation
  B. Clinical signs and symptoms
  1. Nausea, vomiting, and weight loss
  2. Hypotension, tachycardia, and low-grade fever
  3. High-pitched, hyperactive bowel sounds
  4. Distended and tender abdomen
  5. Laboratory test results show mild leukocytosis and low hemoglobin level and hematocrit
  C. Medical management
  1. Insert an NG tube or decompression tube to drain secretions and relieve pressure
  2. Obtain a series of abdominal X-rays to help locate the obstruction
  3. Order a barium enema test or sigmoidoscopy to help locate the obstruction
  4. Order fluid replacement therapy to prevent hypovolemia
  5. Recommend surgery, if indicated, when the cause is diagnosed

D. Nursing management
1. Monitor vital signs (blood pressure, heart rate and rhythm, respiratory rate, and temperature) every 15 minutes until the patient is stable and then every hour
   a. Increases in blood pressure and heart and respiratory rates can result from the release of catecholamines in response to pain and anxiety
   b. Changes in vital signs also may indicate the presence of infection or changes in fluid volume within the bowel
   c. In a patient with bowel obstruction, body temperature seldom rises above 100° F (37.7° C); higher temperatures, with or without guarding and tenderness, and a sustained elevation in pulse rate suggest strangulated obstruction or peritonitis
2. Assess for nonverbal signs of pain, including grimacing, furrowed brow, tachycardia, shallow or rapid respirations, flushing, restlessness, diaphoresis, and facial pallor
   a. Nonverbal signs of pain may indicate a level of pain that the patient can tolerate without medication; however, it is more likely that the pain simply is not recognized as such by the patient
   b. Nonverbal signs of pain should be confirmed with the patient to ensure that the pain exists before deciding on the most appropriate course of action
3. Assess verbal complaints of pain by having the patient identify the location and type of pain, whether it is relieved by the passage of stools, and what measures bring relief; ask the patient to rate the pain on a scale of 1 to 10, with 1 indicating no pain and 10 indicating the greatest pain possible, and compare the level of pain before and after analgesic medication is given
4. Administer I.V. meperidine, as prescribed, and assess its effectiveness in relieving pain; for pain relief in patients with bowel disease, meperidine is preferred to morphine because morphine may decrease peristaltic activity
5. Have the patient lie on one side with knees flexed; this position promotes patient comfort by reducing pressure and tension on the abdomen
6. Work with the patient to determine the most effective methods of decreasing the pain
7. Do not ignore a patient's complaints of pain; a patient who must convince health care providers that he or she is in pain experiences an increased level of anxiety, which can further increase the perception of pain
8. If the patient has bowel obstruction secondary to Crohn's disease, assess his or her understanding of the illness; this chronic disease requires strict adherence to the prescribed medical regimen to prevent or reduce exacerbations

9. Assess for signs and symptoms of infection; a patient with bowel obstruction or perforation associated with Crohn's disease may have a lowered natural resistance as a result of malnutrition, anemia, alterations in the immune system, or long-term corticosteroid treatment

10. Assess for signs and symptoms of dehydration, including decreased skin turgor, dry mucous membranes, thirst, weight loss greater than 0.5 kg/day, low blood pressure, weak and rapid pulse rate, and output less than intake with a urine specific gravity greater than 1.030

    a. Excessive loss of fluid and electrolytes may result from vomiting

    b. Impaired absorption of fluid and electrolytes is associated with inflammation and ulceration of the small intestine, as seen in Crohn's disease

    c. A prolonged, inadequate oral intake may be associated with pain, nausea, fatigue, fear of precipitating an attack of abdominal pain, or prescribed dietary restrictions

11. Monitor potassium level and check for signs and symptoms of hypokalemia, including muscle weakness and cramping, paresthesia, nausea, vomiting, hypoactive or absent bowel sounds, and drowsiness; hypokalemia may result from the loss of potassium-rich intestinal secretions

12. Monitor magnesium and calcium levels and assess for signs and symptoms of hypocalcemia, including changes in mental status, arrhythmias, positive Chvostek's sign, positive Trousseau's sign, muscle cramps, tetany, seizures, and numbness and tingling in fingers, toes, and the circumoral area

    a. Absorption of calcium and magnesium is impaired in patients with Crohn's disease

    b. This impairment occurs because of the lack of absorption of vitamin D and fat from the inflamed small intestine; excess fats then bind calcium and magnesium and are excreted in the stool

13. Assess for signs and symptoms of metabolic acidosis, such as drowsiness, disorientation, stupor, rapid and deep respirations, headache, nausea, and vomiting; obstruction at the end of the small intestine causes loss of bases with fluids and increases the risk of developing metabolic acidosis

14. Assess the patient's pattern of bowel elimination, noting frequency, characteristics, and amount of stool and whether blood, fat, mucus, or pus is present in the stool; identification of the bowel pattern ensures timely intervention when a change from the normal pattern occurs

15. Assess the patient's nutritional status, including total protein and albumin levels, intolerance of certain foods, intake of caffeine-containing drinks and alcohol, appetite, usual weight and recent weight loss, and presence of nausea, weakness, or fatigue

    a. Hypoproteinemia can result from loss of protein through the damaged intestinal epithelium

    b. Weakness results from loss of weight caused by decreased nutrient intake and decreased absorption; cachexia also may occur

16. Assess for signs and symptoms of stress or anxiety, including restlessness, pacing, hand-wringing, and verbal comments indicating concerns

    a. The symptoms of chronic inflammatory bowel disorders, such as Crohn's disease and ulcerative colitis, can be exacerbated by stress or tension

    b. Knowledge of the patient's perception of the effect of stress on the onset of symptoms and the patient's usual coping patterns is useful for planning measures to relieve or reduce stress

17. Monitor for signs and symptoms of intestinal obstruction, including wavelike abdominal pain, abdominal distention, vomiting, and change in bowel sounds (initially hyperactive and then progressing to absent), and assess for impaction

    a. Inflammation, edema, decreased peristalsis, and tumors may cause bowel obstruction

    b. As a result, intestinal contents are propelled toward the mouth instead of the rectum

18. Monitor for signs and symptoms of fistulas, fissures, and abscesses; these signs and symptoms include purulent drainage, fecal drainage from the vagina, increased abdominal pain, burning rectal pain after defecation, signs of sepsis (fever and increased WBC count), cyanotic skin tags, and perianal induration, swelling, and redness

    a. The inflammation and ulceration caused by Crohn's disease can penetrate the intestinal wall and form an abscess or a fistula in other parts of the intestine or skin

    b. Abscesses and fistulas can cause cramping, pain, and fever and may interfere with digestion

    c. Sepsis may arise from seeding of the bloodstream with bacteria from fistula tracts or abscess cavities

19. Monitor for signs and symptoms of GI bleeding, including decreased hemoglobin level and hematocrit, fatigue, irritability, pallor, tachycardia, dyspnea, anorexia, and increased circumference of the abdomen; chronic inflammation of the bowel can erode vessels, resulting in bleeding

20. Monitor for signs of anemia, including decreased hemoglobin level, decreased RBC count, and vitamin B_{12} and folic acid deficiency

    a. Anemia can result from GI bleeding, bone marrow depression (which is associated with chronic inflammatory disease), and inadequate intake or impaired absorption of vitamin B_{12}, folic acid, and iron

    b. Sulfasalazine therapy can cause hemolysis, which contributes to anemia

21. Administer antibiotics and corticosteroids as prescribed

    a. Antibiotics decrease the bacteria count in the bowel and are administered prophylactically in anticipation of rupture or perforation and surgical intervention

    b. Corticosteroids are administered to patients with inflammatory bowel disease to prevent or reduce the inflammatory process

22. Maintain the patency of the NG tube for drainage or suction as prescribed

    a. Maintaining suction on the NG tube allows for decompression of the GI system

    b. Decompression decreases gastric secretions and peristaltic activity above the bowel obstruction, which could contribute to the patient's pain

23. Restrict the patient to bed rest in a quiet environment; this measure helps reduce GI stimulation and secretion, thereby decreasing abdominal pain

24. Turn the patient every 2 hours and encourage range-of-motion exercises as tolerated; even though the patient is restricted to bed rest, these movements are necessary to stimulate peristaltic activity

25. Assist with the insertion of a Miller-Abbot, Cantor, or Harris tube; these tubes, which extend into the small intestine, contain mercury-filled balloons at the end of a lumen that act as a bolus of food to stimulate peristalsis

26. Maintain sterile technique during all invasive procedures to prevent contamination and nosocomial infections; long-term corticosteroid use predisposes the patient to infection because it reduces the immune system response

27. Encourage a fluid intake of 2,500 ml/day in divided doses each shift, with most of the fluid intake during the day; fluids help to soften fecal contents and prevent dehydration

28. Administer I.V. vitamin supplements, particularly when anorexia and nausea are present, until the obstruction is resolved and then advance to a low-residue, high-protein, high-calorie diet; administer iron dextran by the Z-track method as prescribed

    a. Supplemental vitamins are necessary while the patient is on nothing-by-mouth status to prevent malnourishment and maintain immune system functioning

    b. Iron supplements may be necessary to prevent or treat anemia

    c. A low-residue diet promotes bowel rest and is less irritating to the mucosal lining

    d. A diet high in protein and calories replaces nutrients lost through the intestinal wall by way of exudation or bleeding; calories are needed for energy to spare the protein, which is essential for healing

29. Arrange a dietary consultation to plan an adequate nutritional regimen

30. Place the patient in Fowler's position if tolerated, maintain oxygen therapy as prescribed, encourage deep-breathing exercises, and encourage the patient to breathe through the nose and not swallow air

        a. Abdominal distention creates pressure on the diaphragm, inhibiting chest expansion; Fowler's position releases pressure on the diaphragm

        b. Breathing exercises allow maximum expansion of the lungs and help prevent further abdominal distention

        c. Supplemental oxygen maintains optimal tissue perfusion

    31. Encourage the patient to turn, if possible, and deep-breathe every 2 hours; imposed bed rest and immobility cause pooling of secretions in the lungs, which could lead to infection

    32. Organize nursing tasks so that the patient has uninterrupted periods of rest; overactivity can increase patient fatigue and oxygen use

VIII. **Hepatic failure and hepatic coma**

  A. Description

    1. The liver is vital to most bodily processes; even mild disorders of the biliary system can cause life-threatening alterations in body functions

    2. Cirrhosis causes liver cells to degenerate

        a. As the affected liver cells regenerate, nodule formation and scar tissue result; this leads to a resistance to hepatoportal blood flow and to hepatoportal hypertension

        b. Ultimately, cirrhosis causes decreased functioning of the liver, hepatic encephalopathy, and hepatic coma

    3. Fulminant hepatitis is a severe, commonly fatal form of hepatitis in which liver cells fail to regenerate, leading to progression of necrosis

    4. Hepatic failure results from severe hepatic necrosis accompanied by the loss of the liver's synthetic and excretory functions; it eventually leads to multiple organ dysfunction syndrome

  B. Clinical signs and symptoms

    1. Asterixis and hyperactive reflexes

    2. Slurred speech

    3. Generalized seizures

    4. Tachycardia and arrhythmias

    5. Peripheral edema

    6. Rapid, shallow respirations with fetor hepaticus

    7. Jaundice and mucosal bleeding

    8. Hepatomegaly and tenderness in the right upper quadrant of the abdomen

    9. Dark amber urine

  C. Medical management

    1. Place the patient in semi-Fowler's position

    2. Auscultate breath sounds every 2 hours, and administer oxygen as prescribed

    3. Follow universal precautions, and use sterile technique for all invasive procedures

4. Encourage the patient to turn and deep-breathe every 1 to 2 hours

5. Limit the patient's exposure to people with infections

6. Restrict dietary sodium to 200 to 500 mg/day

7. Restrict fluid intake to approximately 1,500 ml/day; space the fluid intake throughout a 24-hour period, with the greatest volume during the day and the least during the night

8. Weigh patient and measure abdominal girth daily; ensure that intake and output are recorded hourly

9. Administer diuretics in combination with an aldosterone antagonist, such as spironolactone

10. Administer dextran or albumin

D. Nursing management

1. Monitor vital signs (blood pressure, heart rate and rhythm, respiratory rate, and temperature) every 5 to 15 minutes until stable and then every 15 to 30 minutes

a. Frequent monitoring of vital signs allows early detection of abnormalities and prompt initiation of treatment to prevent further complications

b. In patients with hepatic failure, blood pressure eventually decreases as a result of fluid transudation and release of vasoactive substances from the damaged liver

2. Monitor CVP every hour

a. Elevated CVP may be a sign of fluid overload, which can directly affect cardiac output

b. Decreased CVP may be a sign of low circulatory volume and leakage of fluid into the third space

3. Monitor for signs of cardiovascular changes, such as flushed skin, hypertension, bounding pulses, and enhanced precordial impulse

a. Cardiovascular symptoms may occur initially because of the patient's hyperdynamic state

b. Arrhythmias can be caused by electrolyte changes; bradycardia may be noted with severe hyperbilirubinemia

4. Monitor ABG and oxygen saturation values

a. Patients with hepatic failure are at risk for respiratory problems related to encephalopathy and altered level of consciousness

b. Additionally, pleural effusion can compress lung tissue as ascitic fluid leaks into the pleural space; if this occurs, the patient may become hypoxemic

5. Monitor the patient's complete blood count and prothrombin time, and assess for signs of impaired coagulation, including bruising, nosebleeds, and petechiae

a. Clotting factors are deficient in patients with hepatic failure

b. Decreased hemoglobin level and hematocrit indicate recent bleeding episodes and the inability of the liver to store hematopoietic factors, including iron, folic acid, and vitamin B_{12}

    c. Decreased WBC and platelet counts are associated with splenomegaly; an elevated WBC count is a sign of infection

6. Monitor sodium, potassium, calcium, and magnesium levels
    a. Initially, sodium and water retention occur in intravascular spaces as a result of the decreased metabolism of antidiuretic hormone (ADH)
        (1) As the liver becomes congested and hepatoportal vein pressure increases, fluid seeps into the peritoneal cavity, causing decreased plasma volume
        (2) This results in release of ADH and aldosterone with activation of the renin-angiotensin system
        (3) As a result, sodium and water retention occur with the eventual development of dilutional hyponatremia
    b. Hypokalemia may result from diarrhea, aldosterone secretion, and the use of diuretics
    c. Hypocalcemia results from decreased dietary intake and decreased absorption of vitamin D
    d. Hypomagnesemia is caused by the inability of the liver to store magnesium

7. Assess serum albumin and total protein levels; these levels decrease as a result of impaired protein synthesis

8. Check the results of liver function tests and monitor bilirubin and ammonia levels
    a. AST, ALT, alkaline phosphatase, and lactate dehydrogenase levels increase in patients with hepatic failure because of damage to hepatocellular or biliary tissue
    b. Bilirubin level increases as a result of liver dysfunction; this rise in bilirubin leads to jaundice
    c. Ammonia level increases as a result of impaired hepatic synthesis of urea

9. Monitor for signs of hepatic encephalopathy by assessing the patient's general appearance, behavior, orientation, and speech patterns (see *Signs of hepatic encephalopathy*); signs of hepatic encephalopathy worsen as a result of the high ammonia level caused by liver dysfunction

10. Monitor GI status by assessing for nausea, vomiting, increased abdominal pain, and decreased or absent bowel sounds
    a. The patient's level of consciousness and fatigue may affect the desire to eat
    b. Increased intra-abdominal pressure caused by ascites compresses the GI tract and reduces its capacity to hold food
    c. Venous congestion in the GI tract can lead to nausea
    d. Pain can result from continued venous engorgement of internal organs and ascites

11. Check for increased abdominal girth, rapid weight loss or gain, asterixis, tremors, confusion, and signs of bleeding

Signs of hepatic encephalopathy

Hepatic encephalopathy progresses as the serum ammonia level increases and the liver continues to fail; it is divided into three stages. Identification of the signs and symptoms of a particular stage can help the nurse determine the extent of encephalopathy and, consequently, hepatic failure.

STAGE	SIGNS
Stage I	Slow thinking, mild disorientation, and difficulty understanding the concepts of a conversation; insomnia; tremors of the extremities; personality changes (usually becoming hostile, uncooperative, and belligerent)
Stage II	Changes in level of consciousness (lethargy, sleepiness, agitation); inappropriate behavior and responses; loss of coordination; speech difficulties (slurred, incoherent speech); bilateral asterixis (flapping of hands accompanied by tremors)
Stage III	Stupor or coma; no response to painful stimuli; abnormal posturing (decorticate or decerebrate); exaggerated deep tendon responses; positive Babinski's reflex

  a. Increased abdominal girth indicates worsening portal hypertension

  b. Rapid weight loss or gain is a sign of negative nitrogen balance; weight gain also may be due to fluid retention

  c. Asterixis (irregular flapping of forcibly dorsiflexed and outstretched hands) indicates worsening hepatic encephalopathy

  d. Tremors result from impaired neurotransmission, which is caused by failure of the liver to detoxify enzymes that act as false neurotransmitters

  e. Confusion results from cerebral hypoxia caused by a high serum ammonia level, which results from the inability of the liver to convert ammonia to urea

  f. Bleeding is a sign of decreased prothrombin time and a deficiency of clotting factors

12. Provide periods of uninterrupted rest

  a. Physical activity depletes the body of the energy needed for healing the damaged liver

  b. Adequate rest may prevent a relapse

13. Give vitamin K as prescribed; vitamin K is required for the synthesis of blood coagulation factors II (prothrombin), VII (proconvertin), IX (plasma thromboplastin component or Christmas factor), and X (Stuart factor or Stuart-Prower factor)

14. Avoid injections, if possible, and apply pressure to all puncture sites for 5 minutes; the patient is at increased risk for bleeding and hemorrhage because of a deficiency in vitamin K-dependent clotting factors

15. Tell the patient to avoid straining or coughing, which may precipitate bleeding of esophageal varices or hemorrhoids that develop secondary to portal hypertension

16. Examine all vomitus and stools for the presence of blood; occult bleeding can be life-threatening because of the patient's volume deficit

17. Maintain a safe environment to prevent such injuries as falling, which could trigger a hemorrhage

18. Provide mouth care and administer antiemetics, such as trimethobenzamide (Tigan) or dimenhydrinate (Dramamine), before meals as prescribed

    a. Accumulation of food particles in the mouth contributes to foul odors and taste, which diminish appetite

    b. Use of prophylactic antiemetics reduces the likelihood of anorexia

19. Administer high-calorie (1,600 to 2,500 calories/day) carbohydrate nutrients with supplemental vitamins by way of an NG tube or I.V. line; when encephalopathy subsides, introduce protein sources, beginning at a rate of 20 g/day

    a. In patients with liver dysfunction, catabolism creates a nutritional deficit that must be counteracted with a high caloric intake

       (1) Proteins must not be given to patients with hepatic encephalopathy because the diseased liver cannot metabolize protein

       (2) Protein intolerance can become chronic, depending on the severity and chronicity of the liver dysfunction

    b. To prevent aspiration, administration by way of a small-bore tube (such as a Dobhoff tube) is necessary in patients with hepatic encephalopathy or coma; I.V. administration is necessary in patients experiencing persistent vomiting

20. Administer I.V. fluids and electrolytes as prescribed

    a. Hepatic failure can cause decreased renal blood flow and reduced glomerular filtration, resulting in renal failure; renal failure in the presence of hepatic failure is called hepatorenal syndrome

    b. Fluids and electrolytes maintain circulating plasma volume and hemodynamic stability

21. Administer lactulose as prescribed

    a. Lactulose passes unchanged into the large intestine, where it is metabolized by bacteria, producing lactic acids and carbon dioxide

    b. This metabolic process decreases the pH to approximately 5.5, which favors the conversion of ammonia to ammonium ions and subsequent excretion in the stool

    c. The laxative action of lactulose further enhances evacuation of ammonia-rich stools

22. Administer enemas, as prescribed, to remove ammonia from the intestine

23. Avoid exposing the patient to ammonia products, which could increase the patient's already high serum ammonia level

24. Use a special mattress that reduces pressure on the skin, turn the patient frequently, and keep the skin clean and moisturized with lotion

    a. Maintaining skin integrity is of utmost importance in a patient with hepatic dysfunction

    b. Jaundice, dry skin, and decreased peripheral circulation can lead to rapid skin breakdown

25. Monitor for adverse effects of medications, and avoid administering opioid analgesics, sedatives, and tranquilizers; in patients with liver dysfunction, metabolism of these drugs is decreased, thereby increasing the risk of drug toxicity

8 Renal disorders

I. **Anatomy**
  A. Kidneys
    1. The kidneys are paired organs located in the retroperitoneal connective tissue of the posterior abdominal wall, with one kidney situated on each side of the vertebral column; an adrenal gland sits atop each kidney
    2. When a person is in the supine position, the kidneys extend from the 12th thoracic level to the 3rd lumbar level, with the right kidney usually a little lower than the left
      a. A single kidney of an adult male weighs 4.4 to 6 oz (125 to 170 g); the kidney of an adult female weighs 4 to 5.5 oz (115 to 155 g)
      b. Each kidney is 1″ to 1.2″ (2.5 to 3 cm) thick, 4.3″ to 4.7″ (11 to 12 cm) long, and 2″ to 3″ (5 to 7.5 cm) wide
    3. The kidneys appear slightly bean-shaped, with their long axis lying approximately vertical; they present anterior and posterior surfaces, medial and lateral margins, and superior and inferior poles
    4. On the medial surface of each kidney is the hilus, through which the renal pelvis, renal artery, renal vein, lymphatics, and nerve plexus pass into the renal sinus
    5. Each kidney is surrounded by a tough, fibrous tissue called the renal capsule
    6. Associated renal structures include the ureters (fibromuscular tubes that transport urine from the renal pelvis to the bladder), urinary bladder (pouch for holding urine), and urethra (tube through which urine passes for excretion)
  B. Kidney cross section
    1. The cortex is a pale, outer region that contains glomeruli, convoluted tubules, and adjacent parts of the loop of Henle; it is the site of aerobic metabolism and formation of ammonia and glucose
    2. The medulla is a darker, inner region that contains collecting tubules and loops of Henle grouped into 8 to 18 renal pyramids; it is the site of anaerobic and glycolytic metabolism needed for active transport
      a. The base of each renal pyramid extends toward the renal pelvis to form a papilla; the tip of the papilla has 10 to 25 small openings that serve as the renal collecting ducts (also called Bellini's ducts)

      b. The cortex, which is about 0.4″ (1 cm) thick, forms a cap over each renal pyramid and lies between each pyramid to form renal columns

   3. The calyxes are cuplike structures that enclose the renal pyramids

      a. The minor calyx receives urine from the collecting tubules

      b. The major calyx directs urine from the renal sinus to the renal pelvis, which then directs urine to the ureter

      c. The walls of the calyxes, renal pelvis, and ureters contain smooth muscle, which helps propel urine to the bladder

C. Microscopic renal structures

   1. The nephron is the structural and functional unit of the kidney; it contains the renal corpuscle and the renal tubule

      a. The renal corpuscle comprises Bowman's capsule and the glomerulus, which lies inside the Bowman's capsule

         (1) Bowman's capsule contains specialized tubules that support the glomerulus

         (2) The glomerulus is a capillary bed that is permeable to water, electrolytes, nutrients, and waste but relatively impermeable to large protein molecules and cells

      b. The renal tubule is divided into the proximal convoluted tubule, loop of Henle, distal convoluted tubule, and collecting duct

   2. At birth, each human kidney contains approximately 1 million nephrons in different stages of development; nephrons mature after birth, but new nephrons are not formed

   3. If nephrons are damaged or destroyed, the remaining functional nephrons compensate by hypertrophy and by filtering a higher solute load

D. Renal blood flow

   1. The kidneys receive 20% to 25% of cardiac output at rest; during physical or emotional stress, the kidneys may receive only 2% to 4% of cardiac output

   2. The abdominal aorta gives rise to the renal artery, which enters the hilus of each kidney and usually divides into anterior and posterior branches

      a. Segmental or lobar arteries from the anterior branch supply the anterior side of the kidney; this supply fans out in the cortex and branches to form afferent arterioles that enter the capillary beds

      b. Efferent arterioles leave the glomerular capillary bed to form a peritubular capillary network; this network becomes progressively larger and leaves the kidney by way of the hilum to join with the inferior vena cava

   3. Each kidney normally is supplied by one artery and one vein, but nearly one-third of all human kidneys have multiple vessels that usually occur on the right side and seldom on the left

4. The juxtaglomerular apparatus is a specialized structure made up of juxtaglomerular cells (smooth-muscle cells that contain inactive renin) and macula densa (a portion of the distal tubule that lies close to the afferent arterioles)

    a. The juxtaglomerular apparatus works by monitoring arterial blood pressure and serum sodium level

    b. It can be triggered by low arterial blood pressure in the afferent and efferent arterioles, low sodium content within the distal tubule, or increased sympathetic stimulation of the kidneys; once the triggers are activated, renin is released to increase blood pressure, and sodium absorption increases

E. Lymphatic system

    1. Interstitial fluid leaves the kidneys by way of the lymphatic system

    2. The renal lymphatic system drains into the aortic and para-aortic nodes of the lumbar lymphatic chain and then into the thoracic duct

F. Innervation

    1. Nerve fibers from the celiac plexus form a renal plexus around the renal artery; this plexus is joined by the lower splanchnic nerve or the renal branch of the lesser splanchnic nerve

    2. These sympathetic, afferent nerve fibers conduct pain impulses and control blood flow to the kidney by means of dilation or constriction of vessels that supply blood to the kidney

II. Physiology

A. Formation of urine

    1. Normal urine volume averages 1 to 1.5 L daily

    2. Urine composition varies slightly from person to person, but all urine contains urea (waste product of protein and amino acid metabolism), uric acid (waste product of purine metabolism by the liver), creatinine (waste product of muscle metabolism), ions (potassium, sodium, calcium, and chloride), hormones and their breakdown products (for example, chorionic gonadotropin), and vitamins (particularly the water-soluble B-complex vitamins and vitamin C)

    a. Certain medications, such as penicillin and aspirin, are excreted in the urine

    b. The presence of glucose, albumin, red blood cells (RBCs), or calculi in the urine is an abnormal finding

    3. The amount of glomerular ultrafiltration is determined by pressure gradients

    a. The glomerular hydrostatic pressure normally is 50 mm Hg, which encourages filtration

    b. A colloid osmotic pressure less than 25 mm Hg and Bowman's capsule pressure less than 10 mm Hg oppose the glomerular hydrostatic pressure to discourage filtration (see *Values for normal glomerular ultrafiltration*)

Values for normal glomerular ultrafiltration

The net filtration pressure is determined by subtracting the colloid osmotic pressure and the Bowman's capsule pressure from the glomerular hydrostatic pressure.

MEASUREMENT	NORMAL VALUE
Glomerular hydrostatic pressure	50 mm Hg
Colloid osmotic pressure	25 mm Hg
Bowman's capsule pressure	10 mm Hg
Net filtration pressure	15 mm Hg

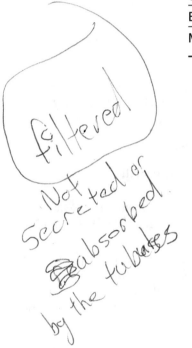

filtered

Not secreted or reabsorbed by the tubules

4. The glomerular filtration rate (GFR) is the volume of plasma cleared of a particular substance per minute
    a. It is calculated as follows: $GFR = (U_x \times V) \ P_x$, where x refers to the substance freely filtered by the glomerulus and not secreted or absorbed by the tubules, U_x is the urine concentration of x, V is the urine flow rate, and P_x refers to the plasma concentration of x
    b. Normal GFR is 125 ml/minute, or 180 L/day
    c. The GFR does not vary enough to affect urine volume, except in certain pathologic conditions
5. The tubular functions of reabsorption and secretion occur through active and passive processes; these processes are directly affected by mean arterial pressure, electrochemical gradients, and hormones
    a. In the active process, ion transport occurs against a gradient, thus requiring energy
    b. In the passive process, diffusion occurs across a concentration gradient, thus requiring no energy
6. The proximal convoluted tubule is the site for reabsorption of glucose, amino acids, phosphates, uric acid, and potassium from the tubular filtrate, which enter the blood through the peritubular capillaries
    a. Reabsorption of these substances occurs mainly through an active process in the tubular epithelium
    b. The proximal tubule also actively reabsorbs sodium (this particular process is stimulated by aldosterone) and passively reabsorbs approximately 80% of water
    c. It also reabsorbs and secretes bicarbonate and hydrogen to help regulate the acid-base balance
7. The loop of Henle is divided into an ascending (thick limb) segment and a descending segment (thin limb); the ascending loop of Henle contains an active sodium pump and is impermeable to water, whereas the descending loop of Henle is permeable to water only

    a. The primary function of the loop of Henle is the concentration or dilution of urine

    b. The loop of Henle performs this function by maintaining a hyperosmolar concentration through the removal of sodium chloride that increases the osmotic force and promotes reabsorption of water in the collecting tubules

8. The distal convoluted tubule is the site for reabsorption of water, sodium chloride, and sodium bicarbonate and the secretion of hydrogen, potassium, ammonia, and other blood-borne substances

    a. Antidiuretic hormone (ADH) controls the amount of water reabsorbed from the distal tubule

    b. The hormone aldosterone controls the reabsorption of electrolytes, especially sodium

9. The collecting duct system comprises the initial collecting tubule, the cortical collecting duct, and the inner and outer medullary segments; the collecting duct system, which is controlled by ADH, is the site of the final osmotic reabsorption of water before urine enters the renal pelvis

B. Excretion of metabolic waste products

    1. The primary function of the kidneys is the excretion of more than 200 metabolic waste products

    2. The effectiveness of the kidneys in excreting metabolic waste is measured by the levels of blood urea nitrogen (BUN) and creatinine

        a. Creatinine, which plays a role in muscle metabolism, is the most sensitive laboratory determinant of kidney function; creatinine normally is excreted at a rate equal to the GFR

        b. Urea is a protein metabolite; its excretion is influenced by urine flow, low blood volume, fever, infection, trauma, drug use, and diet

           (1) Elevated BUN without a concomitant increase in creatinine is a sign of decreased renal perfusion and volume depletion

           (2) Elevated BUN with a concomitant increase in creatinine is an indicator of renal disease

C. Regulation of body water

    1. The principal role of the thirst mechanism is to maintain normal hydration status

        a. The thirst mechanism is located in the anterior hypothalamus

        b. Thirst is triggered when there is a deficit in the intracellular fluid (ICF) volume

    2. Secretion of ADH by the posterior pituitary gland is stimulated by increased serum osmolality and decreased extracellular fluid (ECF) volume

        a. ADH acts on the distal tubule and collecting duct to cause more water to be reabsorbed from the tubular filtrate and to reenter the blood

        b. ADH has an antidiuretic effect

3. Aldosterone is a mineralocorticoid secreted by the adrenal cortex; its primary effect is to increase renal tubular reabsorption of sodium and selective renal excretion of potassium

4. The renal countercurrent mechanism can adjust urine osmolarity for concentration or dilution; this mechanism is a continuous process that occurs in the juxtamedullary nephrons, descending loop of Henle, and vasa recta

D. Renal regulation of the acid-base balance

1. The kidneys minimize variations in the fluid balance through the retention and excretion of hydrogen; fluid balance also is regulated by the lungs, blood, serum bicarbonate level, and plasma protein level

2. Excretion of hydrogen ions occurs after acid is buffered by ammonia or phosphate so that the blood pH level will not drop

3. Reabsorption of bicarbonate (HCO_3^-) begins in the proximal tubule and is completed in the distal tubule; bicarbonate is reabsorbed along with sodium when the bicarbonate level in the filtrate is above 28 mEq/L

   a. Bicarbonate is completely reabsorbed in the glomerulus until the level in the filtrate is less than or equal to 28 mEq/L; phosphate is then secreted to react with hydrogen

   b. Bicarbonate is synthesized in the distal tubule

   (1) Carbonic acid (H_2CO_3) results from the hydration of carbon dioxide (CO_2) by way of carbonic anhydrase

   (2) The carbon dioxide is a product of cellular metabolism

   (3) New bicarbonate is formed as carbon dioxide reacts with water and the resulting carbonic acid dissociates, as shown in the following equation: $H_2O + CO_2 \rightarrow H_2CO_3 \rightarrow H^+ + HCO_3^-$

E. Regulation of blood pressure

1. Normal plasma volume must be maintained for blood pressure control

   a. Decreased plasma volume reduces arterial blood pressure, leading to vasoconstrictrainion that eventually impairs oxygenation

   b. Increased plasma volume raises blood pressure by increasing cardiac preload and cardiac output

2. Vasoconstriction of the circulatory system is controlled by the renin-angiotensin-aldosterone system

   a. As GFR decreases, renin is released from juxtaglomerular cells into the afferent arterioles

   b. Renin then acts on renin substrate to split vasoactive angiotensin

   c. Angiotensin I splits into angiotensin II, which is a potent vasoconstrictor

   d. Fluid response is balanced by angiotensin II, which stimulates aldosterone to increase sodium reabsorption

3. Constriction of the renal arterioles increases ECF volume, thereby increasing blood pressure
4. Dilation of the renal vascular system is stimulated by prostaglandins
   a. Prostaglandins are found in most cells, especially those of the kidneys, brain, and gonads
   b. Prostaglandins inhibit the distal tubule response to ADH; this results in sodium and water excretion and decreased circulating volume
F. Synthesis and maturation of RBCs
   1. The kidneys control the production of RBCs by producing erythropoietin
   2. Erythropoietin is a glycoprotein hormone that stimulates the production of RBCs
      a. Erythropoietin probably is produced in the peritubular interstitial cells of the kidney
      b. It then targets the bone marrow, where synthesis of RBCs occurs

III. Renal assessment
A. Noninvasive assessment techniques
   1. In a patient with renal disease, the medical history often is the most important element in making the diagnosis (see *Components of the medical history in a patient with renal disease*)
   2. The physical examination includes an assessment of vital signs, fluid volume status, and signs of systemic disease, uremia, or obstruction
      a. Vital sign assessment
         (1) Blood pressure
         (2) Heart rate and rhythm
         (3) Temperature
         (4) Respirations
      b. Signs of altered volume status
         (1) Depletion: changes in orthostatic blood pressure and pulse rate as well as decreased skin turgor resulting in tenting
         (2) Overload: jugular venous distention, crackles, ascites, and edema
      c. Possible signs of systemic disease
         (1) Skin: malar rash or butterfly-shaped rash over the nose and cheeks (systemic lupus erythematosus [SLE]), purpura (vasculitis, Henoch-Schönlein purpura), macular rash (acute interstitial nephritis), and scleroderma
         (2) Head, ears, eyes, nose, and throat: alopecia (SLE), uveitis (sarcoidosis or vasculitis), papilledema (malignant hypertension), diabetic retinopathy, hypertension, throat infection, and hearing loss (Alport's syndrome)
         (3) Pulmonary system: consolidation (glomerulonephritis secondary to pneumonia)

Components of the medical history in a patient with renal disease

Obtaining a thorough history is important in assessing the cause of renal disease and in determining its subsequent treatment. The outline below details what to look for when performing a health history interview and a physical assessment.

A. Previous evidence of renal disease
 1. Previous elevated blood urea nitrogen or creatinine level
 2. History of albuminuria (foamy urine), hematuria (dark urine), edema, or urinary tract infections
 3. Evidence of renal disease during previous medical examinations
 4. History of hypertension
 5. Symptoms of lower urinary tract infection (urinary frequency, burning, hesitancy, urgency)
 6. Oliguria, polyuria, nocturia
 7. History of infections (throat, skin)
 8. Family history of renal disease (polycystic disease, Alport's disease [hearing loss])
B. History of systemic diseases
 1. Diabetes mellitus
 2. Collagen vascular diseases (systemic lupus erythematosus, periarteritis, Sjögren's disease, Wegener's granulomatosis, Henoch-Schönlein purpura)
 3. Cancer (myeloma, breast, lung, colon, lymphoma)
 4. Essential hypertension
 5. Sickle cell disease
 6. Primary or secondary amyloidosis
C. History of drug exposure
 1. Nonsteroidal anti-inflammatory drugs
 2. Penicillins
 3. Aminoglycosides
 4. Chemotherapeutic drugs
 5. Abuse of opioid drugs
 6. Recent use of drugs associated with temporary renal failure (such as angiotensin-converting enzyme inhibitors)
 7. Exposure to heavy metals (lead, gold, cadmium)
D. History of factors contributing to prerenal or postrenal azotemia
 1. Heart failure
 2. Diuretic use
 3. Nausea and vomiting, diarrhea, high fever, GI bleeding
 4. Salt-restricted diet
 5. Cirrhosis of the liver
 6. Lower urinary tract infections
 7. Pelvic disease
E. Uremic symptoms
 1. Nausea and vomiting, anorexia
 2. Weight loss
 3. Pruritus
 4. Weakness, fatigability
 5. Lethargy, drowsiness

(4) Heart: murmurs (endocarditis)

(5) Abdomen: bruits (renal artery stenosis)

(6) Extremities: livedo reticularis (vasculitis), blue extremities (embolic events), Janeway's lesions, Osler's nodes, and angiokeratomas

   d. Signs of uremia

(1) Skin: uremic frost and ecchymosis

(2) Heart: pericardial rub and paradoxical pulse (tamponade)

(3) Extremities: asterixis, Trousseau's sign, and Chvostek's sign

(4) Lungs: Kussmaul's respirations (metabolic acidosis)

   e. Signs of obstruction

(1) Percussible bladder

(2) Enlarged prostate

(3) Phimosis

B. Noninvasive imaging techniques

   1. Ultrasonography is used to determine the size and symmetry of the kidneys and to pinpoint the location of cysts, fluid collection, and calculi; prevoiding and postvoiding imaging is helpful in making the diagnosis

   2. Renal radionuclide scan (renogram) is used to assess glomerular filtration, renal plasma flow, arterial occlusion, and obstruction of outflow

   3. Renal arteriography is used to assess renal arterial vasculature; the dye used in this test is nephrotoxic, and all patients receiving this test should be monitored closely

   4. Computed tomography is used to identify tumors and lymphoceles

   5. Cystoscopy can detect bladder or urethral problems

   6. Retrograde pyelography, retrograde urethrography, and voiding cystourethrography are specialized X-rays that show specific renal deficits

   7. Intravenous pyelography (IVP) is used less often since the advent of ultrasonography, but it remains useful for detecting papillary necrosis and abnormalities of the renal calyxes and collecting ducts

C. Invasive assessment technique

   1. A kidney biopsy is the most direct method of determining the cause of intrinsic parenchymal disease

   2. Biopsies can be open (by way of surgery) or closed (by way of a percutaneous method)

D. Key laboratory values

   1. Blood

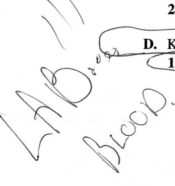

     a. Serum abnormalities are found in patients with acute or chronic renal failure

     b. BUN level (normal value: 10 to 20 mg/dl) may be elevated

     c. Creatinine level (normal value: 0.7 to 1.4 mg/dl) may be elevated

     d. Ratio of BUN level to creatinine level (normal value is 10:1)

e. Potassium level (normal value: 3.5 to 5.5 mg/dl) may be elevated

2. Urine

    a. Normal urine specific gravity ranges from 1.010 to 1.030

        (1) A specific gravity less than 1.010 is consistent with a defect in the kidneys' ability to concentrate urine and may be due to diabetes insipidus

        (2) A specific gravity greater than 1.030 indicates severe dehydration, which may result from proteinuria

    b. Normal urine pH ranges from 4.5 to 8

    c. Normal creatinine clearance is 110 to 120 ml/minute

    d. Glucose in the urine is an abnormal finding and may be related to diabetes

    e. Acetone in the urine is seen in diabetic ketoacidosis

    f. Protein in the urine is diagnostic for nephrotic syndrome

3. Urine electrolyte profile

    a. A 24-hour urine examination (in which all urine voided during a 24-hour period is saved) is used to determine the urine electrolyte profile and can be used to differentiate between prerenal causes and postrenal causes of renal failure; prerenal causes of renal failure are indicated by decreased renal perfusion, whereas postrenal causes of renal failure generally stem from obstruction

    b. Urine sodium concentration (normal value: 130 to 200 mEq/24 hours) indicates water and salt balance

    c. Urea nitrogen (normal value: 9 to 16 g/24 hours); an increase in this value indicates impaired renal function

4. Culture and sensitivity tests

    a. These tests may reveal the presence of hyaline, blood, granular, fatty, or renal tubular casts in the urine

        (1) RBC casts are a sign of active glomerulonephritis

        (2) The presence of white blood cells (WBCs) and casts indicate renal infection

        (3) Granular casts can indicate acute tubular necrosis, interstitial nephritis, acute or chronic glomerulonephritis, chronic renal disease, or proteinuric states

        (4) Fatty casts may indicate nephrotic syndrome or proteinuric states

        (5) Renal tubular casts may indicate renal failure

    b. These tests also are used to check for the presence of bacteria, WBCs, RBCs, crystals, and eosinophils in the urine

IV. Acute renal failure

  A. Description

    1. Acute renal failure is a syndrome that can be broadly defined as rapid deterioration of renal function resulting in the accumulation of nitrogenous wastes

2. Acute renal failure typically occurs when the GFR is decreased by 50% or more; six major syndromes are associated with decreased GFR

   a. *Prenenal azotemia* results from renal hypoperfusion that is immediately reversed by the return of blood flow and does not damage the renal structures

      (1) The renal response to prerenal azotemia is multiphasic

      (2) Decreased renal blood flow from the cortex to the medulla leads to decreased afferent glomerular arterial pressure, which decreases GFR and causes fluid reabsorption in the tubules

   b. *Acute (intrinsic) renal failure* (also called acute tubular necrosis) is caused by renal hypoperfusion or a nephrotoxin; it cannot be immediately reversed and results in some damage to tubular cells

      (1) Renal hypoperfusion may be caused by intravascular volume depletion (resulting from trauma, burns, or hemorrhage), decreased cardiac output (caused by severe heart failure, pulmonary hypertension, or positive-pressure mechanical ventilation), or an increase in the renal-systemic vascular resistance ratio

         (a) Renal vasoconstriction, which may cause acute renal failure if it occurs for an extended period, results from the use of amphotericin B or alpha-adrenergic agents (for example, norepinephrine) or from hypercalcemia

         (b) Systemic vasodilation results from decreased afterload, use of antihypertensive medications, anaphylactic shock, sepsis, drug overdose, or liver failure; it decreases blood pressure, thereby causing decreased renal blood flow and acute renal failure

      (2) Nephrotoxic acute renal failure usually is reversible if identified early

         (a) Exogenous nephrotoxins can cause tubule destruction, papillary necrosis, and interstitial nephritis

         (b) Common nephrotoxins include aminoglycosides and other antibiotics, contrast agents, anesthetics, and chemotherapeutic agents

   c. *Acute interstitial nephritis* is caused by interstitial inflammation

   d. *Acute glomerulonephritis or vasculitis* results from glomerular or vessel inflammation

   e. *Acute renovascular disease* is caused by obstruction of the renal artery or vein in a single kidney or by bilateral kidney disease

   f. *Obstructive uropathy* results from obstruction of the urinary collecting system

      (1) Extraureteral obstruction may be caused by a tumor or an inflammatory aortic aneurysm

        (2) Intraureteral obstruction may be caused by blood clots, calculi, or edema

        (3) Bladder outlet obstruction can result from calculi, blood clots, prostatic hypertrophy, or bladder infection

        (4) Urethral obstruction may be caused by a congenital valve defect, stricture, phimosis, or tumor

B. Clinical signs and symptoms

  1. Pruritus (the most common symptom), poor skin turgor, anorexia, nausea, vomiting, weight loss (resulting from decreased food intake or increased catabolism) or weight gain (resulting from edema or ascites), and generalized weakness and fatigue

  2. Metallic taste, stomatitis, and GI hemorrhage

  3. Hypertension or hypotension, pericarditis, and cardiomyopathy

  4. Pulmonary edema, pleural effusion, and dyspnea

  5. Encephalopathy and stupor

  6. Osteodystrophy

C. Diagnostic tests

  1. Laboratory tests of blood and urine samples may show abnormal values

  2. Ultrasonography is used to assess the size and symmetry of the kidneys

  3. Renal arteriography is used to check the renal vasculature

  4. Kidney biopsy is the most definitive diagnostic test for a renal disorder

D. Medical management

  1. Individualize treatment according to the patient's condition

  2. Determine whether the patient is a candidate for dialysis

  3. Prescribe medications, as indicated, to control blood pressure, metabolic disturbances, fluid balance, and anemia

  4. Restrict the patient's intake of sodium, phosphorus, potassium, protein, magnesium, and caffeine; fluid intake usually is restricted to 500 ml/day plus the previous day's output

E. Nursing management

  1. Record the patient's weight at admission to determine the baseline hydration status; weigh the patient daily thereafter

    a. Weight is an indicator of overhydration or dehydration

    b. Assessment of fluid intake and output must take into account insensible losses by way of the skin, lungs, and intestines (which average 700 to 800 ml/day) and the catabolic rate (which averages 350 ml/day and includes fluids derived from ingested food)

  2. Monitor vital signs every 1 to 4 hours, and check for signs and symptoms of hypervolemia and hypovolemia

3. Perform a review of all body systems, which should include heart and breath sounds to determine cardiac and pulmonary response to volume status and laboratory values to determine the effectiveness of the treatment plan

4. Restrict fluid intake as prescribed; fluid intake usually is limited to 500 ml/day plus the previous day's output

5. Restrict the patient's intake of sodium, phosphorus, potassium, protein, magnesium, and caffeine; these substances are excreted by the kidneys and can accumulate in toxic levels when the kidneys are not functioning properly

6. Administer fluid challenges (normal saline solution or albumin), as prescribed, to help control hypotension secondary to volume depletion

7. Encourage the patient to participate as much as possible in dietary and fluid management; patient compliance is the most important factor in the successful treatment of renal disease

8. Monitor potassium, sodium, calcium, phosphate, and magnesium levels for indications of electrolyte imbalance

9. Monitor for conditions that may produce electrolyte imbalance, such as vomiting, diarrhea, nasogastric tube suctioning, and tissue destruction resulting from trauma or burns

10. Administer antihypertensive medications, as prescribed, and monitor their effects; hypertension is a common complication of renal failure

11. Administer such medications as dopamine and digoxin, as prescribed, for renal hypoperfusion; by increasing cardiac output, these medications indirectly increase renal perfusion

12. Monitor the effects of dialysis, and recommend changes in ideal body weight after consultation with dialysis unit personnel and dietitian; because long-term dialysis causes a breakdown in muscle mass or decreases "dry" or "ideal" body weight, most dialysis patients retain fluids and their weight seems to stay the same

V. **Electrolyte imbalance**

A. Description

1. Electrolyte imbalance results when an electrolyte value lies outside safe parameters

2. In a patient with a renal disorder, sodium, potassium, calcium, and phosphate levels must be monitored closely

a. Sodium

(1) Hyponatremia (serum sodium concentration less than 135 mEq/L)

(2) Hypernatremia (serum sodium concentration greater than 145 mEq/L)

b. Potassium

(1) Hypokalemia (serum potassium level less than 3.5 mEq/L)

(2) Hyperkalemia (serum potassium level greater than 5.5 mEq/L)

  c. Calcium

    (1) Hypocalcemia (serum calcium level less than 8.5 mg/dl)

    (2) Hypercalcemia (serum calcium level greater than 10.5 mg/dl)

  d. Phosphorus

    (1) Hypophosphatemia (serum phosphate level less than 2.5 mg/dl)

    (2) Hyperphosphatemia (serum phosphate level greater than 5 mg/dl)

B. Clinical signs and symptoms

  1. Hyponatremia

    a. The severity of symptoms is related to the degree and rate of sodium loss

    b. The most serious symptoms (ranging from lethargy and confusion to seizures and coma) occur when the serum sodium level is less than 120 mEq/L

  2. Hypernatremia

    a. Neurologic deficits result from shrinking brain cells, which occur in proportion to the degree of hypernatremia

    b. Severe symptoms are seen when the serum sodium level is greater than 155 mEq/L

    c. The expected normal renal response to hypernatremia is the excretion of a minimal volume of maximally concentrated urine; a lack of ADH, neurohypophysial insufficiency (diabetes insipidus), hypercalcemia, osmotic diuretic therapy, and uncontrolled diabetes mellitus can cause polyuria and lead to hypernatremic dehydration

  3. Hypokalemia

    a. The most important symptoms are muscle weakness leading to flaccid paralysis and increased susceptibility to arrhythmias

    b. Severe hypokalemia can lead to respiratory arrest

  4. Hyperkalemia

    a. The initial patient complaint usually is numbness of the extremities

    b. Electrocardiogram (ECG) changes indicate the severity of the condition; peaked and elevated T waves, widening QRS complex, prolonged PR interval, and loss of P wave and sine wave formation may be seen

  5. Hypocalcemia

    a. Acute hypocalcemia must be distinguished from protein-bound calcium secondary to hypoalbuminemia and from surgical correction of primary hyperparathyroidism

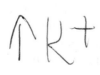
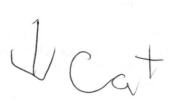

(handwritten margin notes: ↓Ca, ↑Ca, Medical Management)

b. In true hypocalcemia, neuromuscular symptoms (paresthesia and tetany) predominate, and the ECG may show a prolonged QT interval

c. Chvostek's sign (facial twitching in response to tapping on the facial nerve) and Trousseau's sign (carpal spasm after 3 minutes of inflation of a blood pressure cuff to above the systolic pressure) are indicative of hypocalcemia

6. Hypercalcemia

a. The most common symptoms of severe hypercalcemia are nausea, vomiting, confusion, somnolence, polyuria, and polydipsia

b. Hypercalcemia places the patient at increased risk for metastatic calcification and renal calculi

7. Hypophosphatemia

a. Severe hypophosphatemia manifests as skeletal muscle weakness and cardiomyopathy; rhabdomyolysis and hemolysis also have been reported

b. This condition commonly is seen in alcoholic patients, patients in the recovery phase of diabetic ketoacidosis, and those receiving total parenteral nutrition (TPN); it also can result from the excessive use of phosphate binders

8. Hyperphosphatemia

a. Hyperphosphatemia usually is correlated with hypocalcemia, which stimulates the secretion of parathyroid hormone and the resorption of calcium from bone

b. Osteoporosis, bone pain, and pathologic fractures are signs and symptoms of hyperphosphatemia

C. Medical management

1. Hyponatremia

a. In patients with hyponatremia, the goal is to increase the sodium concentration to a safe level and reduce free water intake

b. A hypovolemic patient should receive I.V. isotonic saline solution and albumin if hypoalbuminemia is present

c. If neurologic symptoms develop, the saline infusion rate should be increased at a rate of 1 to 2 mEq/L/hour

d. In patients with chronic hyponatremia (hyponatremia persisting for more than 48 hours), the saline infusion rate should be increased to a maximum of 0.6 mEq/L/hour

e. If the patient has water excess, a hypertonic saline solution (such as 3% sodium chloride) should be infused at a rate of 50 mg sodium per hour

2. Hypernatremia

a. The causative factors of hypernatremia must be determined before treatment can begin

b. Water loss can be replaced with hypotonic sodium chloride solution and dextrose 5% in water (D_5W) if the patient has moderate volume depletion or with isotonic saline solution if the patient has severe volume depletion

3. Hypokalemia

   a. The management of hypokalemia begins with monitoring for cardiac changes

   b. Oral or I.V. potassium is administered to raise the potassium level to within a normal range

4. Hyperkalemia

   a. As with hypokalemia, initial management of hyperkalemia begins with monitoring for cardiac changes

   b. When the potassium level is above 6 mEq/L, the patient should receive I.V. calcium gluconate to stabilize the myocardium

   c. Potassium can be shifted into the cells through the administration of I.V. sodium bicarbonate, glucose, or insulin

   d. Hemodialysis may be the quickest treatment for hyperkalemia if dialysis access is intact

   e. Potassium can be removed less quickly through the use of potassium-binding resins (such as sodium polystyrene sulfonate [Kayexalate] or sorbitol) or diuretics

     (1) Kayexalate works by exchanging potassium for sodium in a 1:1 ratio in the bowel cell wall

     (2) Sorbitol induces diarrhea to remove potassium

5. Hypocalcemia

   a. In patients with hypocalcemia, urgent treatment usually is required to relieve tetany and prevent arrhythmias and seizures

   b. Administer I.V. calcium gluconate for short-term treatment of hypocalcemia; administer oral calcium carbonate for long-term therapy

6. Hypercalcemia

   a. An isotonic sodium chloride infusion is used to control hypercalcemia through volume expansion

   b. Corticosteroids are administered to decrease calcium absorption in the intestines; if indicated, the patient may receive calcitonin therapy to regulate calcium level

   c. A low phosphate level also may need to be corrected in patients with hypercalcemia

7. Hypophosphatemia

   a. Hypophosphatemia can be managed by administering I.V. phosphorus at a rate of 1 mmol/L/kg over 24 hours

   b. Hypophosphatemia secondary to TPN or acute respiratory alkalosis does not require replacement therapy

8. Hyperphosphatemia

   a. Hyperphosphatemia is treated with phosphate binders to decrease GI absorption of phosphorus

   b. Fluid intake may be increased if adequate renal function exists

D. Nursing management

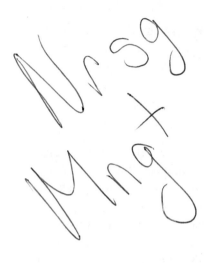

1. Monitor the patient for various signs and symptoms of electrolyte imbalance; electrolyte abnormalities are potentially fatal if left untreated
2. Observe for central pontine myelinolysis, which may result from too rapid correction of hyponatremia
3. Dilute oral potassium supplements before administration; this step is necessary for proper absorption and for alleviation of GI distress
4. Infuse I.V. potassium supplements slowly to prevent hyperkalemia and, possibly, ventricular fibrillation
5. Ensure that the patient is connected to a heart monitor after potassium replacement therapy is completed; electrolyte replacement therapies can affect cardiac functioning
6. Monitor for ECG changes, record the patient's intake and output, and check neurologic status frequently; these assessments are necessary to identify complications of treatment
7. Check whether the patient is receiving digitalis glycoside therapy; electrolyte abnormalities, especially abnormalities in the potassium level, increase the risk of digitalis toxicity

VI. Kidney transplantation

  A. Description

  1. Patients with end-stage renal disease are candidates for kidney transplantation
  2. The transplanted kidney may be donated by a living relative or taken from a cadaver
  3. To prevent rejection of the transplanted organ, the patient is given immunosuppressant medications

  B. Contraindications

  1. Contraindications to kidney transplantation vary among transplant centers
  2. The three absolute contraindications are incurable cancer or infection, refractory noncompliance, and patient refusal to provide informed consent

  C. Medical management

  1. Determine whether the patient is a candidate for kidney transplantation
  2. Maintain potential recipients on dialysis before surgical transplantation of the kidney

  D. Nursing management

  1. Determine the patient's level of knowledge about the transplant procedure and its implications; a patient-teaching plan that covers all aspects of transplantation is necessary for the success of the procedure

2. Before the transplant procedure, monitor the patient's vital signs; check when the patient last underwent dialysis; perform a physical assessment; assess for recent exposure to infection; review laboratory test results, including blood crossmatching and baseline values; ensure that a chest X-ray was taken; maintain the patient on nothing-by-mouth status; teach the patient how to turn, cough, and deep-breathe; and initiate immunosuppressant therapy

3. After the transplant procedure, maintain adequate respiratory function, maintain fluid volume status, monitor for signs and symptoms of rejection or infection, and assess renal transplant function

   a. Immunosuppressant medications leave the patient vulnerable to infections

   b. The initial signs and symptoms of rejection typically are decreased urine output, abdominal pain, and low-grade fever

4. Help the patient manage the emotional aspects of the procedure; after major surgery involving transplantation of an organ from another person, many patients have difficulty coping emotionally

5. Before discharge, educate the patient about diet, fluid intake, medications, activity level, signs and symptoms of infection and rejection, and follow-up appointments

VII. Continuous arteriovenous hemofiltration

  A. Description

    1. In continuous arteriovenous hemofiltration (CAVH), arterial blood is diverted through a small artificial kidney filter

      a. An arterial port and a venous port are placed on opposite sides of the filter to connect the filter to a larger artery and a major vein

      b. Blood flows through the filter and back through the venous system

      c. Ultrafiltrate is removed by means of a drain port

    2. The patient's systolic blood pressure must be at least 80 mm Hg for CAVH to function properly

    3. CAVH is used to manage short-term renal problems in hemodynamically unstable patients who cannot tolerate hemodialysis or peritoneal dialysis

  B. Medical management

    1. Determine the patient's suitability for CAVH

    2. Obtain vascular access

    3. Determine the appropriate length of treatment

  C. Nursing management

    1. Frequently monitor the filter site and connections for clots, leaks, and kinks; these common complications prevent the device from working properly

    2. Do not allow the patient to lay on the filter, which can kink the tubes or damage the filter

       3. Use aseptic technique when handling the filter and tubes because infectious organisms can easily be introduced into the bloodstream with this type of filter

VIII. Hemodialysis

    A. Description

       1. Hemodialysis is the removal of waste products or toxins from the blood by diffusion across a semipermeable membrane while the blood is circulated outside the body

       2. Hemodialysis is indicated for chronic renal failure and acute renal failure resulting from trauma or infection; it also is used to rapidly remove toxic substances, including alcohol, barbiturates, and poisons

       3. There are no absolute contraindications to hemodialysis

    B. Medical management

       1. Determine the patient's suitability for hemodialysis

       2. Obtain vascular access by means of surgical insertion of a double-lumen subclavian catheter, atrioventricular fistula, or atrioventricular graft

       3. Determine the length of treatment, and select the pressure settings on the dialysis machine

    C. Nursing management

       1. Educate the patient about hemodialysis and the associated vascular access procedures

       2. Before hemodialysis is started, monitor the patient's vital signs, including heart rate and rhythm; assess volume status by checking the patient's weight, neck vein distention, pulmonary artery wedge pressure, central venous pressure, and intake and output; and review laboratory and X-ray reports

          a. These assessments are necessary to determine the settings on the dialysis machine

          b. They also provide baseline parameters for assessing postdialysis data

       3. Assist the doctor with vascular access placement; this procedure may be done in the patient's room but usually is performed in the operating room

       4. After vascular access is obtained, secure all connections and verify placement before beginning hemodialysis; patency of the vascular access device is critical to successful hemodialysis

       5. Follow anticoagulant protocols to prevent dialyzer clotting complications; patients with active bleeding or contraindications to heparin can be dialyzed on a heparin-free or citrate anticoagulant regimen

       6. Check activated clotting times to monitor the effects of heparin administration

          a. Activated clotting times should be determined 1 hour after dialysis is started and 30 minutes before dialysis is discontinued or if clots are seen

b. Activated clotting times should be determined every $3\frac{1}{2}$ to 4 minutes during dialysis in patients with subclavian catheters, Hemocaths, or external shunts

7. Do not perform venipuncture, administer I.V. therapy or injections, or take a blood pressure reading with a cuff on the extremity having vascular access; all these activities can damage the vascular access and impede hemodialysis

8. Instruct patients not to lie on the extremity having vascular access, wear tight clothing, or injure the extremity in any way

9. Monitor access sites for bleeding, which is one of the most serious complications related to vascular access

IX. Peritoneal dialysis

A. Description

1. In peritoneal dialysis, the peritoneum surrounding the abdominal cavity serves as a dialyzing membrane

2. Peritoneal dialysis is indicated for acute renal failure, chronic renal failure, refractory heart failure, and intraperitoneal chemotherapy

3. There are three forms of peritoneal dialysis: continuous ambulatory peritoneal dialysis, continuous cyclic peritoneal dialysis, and intermittent peritoneal dialysis

a. Continuous ambulatory peritoneal dialysis is the peritoneal dialysis treatment of choice; it involves exchanges over a 24-hour period, 7 days a week

b. Continuous cyclic peritoneal dialysis uses a cycling machine that infuses and drains dialysate fluid while the patient sleeps at night; during the day, the patient does not have any dialysate fluid in the peritoneal cavity

c. Intermittent peritoneal dialysis (also called automated peritoneal dialysis) can be performed manually or with a cycling machine; typically, it is done at night, and the dialysate from the last exchange remains in the peritoneal cavity during the day and is drained at the initiation of the next exchange

B. Contraindications

1. An absolute contraindication to peritoneal dialysis is significant loss of peritoneal surface resulting from adhesions or recurrent peritonitis

2. Relative contraindications include the presence of ostomies, extreme obesity, recent abdominal surgery or trauma, and tuberculous or fungal peritonitis

3. Continuous ambulatory peritoneal dialysis and continuous cyclic peritoneal dialysis may be contraindicated when the patient has a condition that is exacerbated by intraperitoneal pressure, such as hernia, hemorrhoids, and low back pain

C. Medical management

1. Determine the patient's suitability for peritoneal dialysis

2. Surgically insert an abdominal catheter

3. Determine the solution concentration based on laboratory values

D. Nursing management
1. Educate the patient about peritoneal dialysis, including peritoneal catheter placement, what to expect before and after the procedure, the importance of aseptic technique, the use of local anesthetics, anticipated discomfort, and postprocedure activity; after the catheter is inserted, the patient is responsible for much of his or her care and must thoroughly understand the dialysis procedure
2. Assist the doctor with catheter placement; a patient undergoing peritoneal dialysis typically has a trocar catheter inserted surgically into the peritoneum
3. Before peritoneal dialysis is started, monitor the patient's vital signs, including heart rate and rhythm; assess volume status by checking the patient's weight, neck vein distention, pulmonary artery wedge pressure and central venous pressure, and intake and output; and review laboratory and X-ray reports; because the patient has some degree of renal failure, the patient must be monitored closely before dialysis begins
4. Inspect the catheter and exit site for dialysate leaks and signs and symptoms of infection; these complications commonly are seen after the catheter is inserted
5. Review with the patient the use of the manual or automated dialysis system, dialysate volume, dialysate dextrose concentration, and fill, dwell, and drain times
6. Explain to the patient how medications are added to the dialysate, and ensure that the patient understands the parameters for adjusting dialysate dextrose concentrations and knows how to care for the catheter exit site; this information is crucial for preventing infections
7. Teach the patient how to perform the peritoneal dialysis procedure; ascertain patency by draining the first dialysate solution and then allowing other infusions to fill, dwell (usually for 20 to 45 minutes), and drain
8. Check the color and consistency of the drainage
   a. Normal drainage is clear and pale yellow
   b. Bleeding or bloody drainage is not unusual during the first to fourth exchanges
   c. Cloudy fluid usually indicates peritonitis, which requires immediate treatment
9. Teach the patient to monitor vital signs and record total body intake and output (have the patient record the measured amount of fluid removed for each exchange and record the negative and positive balance); make sure that diabetic patients are aware that dialysate contains glucose and that some absorption may occur and that they know how to monitor blood glucose level
10. Teach the patient how to obtain outflow fluid samples for baseline culture and sensitivity tests

9 Multisystem disorders

I. Asphyxia

    A. Description

        1. Asphyxia is a general term used to describe low oxygen level in the blood with a corresponding increase in the level of carbon dioxide

        2. Anything that interrupts normal gas exchange in the respiratory system can produce asphyxia

        3. Common causes of asphyxia include near drowning; trauma to the face, neck, larynx, or trachea; trauma to the lungs; foreign body obstruction of the airways; electric shock; inhalation of toxic gases or smoke; and any severe disease of the lungs

        4. Almost all patients who experience an episode of asphyxia are cared for in the critical care unit

        5. Because of the cerebral and general systemic anoxia resulting from asphyxia, these patients are in critical condition, commonly are unresponsive, and have multiple organ dysfunction syndrome

    B. Medical management

        1. Insert an endotracheal tube if indicated

        2. Insert an arterial and a central line for pressure monitoring

        3. Administer appropriate vasoactive, cardiotonic, and bronchodilating medications as indicated

    C. Nursing management

        1. Monitor the patient's respiratory capabilities continuously or at least every hour; note the rate, depth, and spontaneity of respirations and assess breath sounds; the data provided by continual respiratory system assessment are essential for developing a plan of care

        2. Determine whether the injury that caused the asphyxia has resulted in other complications; traumatic injuries commonly affect other body systems

        3. Check for conditions that contribute to asphyxia, such as lung disease, obesity, chest wall injuries, and neuromuscular dysfunction resulting from fractures of the spine; the presence of these conditions can complicate attempts to maintain adequate respiration

        4. Continuously monitor vital signs, output, and hemodynamic pressures; the invasive monitoring techniques that almost always are used in these critically ill patients provide important information about changes in the patient's status

5. Assess neurologic function every hour until the patient is stable; the use of a neurologic assessment sheet or the Glasgow Coma Scale provides important information about the oxygenation of cerebral tissues

6. Place the patient in Fowler's or semi-Fowler's position to facilitate full expansion of the lungs

7. Change the patient's position every 1 to 2 hours to prevent skin breakdown and to help mobilize secretions

8. Check the settings, functioning, and effect of the mechanical ventilator; the patient is mechanically ventilated until spontaneous respirations resume

9. Check the position, cuff pressure, and patency of the endotracheal tube; aeration of the patient is impeded if the endotracheal tube is not patent or is improperly positioned

10. Suction the patient, as indicated, if dyspnea, coughing, rhonchi, or visible secretions in the tubing occur; the buildup of secretions in the endotracheal tube can cause airway obstruction

11. During suctioning, monitor the patient's blood pressure, heart rate, and electrocardiogram (ECG); suctioning can cause a number of complications, ranging from hypotension to bradycardia and ventricular tachycardia

12. Obtain arterial blood gas (ABG) samples immediately if the patient's condition significantly deteriorates; ABG analysis can identify subtle changes in oxygenation

13. Monitor the patient for pulmonary infections; intubation and mechanical ventilation place the patient at increased risk for pulmonary infections

14. Administer medications, as indicated, to maintain tissue perfusion because asphyxia commonly is accompanied by generalized multiple organ dysfunction syndrome; such medications include vasoactive drugs, sympathetic stimulants, antibiotics, steroids, and plasma expanders

15. Monitor the patient for related complications, such as adult respiratory distress syndrome (ARDS), disseminated intravascular coagulation (DIC), renal failure, hepatic failure, and heart failure; asphyxia has many potential complications that may prevent the patient's recovery

II. **Burns**

A. Integumentary anatomy

1. The epidermis is the outermost layer of the skin; it consists of the stratum corneum and the cellular stratum

a. The stratum lucidum is a thick layer of skin found only in the palms and soles

b. The basement membrane lies beneath the cellular stratum and connects the epidermis with the dermis

2. The dermis is a layer of connective tissue that supports and separates the epidermis from the subcutaneous adipose tissue

        a. It has a rich vascular supply

        b. The dermis contains elastin, collagen, and reticulum fibers for strength and sensory nerve fibers for pain, touch, and temperature

        c. It also contains the autonomic motor nerves for innervation of blood vessels, glands, and arrectores pilorum muscles

    3. The hypodermis is a subcutaneous layer that connects the dermis with the underlying organs

        a. It is composed of loose connective tissue filled with fatty cells

        b. The fat cells provide insulation, absorb shocks, and store calories

    4. Appendages of the skin

        a. Eccrine sweat glands open directly on the surface of the skin and regulate body temperature by secreting water

        b. Apocrine glands are found only in the axillae, nipples, areolae, genital area, eyelids, and external ears; these glands secrete fluids in response to intense emotional or physiologic stimulation

        c. Sebaceous glands respond to sex hormones and secrete sebum to keep the skin and hair moist

B. Integumentary physiology

    1. The skin forms an elastic, rugged, self-regenerating, protective covering for the body

    2. It protects the internal structures of the body from invasive microorganisms and from minor physical trauma

    3. It maintains internal fluid balance by preventing fluid loss

    4. The skin regulates body temperature through radiation, conduction, convection, and evaporation

    5. It conveys sensory input to the central nervous system through nerve endings and specialized receptors

    6. It helps regulate blood pressure through vasoconstriction and vasodilation

    7. It helps eliminate waste products from the body by excreting sweat, urea, lactic acid, bilirubin, and the metabolites of many medications

C. Integumentary assessment

    1. Patient history

        a. Note skin care habits, including the use of soaps, sunscreens, and lotions

        b. Note hair care habits, including the use of shampoos, coloring, and permanents, and changes in care procedures

        c. Note nail care habits, including instruments used, procedures used, and difficulties encountered in care

        d. Assess exposure to environmental or occupational hazards, chemicals, and sunlight

    2. Physical examination

        a. Inspect and palpate the skin for coloration, lesions, temperature, texture, turgor, and mobility

      b. Inspect the hair for texture, color, distribution, quantity, abnormal location, and abnormal destruction

      c. Inspect the nails for color, length, configuration, symmetry, and cleanliness

      d. Take culture samples from the skin and skin lesions to determine bacteria growth and sensitivity to medications

D. Description

  1. Burns are injuries to the skin caused by exposure to heat, chemicals, electricity, or radiation

  2. The severity of the burn depends on the depth of the injury and the amount of body surface area (BSA) affected

  3. Burns are classified according to the depth of the injury

      a. In a first-degree burn, damage is limited to the epidermis, causing erythema and pain

      b. In a second-degree burn, the epidermis and part of thedermis are damaged, producing blisters and mild-to-moderate edema and pain

      c. In a third-degree burn, the epidermis and dermis are damaged; although no blisters appear, white, brown, or black leathery tissue and thrombosed vessels can be seen

      d. In a fourth-degree burn, damage extends from deeply charred subcutaneous tissue to muscle and bone

  4. Burns also are classified according to the amount of BSA affected; they may be categorized as minor, moderate, or major

      a. Minor burns are those that involve less than 2% of BSA, second-degree burns on less than 15% of an adult's BSA, or second-degree burns on less than 10% of a child's BSA; patients with minor burns usually are treated at home or in a doctor's office or hospital emergency department

      b. Moderate burns are those that involve third-degree burns on 2% to 10% of BSA, second-degree burns on 15% to 25% of an adult's BSA, or second-degree burns on 10% to 20% of a child's BSA; patients with moderate burns may be treated in a general critical care unit if no complications or related injuries are present

      c. Major burns include third-degree burns on more than 10% of BSA; second-degree burns on more than 25% of an adult's BSA; second-degree burns on more than 20% of a child's BSA; burns of the hands, face, feet, or genitalia; electrical burns; and all burns in poor-risk patients

      d. Patients with major burns are best cared for at specialized burn centers

  5. Burns over large areas of the body produce significant changes in all body systems, including changes in temperature regulation, fluid volume shifts, increased susceptibility to infections, and loss of self-image

6. Recovery from a burn injury can take months or even years

E. Medical management

    1. Begin fluid replacement with appropriate I.V. colloid or crystalloid solutions

    2. Administer appropriate antibiotic therapy

    3. Determine the appropriate treatment method (open, closed, or semi-open)

        a. *Open treatment* involves the application of an antimicrobial cream (such as Silvadene) to the burn area and leaving it exposed to the air; this method allows for better detection of infection and improved ambulation

        b. *Closed treatment* uses an occlusive dressing to cover the burn, which is left on for several days; it is used for burns of the hands and feet

        c. *Semi-open treatment* involves the application of an antimicrobial cream and a fine-mesh gauze cover on the burn area

    4. Debride the injured area and perform skin grafting and other surgical procedures as indicated

    5. Order a diet that meets the patient's caloric needs

F. Nursing management

    1. Assess the patient's airway for patency, and check for signs of respiratory complications, such as wheezing, increased respiratory rate, smoke-colored sputum, hoarseness, stridor, and burned facial hairs, nostril hairs, or eyebrows

        a. Burns that occur in closed areas or affect the head and neck are likely to cause airway obstruction by causing edema of the respiratory tract passages

        b. Respiratory complications can occur several hours after the burn injury

    2. Assess the depth and extent of the burn; use the Rule of Nines to determine an adult's total BSA burned (see *Rule of Nines,* page 234); the more extensive the burn and the greater its depth, the more likely the patient will experience multisystem complications during recovery

    3. Assess the burned areas for blisters, edema, charring, and open tissue or exposed bone; burns with these characteristics promote loss of large amounts of fluid by way of evaporation, contribute to dehydration, and leave the patient vulnerable to infections

    4. Check the burn wound for contamination, including burned clothing, dirt, ash, soot, and other foreign matter; these substances can cause invasive infections

    5. Obtain a complete health history, including allergies, chronic health problems (including prior skin conditions), current medications, and recent operations or injuries; because burn injuries stress the whole body, prior existing diseases can complicate the recovery process

Rule of Nines

To quickly estimate the extent of an adult's burns, the nurse can use the Rule of Nines, which divides the body into percentages. To use this method, mentally transfer the patient's burns to the body chart shown here. Then add up the corresponding percentages for each burned body section. The total is a rough estimate of the extent of the patient's burns.

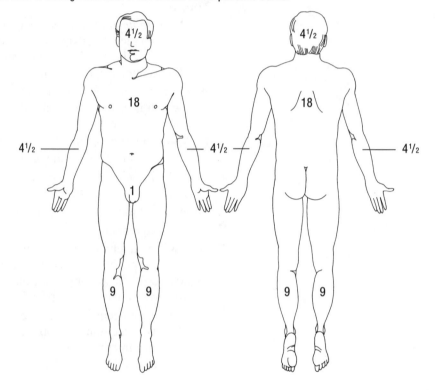

6. Assess the patient's urine output hourly; burns are a leading cause of acute renal failure, and urine output also provides an indication of hydration status

7. Monitor vital signs continuously during the immediate postburn period; sudden changes in vital signs may indicate impending shock

8. Assess the location, type, and severity of pain; first- and second-degree burns and some third-degree burns can be extremely painful; pain is a stressor in all types of trauma

9. Monitor the patient's neurologic status, noting agitation, memory loss, confusion, headache, and mental changes; changes in neurologic status commonly are the first indication of changes in oxygenation, tissue perfusion, and cardiac output

10. Assess the abdomen for bowel sounds, distention, and tenderness; burn injuries commonly result in paralytic ileus, bowel obstruction, and sloughing of the lining of the intestines

11. Maintain a patent airway through intubation or tracheostomy, positioning, or mechanical ventilation; airway obstruction is a common complication in the immediate postburn period

12. Identify vascular access sites and start I.V. lines with large-gauge needles or assist the doctor with central lines; adequate hydration during the first 72 hours is essential for the survival of patients with severe burns

13. Ensure that the patient receives the proper type and amount of fluids; both dehydration and fluid overload are potential problems in the early treatment period

14. Administer tetanus prophylaxis; patients with burn injuries are at high risk for tetanus

15. Maintain the patient on nothing-by-mouth status and insert a nasogastric tube
    a. Gastrointestinal shutdown usually occurs after severe burns
    b. Giving the patient fluid or food by mouth can lead to vomiting and aspiration

16. Administer medications, including antibiotics, plasma expanders, steroids, histamine$_2$-receptor antagonists, and analgesics, as prescribed; all medications should be given I.V.

17. Check the data from invasive hemodynamic monitoring equipment; central venous pressure, pulmonary artery pressure, and cardiac output commonly are monitored to help regulate fluid administration in severely burned patients

18. Assist with or perform burn wound care using strict aseptic technique
    a. Although sometimes reverse isolation is used, strict aseptic technique is effective in preventing infections from outside sources
    b. The patient's own body is the primary source of infective organisms

19. Monitor for hypothermia, using a continuous temperature monitoring device; patients can lose large amounts of heat through open burn wounds

20. Maintain the patient's room at 80° F (26.6° C) with 50% to 60% humidity; these measures help prevent hypothermia and reduce fluid loss through evaporation

21. Begin active and passive range-of-motion exercises as soon as possible; the sooner physical therapy is started, the less likely that contractures and circulatory complications will develop

22. Reposition the patient every 2 hours to prevent pressure ulcers

23. Provide a diet high in calories and protein and include vitamin supplements, especially B-complex vitamins and vitamin C; provide frequent, small meals or supplemental feedings if required
    a. Severe burns cause a negative nitrogen balance (catabolism)
    b. Extra calories (5,500 calories/day for an adult) are required to prevent muscle tissue breakdown

  c. Vitamin supplements play an important role in the healing process

24. Assess burn wounds for healing or signs of infection
  a. Healing is marked by the development of pink, healthy tissue
  b. Infection is characterized by redness, tenderness, and purulent drainage
  c. Obtain tissue culture samples from burn wounds, as prescribed, to determine bacterial growth and sensitivity to medications

25. Assist the patient during whirlpool debridement, dressing changes, and surgical procedures; the necrotic burned skin (eschar) must be removed before healing can take place

26. Check skin grafts used on the burn wound for signs of infection
  a. Autologous skin grafts are taken from unburned areas of the patient's body; these grafts are surgically attached and will grow new skin
  b. Homologous skin grafts are taken from human cadavers; these grafts are surgically attached and do not grow, but they allow new skin to develop underneath; homologous grafts remain in place until they slough off
  c. Animal skin grafts form a type of biologic dressing using the skin of cows (bovine grafts) or pigs (porcine grafts); these grafts remain on the wound for 3 to 4 days before they are changed

27. Monitor the patient's psychological status and progression through the stages of grief
  a. Burn injuries produce profound changes in body image
  b. Patients who are severely burned commonly experience denial, anger, depression and ultimately, acceptance

28. Teach the patient and family about the hospital plan of care and about home care after discharge; providing this information allows the patient and family to participate in the recovery process, increases the patient's sense of security, and promotes continued family communication

29. Contact social services to help the patient cope with financial and rehabilitation concerns; the prolonged recovery period of many burn patients often decimates their financial resources, may cause loss of employment, and is stressful to the family

30. Monitor the patient for long-term complications of burn injuries
  a. Severe burn injuries can trigger numerous complications, which can develop at any time during the recovery period
  b. These complications include ARDS, DIC, heart failure, renal failure, hepatic failure, infections, pulmonary emboli, contractures, stress ulcers, pulmonary fibrosis, drug dependence, and depression

III. Shock

   A. Description

    1. In shock, an insufficient amount of circulating blood volume results in less than adequate perfusion of cells and vital organs

    2. No matter what the cause, the result of prolonged shock is the same—cell death due to lack of adequate nutrition and lack of oxygenation to the tissues

    3. The severely ill patient typically seen in the critical care unit always is at risk for some type of shock

    4. There are five types of shock: anaphylactic, cardiogenic, neurogenic, hypovolemic, and septic

    5. Many of the nursing assessments and basic nursing care are similar for each type of shock

   B. Septic shock

    1. Sepsis occurs when large numbers of pathogenic microorganisms or their toxins are present in the blood or other tissues

    2. Although it does not always lead to septic shock, sepsis almost always is fatal if left untreated

    3. Septic shock results when massive vasodilation occurs secondary to the release of toxins by certain bacteria

    4. Septic shock is most common in patients with sepsis caused by gram-negative organisms (such as *Escherichia coli, Klebsiella, Proteus,* and *Pseudomonas*) or by some gram-positive organisms (such as *Streptococcus* and *Staphylococcus*)

    5. Sepsis and septic shock may be caused by peritonitis, urinary tract infection, toxic shock syndrome, food poisoning, lacerations, compound fractures, major burn injuries, and conditions that cause debilitation, such as cancer and cerebrovascular accident

    6. The clinical signs and symptoms of early septic shock differ from those of late septic shock (see *Assessment findings in early and late septic shock,* page 238)

   C. Medical management

    1. Rapidly infuse I.V. solutions

    2. Administer I.V. antibiotics

    3. Maintain the patient on strict bed rest

    4. Use the shock position (patient in supine position with legs elevated 10 to 30 degrees) or modified Trendelenburg's position as needed

    5. Administer volume expanders, plasma, dextran, and albumin, as indicated, and monitor for fluid overload

    6. Insert arterial and central venous lines for pressure monitoring

   D. Nursing management

    1. Monitor for restlessness, anxiety, apprehension, and decreased level of consciousness; decreased cerebral perfusion secondary to the shock state causes changes in neurologic status

    2. Assess for changes in skin temperature and color

Assessment findings in early and late septic shock

In early septic shock, the body's compensatory mechanisms attempt to fight the widespread systemic infection. As septic shock progresses, it is complicated by the inadequate perfusion of cells and vital organs. Early septic shock can be characterized as the hyperdynamic phase of septic shock; late septic shock can be characterized as the hypodynamic phase of septic shock. The assessment findings for each stage are shown below.

SYSTEM	EARLY SEPTIC SHOCK	LATE SEPTIC SHOCK
Respiratory	Tachypnea, deep breaths	Tachypnea, shallow breaths
Cardiovascular	Mild hypotension, decreased afterload, decreased preload, increased cardiac output, sinus tachycardia	Severe hypotension, increased afterload, decreased preload, decreased cardiac output, ventricular arrhythmias
Neurologic	Anxiety, alertness, mild confusion	Decreased level of consciousness, severe confusion
Renal	Near-normal urine output	Decreased or absent urine output
Hematologic (as evidenced by blood pH)	Normal or respiratory alkalosis	Metabolic acidosis

    a. Decreased oxygenation and the stress response lead to vasoconstriction, causing the skin to become cold, pale, and diaphoretic
    b. A gray color to the skin often indicates gram-negative sepsis; a ruddy color may indicate a gram-positive infection
  3. Monitor vital signs, including heart and respiratory rates, blood pressure, and temperature
    a. The shock state reduces the circulating blood volume and typically lowers the blood pressure (mean arterial pressure less than 70 mm Hg) and increases the pulse rate (above 100 beats/minute) as a compensatory mechanism
    b. The respiratory rate tends to increase to help maintain oxygenation
    c. Body temperature may increase as a result of the bacterial infection, although the temperature may remain normal in patients with overwhelming infections and in older patients
  4. Control the patient's temperature with hypothermia blankets, light covers, tepid soaks, and alcohol baths; high fevers must be lowered to prevent brain damage
  5. Monitor for decreased urine output (less than 25 ml/hour); a mean arterial pressure less than 70 mm Hg can lead to inadequate renal perfusion and decreased urine output
  6. Monitor ABG values for metabolic acidosis; many organisms produce toxins that cause lactic acidosis, thereby lowering the pH below 7.35 and the bicarbonate below 22 mEq/L

7. Assess for thirst; as the circulating fluid volume decreases, the hydration mechanism attempts to compensate by increasing the patient's need for oral fluid intake

8. Check data from pulmonary artery catheters or central venous pressure lines every 1 to 4 hours; these generally are inserted in patients with septic shock and are useful for monitoring cardiac output, fluid volume, and hydration status

9. Monitor oxygenation using pulse oximetry, ABG measurements, or other means; shock state decreases partial pressure of oxygen, oxygen saturation, and pH levels

10. Observe and report changes in the patient's condition that indicate worsening infection
    a. Sepsis and septic shock progress rapidly to overwhelming infection that often is irreversible
    b. Any deterioration in the patient's condition requires aggressive treatment

11. Maintain a patent airway, and administer supplemental oxygen to lessen the effects of cerebral anoxia

12. Monitor for potential complications of septic shock, which include pulmonary edema, metabolic acidosis, and DIC

13. Monitor the rapid infusion of I.V. solutions; large amounts of I.V. solutions are needed to lessen the effects of hypovolemia caused by vasodilation and blood pooling

14. Maintain the patient on strict bed rest to decrease cellular oxygen demands

15. Monitor the patient closely if the shock position or modified Trendelenburg's position is used; elevating the foot of the bed 45 degrees with the head of the bed slightly elevated increases peripheral venous return and permits adequate respiratory exchange

16. Reposition the patient every 2 hours or more frequently if necessary to reduce the risk of skin breakdown resulting from immobility

17. Monitor the effects of I.V. antibiotic therapy
    a. Patients with septic shock typically receive large doses of several broad-spectrum I.V. antibiotics
    b. Allergic reactions, renal failure, aplastic anemia, and other adverse effects may result from antibiotic therapy

18. Monitor the effects of volume expanders, plasma, dextran, and albumin, if prescribed, and check for fluid overload
    a. Hypertonic volume expanders draw fluid from the tissues into the vascular system
    b. Heart failure is a potential adverse effect of volume expanders, particularly in elderly patients

19. Administer and monitor the effects of other commonly used medications
    a. High doses of dopamine, epinephrine, norepinephrine, and metaraminol bitartrate are used as sympathetic stimulants

      b. Low doses of dopamine and nitroglycerin are used as vasodilators

      c. High doses of steroids may be used to decrease inflammation and stabilize cell membranes; long-term steroid use suppresses the immune system

IV. Toxic ingestions

  A. Description

      1. Toxic ingestions include all types of drug overdoses, whether accidental or intentional; this category also encompasses accidental ingestion of common household chemicals by children and withdrawal from addictive substances, including alcohol and such drugs as cocaine and heroin

      2. Patients who have ingested toxic substances of any type often are monitored and managed in the critical care unit

      3. Although each substance causes unique problems and complications, nursing care for all types of toxic ingestion is similar

      4. Critical care nurses most often care for patients who have ingested common drugs, such as aspirin and acetaminophen; patients who have taken an overdose of these medications often have made an intentional attempt at suicide, thereby complicating their care

      5. Critical care nurses also commonly care for patients who have overdosed on illicit drugs; in many cases, such overdoses are accidental

        a. Critical care units frequently are used as detoxification units for people who abuse illicit drugs

        b. These patients can be difficult to manage, commonly are mentally unstable, and have a tendency to be violent

      6. Patients who have intentionally or accidentally ingested substances other than drugs also may be cared for by critical care nurses

        a. These substances range from cleaning products, such as furniture polish, liquid detergents, and window cleaners, to industrial chemicals, such as antifreeze, lye-based compounds, and petroleum products

        b. The care of children and of adults who ingest these substances is similar

      7. Another group of patients who may be cared for in the critical care unit are those who have accidentally overdosed on prescription medications

        a. Elderly patients are particularly susceptible to this type of poisoning

        b. Many of the medications that older patients are routinely prescribed have narrow therapeutic ranges and are potentially toxic; even small overdoses of cardiac medications, such as digitoxin (Lanoxin), diltiazem (Cardizem), propranolol, and disopyramide, can cause severe arrhythmias or even cardiac arrest

      c. Other categories of medications, including antibiotics, steroids, antihypertensive agents, and hypoglycemic agents, can be lethal in large doses for elderly patients

B. Medical management

    1. Contact the regional poison control center to determine how to counteract the effects of the substance or eliminate it from the body

    2. Dilute the substance by giving the patient milk or water—as indicated by the poison control center—unless the patient is unresponsive

    3. If indicated, perform gastric lavage using a large-bore orogastric tube; gastric lavage is particularly important in patients who have ingested caustic substances (strong bases) or hydrocarbons (petroleum products or cleaning solutions)

    4. Use a peristaltic pump to wash out the patient's gut with warmed electrolyte solutions

    5. If the substance is a drug or noncaustic substance, induce emesis with 30 ml of ipecac syrup followed by 240 ml of water; vomiting should occur within 15 to 30 minutes

    6. Administer 25 to 50 g of activated charcoal by evacuator tube after the ipecac syrup has induced vomiting

    7. Administer antidotes or antagonist medications as appropriate

C. Nursing management

    1. Monitor vital signs at least every 15 minutes until the patient is stable; most drug overdoses produce significant changes in vital signs, including increased pulse rate and decreased blood pressure, respiratory rate, and temperature

    2. Assess neurologic signs, using the Glasgow Coma Scale or another appropriate neurologic assessment tool, every hour until the patient is stable; many drugs, particularly those that affect the central nervous system (CNS), alter neurologic signs

    3. Obtain as complete a history as possible concerning the type and amount of substance ingested, when the ingestion occurred, current medication use, and whether the patient has associated health problems or long-term health problems; many factors influence how substances act in the body and a complete history can be valuable for determining appropriate treatment

    4. Maintain a patent airway; many medications can suppress the CNS and the respiratory center

    5. Position the patient on his or her side and keep suction equipment at the bedside; the side-lying position promotes drainage of secretions, and suction equipment may be needed if the patient vomits

    6. Monitor ABG values as prescribed; changes in ABG values may be the first warning sign of alterations in the respiratory system

    7. Monitor urine output every hour; report outputs that are less than 25 ml/hour or any sudden changes in output; changes in output may indicate impending renal failure or changes in hydration status

8. Monitor and maintain invasive lines, such as those used for central venous pressure and pulmonary artery pressure monitoring, and arterial or subclavian I.V. lines; patients who are treated in the critical care unit often have one or more of these devices in place to maintain hydration and facilitate monitoring

9. Monitor for complications of acetaminophen overdose, including hepatic failure, coagulation defects, renal failure, hepatic encephalopathy, and shock

10. Monitor for complications of salicylate overdose, including respiratory failure, arrhythmias, acid-base imbalances, renal tubular necrosis, GI bleeding, hepatotoxicity, pulmonary edema, and shock

11. Monitor for signs of alcohol toxicity, including respiratory depression, aspiration, hepatic failure, and GI bleeding

12. Monitor for complications of barbiturate overdose, including arrhythmias, respiratory arrest, seizures, pulmonary edema, and shock

13. Monitor for signs of benzodiazepine overdose, including respiratory depression, tachycardia, hypotension, and coma

14. Monitor for cocaine toxicity, which can cause myocardial infarction, tachyarrhythmias, cerebral hemorrhage, respiratory arrest, and status epilepticus

15. Monitor for opioid overdose, which can result in respiratory arrest, arrhythmias, and shock

16. Monitor for complications of tricyclic antidepressant overdose, including arrhythmias, complete heart block, heart failure, paralytic ileus, and shock

17. Initiate and maintain good therapeutic communication with patients who have attempted suicide
    a. After a suicide attempt, many patients feel shame, guilt, hopelessness, and helplessness
    b. Allowing these patients to express their feelings in a noncondemning environment can aid in their recovery

18. Check the environment for items that could be used in future suicide attempts; although most patients do not make another suicide attempt while in the hospital, the critical care unit is not an especially safe place for such patients

Appendix A: Common drugs used in critical care

The following chart identifies drugs by class and summarizes their action, indications, and nursing implications.

COMMON DRUGS	ACTION	INDICATIONS	NURSING IMPLICATIONS
Antihistaminic drugs			
astemizole (Hismanal), azatadine maleate (Optimine), chlorpheniramine maleate (Chlor-Trimeton), diphenhydramine hydrochloride (Benadryl)	These drugs compete with histamines for histamine$_1$-receptor sites.	• Allergies • Pruritus • Sinusitis • Central nervous system (CNS) depression	• Do not administer to a patient with acute asthma. • Use with caution in a patient with lower respiratory tract disease. • Evaluate therapeutic response and intake and output. • Implement oral care for dry mouth. • Know that these drugs may cause urine retention.
Anti-infective drugs			
Antibacterial drugs			
aminoglycosides: amikacin sulfate (Amikin), gentamicin (Garamycin), streptomycin sulfate	Aminoglycosides inhibit protein synthesis in the pathogen.	• Aerobic gram-negative bacilli, bacteremia, peritonitis, and pneumonia	• Assess blood urea nitrogen (BUN) and creatinine levels. • Evaluate therapeutic response. • Monitor for signs and symptoms of superinfection. • Know that these drugs may cause irreversible ototoxicity and nephrotoxicity.
penicillins	Penicillins kill bacteria.	• Respiratory tract infections • Scarlet fever • Otitis media • Pneumonia • Gonorrhea	• Report hematuria to the doctor. • Monitor kidney and liver function test results. • Administer drug on an empty stomach for maximum absorption. • Know that these drugs may cause nausea, vomiting, diarrhea, elevated liver enzyme levels, and superinfection.
Antifungal drugs			
amphotericin B (Fungizone), fluconazole (Diflucan)	Amphotericin B changes cell membrane permeability; fluconazole directly damages the cell membrane phospholipids.	• Severe systemic fungal infections	• Premedicate with anti-inflammatory drugs and antihistamines. • Monitor for immediate hypersensitivity. • Monitor liver enzyme values and intake and output. • Know that these drugs may cause nephrotoxicity, electrolyte imbalances, fever, and weight loss.

(continued)

Common drugs used in critical care *(continued)*

COMMON DRUGS	ACTION	INDICATIONS	NURSING IMPLICATIONS
Anti-infective drugs *(continued)*			
Antiviral drugs			
acyclovir (Zovirax), ganciclovir (Cytovene)	These drugs interfere with viral replication.	• Herpes simplex virus types 1 and 2 • Cytomegalovirus retinitis	• Use with caution in a patient with a history of pancreatitis. • Monitor all laboratory test results carefully. • Administer drug 30 minutes before morning and evening meals. • Know that these drugs may cause blood dyscrasias, coma, arrhythmias, hypotension, and hypertension.
ritonavir (Norvir)	This drug inhibits human immunodeficiency virus (HIV) protease, thereby inhibiting the virus's ability to form functional proteins in infected cells.	Treatment of HIV infection	• Administer the drug with food. • Store the drug in the refrigerator in a light-resistant container. • Use the drug with caution in patients with a history of liver disease. • This drug may cause paresthesia, chest pain, bleeding, hypotension, diarrhea, muscle weakness, seizures, and loss of vision or hearing. • Teach the patient that this drug does not cure the disease or reduce the risk of transmission to others through blood contamination or sexual contact.
saquinavir mesylate (Invirase)	This drug inhibits HIV protease, thereby inhibiting the virus's ability to form functional proteins in infected cells.	Treatment of HIV infection	• Administer this drug within 2 hours of a full meal. • Use with caution in patients with a history of liver disease. • This drug may cause syncope, bleeding, hypotension, abdominal bloating, muscle weakness, seizures, and loss of coordination. • Teach the patient that this drug does not cure the disease or reduce the risk of transmission to others through blood contamination or sexual contact.

Common drugs used in critical care *(continued)*

COMMON DRUGS	ACTION	INDICATIONS	NURSING IMPLICATIONS
Antidote			
flumazenil (Romazicon)	This drug blocks benzodiazepine receptors and antagonizes the actions of benzodiazepine on the CNS.	Complete or partial reversal of the sedative effects of benzodiazepine compounds, including general anesthesia, sedation, and management of overdose	• This drug is most effective if used just after mixing. • Administer the drug through a freely flowing I.V. line in a large vein. • Monitor the patient's level of consciousness during and after administration. Because the half-life of many benzodiazepine drugs is longer than that of flumazenil, resedation may occur in 15 to 30 minutes. • This drug does not reverse the amnesia associated with benzodiazepine drugs. Patient teaching may need to be repeated after surgical procedures. • This drug may cause seizures, headache, dizziness, agitation, emotional lability, blurred vision, vomiting, and injection site pain.
Autonomic drugs			
Parasympathomimetic (cholinergic) drugs			
neostigmine methylsulfate (Prostigmin)	This cholinesterase inhibitor blocks destruction of corticotropin (also known as adrenocorticotropic hormone).	• Myasthenia gravis • Antidote for nondepolarizing neuromuscular blocker overdose • Postoperative abdominal distention and bladder atony	• Monitor vital signs, intake and output, and respiratory pattern. • Know that this drug may cause bradycardia, reflex tachycardia, hypotension, seizures, and bronchospasm.
Anticholinergic drugs			
atropine sulfate	This drug blocks corticotropin at the neuroeffector site, increases cardiac output and heart rate by blocking vagal stimulation, and dries oral secretions.	• Bradyarrhythmias • Suppression of oral secretions • Urine retention • Adjunct treatment of peptic ulcers • Treatment of functional GI disorders	• Do not administer to a patient with acute angle-closure glaucoma, myasthenia gravis, or paralytic ileus. • Use with caution in a patient with heart failure, coronary artery disease, or Down syndrome. • Additive cholinergic effects may occur when this drug is administered concurrently with antiarrhythmic drugs, meperidine, or antiparkinsonian drugs. • Monitor intake and output and electrocardiogram (ECG). • Know that this drug may cause dry mouth, headache, and tachycardia.

(continued)

Common drugs used in critical care *(continued)*

COMMON DRUGS	ACTION	INDICATIONS	NURSING IMPLICATIONS
Autonomic drugs *(continued)*			
Sympathomimetic (adrenergic) drugs			
albuterol (Proventil)	This noncatecholamine relaxes smooth muscle.	• Bronchospasm	• Use with caution in a patient with a cardiovascular disorder, diabetes mellitus, or hyperthyroidism. • Monitor cardiovascular and pulmonary values. • Know that this drug may cause arrhythmias, hypertension, and paradoxical bronchospasm.
dobutamine hydrochloride (Dobutrex)	This catecholamine acts as a beta stimulator and produces a positive inotropic effect.	• Acute heart failure • Coronary bypass graft surgery • Insufficient cardiac output	• Do not administer to a patient with hypertrophic cardiomyopathy. • Use with caution in a patient with a history of hypertension. • Monitor the patient's ECG and blood pressure. • Use a pulmonary artery catheter, if present, to monitor cardiac parameters. • Know that this drug may cause tachycardia and hypertension.
dopamine hydrochloride (Intropin)	A chemical precursor of norepinephrine, this drug has alpha-, beta-, and dopaminergic-receptor stimulating actions. It also dilates renal and mesenteric blood vessels (at low dosages).	• Increased BUN and serum creatinine levels (indicating impending renal failure) • Acute renal failure • Hypotension caused by myocardial infarction (MI), trauma, sepsis, or open-heart surgery • Shock	• Do not administer to a patient with tachyarrhythmias or ventricular fibrillation. • Monitor ECG; monitor blood pressure continuously. • Also monitor hemodynamic parameters, if available. • Know that this drug may cause hypotension and vasoconstriction; vasoconstriction is more likely to occur at doses greater than 10 mcg/kg/minute.
epinephrine (Adrenalin, Bronkaid Mist)	A catecholamine, this drug produces vasoconstriction and dilates bronchial smooth muscles.	• Bronchospasm • Hypotension • Cardiac arrest	• Do not administer to a patient with acute angle-closure glaucoma. • Use with caution in a patient with hyperthyroidism or bronchial asthma. • Monitor hemodynamic variables, including ECG, blood pressure, and fluid status. • Know that this drug may cause hypertension and vasoconstriction-induced tissue sloughing.

Common drugs used in critical care *(continued)*

COMMON DRUGS	ACTION	INDICATIONS	NURSING IMPLICATIONS
Autonomic drugs *(continued)*			
Sympathomimetic (adrenergic) drugs *(continued)*			
isoproterenol (Isuprel)	This catecholamine has positive inotropic and chronotropic effects; it increases atrioventricular (AV) node conduction and relaxes bronchial smooth muscles.	• Asthma and bronchospasm • Heart block • Ventricular arrhythmias	• Do not administer to a patient with digitalis toxicity or preexisting arrhythmias. • Know that this patient requires continuous respiratory and cardiovascular monitoring. • Monitor intake and output. • Know that this drug may cause tachycardia, hypertension, hypotension, bronchial edema and inflammation, and ventricular arrhythmias.
norepinephrine bitartrate (Levophed)	This catecholamine increases cardiac output and heart rate; it also produces vasoconstriction.	• Acute hypotension	• Do not administer to a patient with peripheral vascular thrombosis. • Use with caution in a patient with heart disease. • Monitor the patient's cardiovascular status, central venous pressure, pulmonary artery pressure, and intake and output. • Know that this drug may cause hypertension, arrhythmias, ventricular tachycardia, and ventricular fibrillation.
Sympatholytic (adrenergic-blocking) drugs			
esmolol hydrochloride (Brevibloc)	A beta-adrenergic blocker with antiarrhythmic effects, this drug decreases heart rate, blood pressure, supraventricular tachycardia, and noncompensatory tachycardia.	• Supraventricular tachycardia • Atrial flutter or fibrillation • Hypertension	• Do not administer to a patient with sinus bradycardia or cardiogenic shock. • Use with caution in a patient with bronchospasm or impaired renal function. • Monitor cardiovascular status continuously. • Compare liver and kidney function test results to baseline values, and then monitor liver and kidney function daily. • Know that this drug may cause hypotension.
labetalol hydrochloride (Normodyne)	A beta-adrenergic blocker, this drug decreases blood pressure without producing reflux tachycardia.	• Mild, moderate, or severe hypertension	• Do not administer to a patient with bronchial asthma. • Use with caution in a patient with heart failure, hepatic failure, or preexisting peripheral vascular disease. • Monitor the patient's cardiovascular status and intake and output. • Compare liver and kidney function test results to baseline values, and then monitor liver and kidney function daily.

(continued)

Common drugs used in critical care *(continued)*

COMMON DRUGS	ACTION	INDICATIONS	NURSING IMPLICATIONS
Autonomic drugs (continued)			
Sympatholytic (adrenergic-blocking) drugs (continued)			
labetalol hydrochloride (Normodyne) *(continued)*			• Know that this drug may cause heart failure, ventricular arrhythmias, AV block, hypotension or orthostatic hypotension, dizziness, and peripheral vascular disease.
propranolol hydrochloride (Inderal)	This beta-adrenergic blocker produces antihypertensive and antianginal effects.	• Hypertension • Supraventricular tachycardia • Migraine, vascular headache • Chronic stable angina • Essential tremor	• Compare vital signs with baseline values. • Weigh the patient daily. • Monitor intake and output, liver enzyme levels, and ECG. • Know that this drug may cause bradycardia, bronchospasm, and hypotension.
Skeletal muscle relaxants			
nondepolarizing blocking drugs: atracurium besylate (Tracrium), pancuronium bromide (Pavulon), vecuronium bromide (Norcuron)	These drugs compete with corticotropin at cholinergic receptor sites and prevent the muscle from depolarizing.	• Skeletal muscle relaxation during mechanical ventilation, surgery, or intubation	• Monitor for electrolyte imbalance, which may potentiate the action of these drugs. • Monitor intake and output and vital signs. • Assess motor reflexes regularly. • Administer sedative concurrently when also using a paralytic drug. • Know that these drugs may cause bradycardia or tachycardia, increased or decreased blood pressure, and bronchospasm.
depolarizing blocking drugs: succinylcholine chloride (Anectine)	An ultra-short-acting neuromuscular blocker, this drug inhibits nerve impulse transmission by binding with cholinergic receptor sites.	• Facilitation of intubation • Skeletal muscle relaxation during orthopedic manipulation	• Monitor electrolyte levels and vital signs until the patient has recovered from drug administration. • Know that this drug may cause sinus arrest, bradycardia, hypertension, hypotension, and prolonged apnea.
Hematinic drugs			
Anticoagulant drugs			
heparin	This anticoagulant enhances inhibitory effect of antithrombin III; it prevents clots from enlarging but cannot dissolve already existent clots.	• Deep vein thrombosis • Open-heart surgery • MI • Disseminated intravascular coagulation • Atrial fibrillation with embolization	• Watch for bleeding. • Monitor partial thromboplastin time for therapeutic effect of drug. • Know that this drug may cause hematuria, hemorrhage, and thrombocytopenia.

Common drugs used in critical care *(continued)*

COMMON DRUGS	ACTION	INDICATIONS	NURSING IMPLICATIONS
Hematinic drugs *(continued)*			
Anticoagulant drugs *(continued)*			
warfarin sodium (Coumadin)	An anticoagulant, this drug alters synthesis of vitamin K clotting factors.	• Deep vein thrombosis • Pulmonary emboli	• Monitor for therapeutic prothrombin time. • Know that this drug may cause bleeding, bruising, and allergic response.
Thrombolytic drug			
streptokinase (Streptase)	This thrombolytic drug converts plasminogen to the enzyme plasmin; lysis of thrombin subsequently occurs.	• Deep vein thrombosis • Pulmonary and arterial embolism • Arterial thrombosis • Lysis of coronary artery thrombi after MI	• Be aware that this drug is not effective in managing thrombi over 1 week old. • Monitor cardiovascular, pulmonary, and neurologic status carefully. • Know that this drug may cause bronchospasm, bleeding, and anaphylaxis.
Blood coagulation drugs			
desmopressin acetate (DDAVP)	This drug contains coagulation factor XIII and has antidiuretic properties.	• Hemophilia A • von Willebrand's disease	• Use with caution in a patient with coronary artery disease or hypertension. • Monitor coagulation studies (for continued bleeding), vital signs, and intake and output. • Know that this drug may cause hypertension or hypotension.
protamine sulfate	This antidote binds with heparin, thus making heparin ineffective.	• Postoperative bleeding • Heparin overdose	• Monitor coagulation studies (for continued bleeding) and vital signs. • Know that this drug may cause nausea and vomiting, hypertension, and hypotension.
vitamin K_1 [phytonadione] (AquaMEPHYTON), vitamin K_3 (Synkayvite)	These drugs stimulate hepatic synthesis of clotting factors.	• Hypoprothrombinemia	• Monitor coagulation studies (for indications of continued bleeding) and vital signs. • Know that these drugs may cause bronchospasm, anaphylaxis, and hypotension.
Cardiovascular system drugs			
Antihypertensive drugs			
angiotensin-converting enzyme (ACE) inhibitors: captopril (Capoten), enalapril maleate (Vasotec), ramipril (Altace), lisinopril (Prinivil, Zestril)	ACE inhibitors prevent conversion of angiotensin I to angiotensin II, thus resulting in dilation of arteries and veins.	• Hypertension • Heart failure • Diabetic neuropathy	• Use with caution in a patient with renal insufficiency. • Monitor blood studies, blood pressure, ECG, intake and output, and renal status. • Know that these drugs may cause heart failure and hypotension.

(continued)

Common drugs used in critical care *(continued)*

COMMON DRUGS	ACTION	INDICATIONS	NURSING IMPLICATIONS
Cardiovascular system drugs *(continued)*			
Antihypertensive drugs *(continued)*			
nitroprusside sodium (Nipride)	A vasodilator, this drug directly relaxes arteriolar and venous smooth muscle and decreases afterload and preload.	• Hypertension • To produce controlled hypotension	• Use with caution in a patient with hypothyroidism, hepatic disease, or renal disease. • Monitor thiocyanate levels daily if the patient is on long-term therapy. • Monitor blood pressure and ECG continuously; also monitor pulmonary, kidney, and liver function. • Know that this drug may cause severe hypotension and altered level of consciousness.
Antiarrhythmic drugs			
adenosine (Adenocard)	This drug slows electrical conduction in the AV node and interrupts the reentry circuit.	• Supraventricular tachycardia	• Do not administer to a patient with AV block. • Monitor the patient's ECG and blood pressure. • Know that this drug may cause bronchial constriction and AV block.
bretylium tosylate (Bretylol)	After a transient release of norepinephrine, this drug inhibits further release of norepinephrine, prolongs the action potential, and acts as an antiarrhythmic.	• Supraventricular tachycardia • Ventricular fibrillation	• Use with caution in a patient receiving digitalis glycoside therapy or one with aortic stenosis or pulmonary hypertension. • Monitor the patient's ECG and blood pressure continuously. • Know that this drug may cause hypotension and bradycardia.
lidocaine hydrochloride (Xylocaine)	This antiarrhythmic decreases ventricular excitability and the force of ventricular contraction.	• Premature ventricular contractions • Ventricular tachycardia • Ventricular fibrillation	• Use with caution in a patient with liver or kidney disease. • Monitor ECG and blood pressure. • Watch for change in level of consciousness, which may indicate toxicity. • Know that this drug may cause confusion, hypotension, bradycardia, and anaphylaxis.
procainamide hydrochloride (Procan SR)	An antiarrhythmic that depresses electrical stimulation and slows conduction.	• Life-threatening ventricular arrhythmias	• Monitor ECG (especially length of PR interval and QRS complex), blood pressure, electrolyte status, and serum drug level. • Know that this drug may cause heart block, systemic lupus erythematosus, and ventricular arrhythmias.

Common drugs used in critical care *(continued)*

COMMON DRUGS	ACTION	INDICATIONS	NURSING IMPLICATIONS
Cardiovascular system drugs *(continued)*			
Antiarrhythmic drugs *(continued)*			
quinidine	This antiarrhythmic decreases myocardial excitability.	• Atrial fibrillation • Atrial flutter • Ventricular tachycardia • Paroxysmal atrial tachycardia • Premature ventricular contractions	• Monitor ECG (especially length of PR interval and QRS complex), blood pressure, electrolyte status, and serum drug level. • Know that this drug may cause heart block, cardiovascular collapse, thrombocytopenia, and respiratory depression.
Digitalis glycosides and bipyridines			
amrinone lactate (Inocor)	A positive inotropic drug that reduces preload and afterload by causing vasodilation.	• Heart failure	• Know that this patient requires continuous monitoring of cardiovascular and pulmonary status. • Monitor electrolyte status and renal function. • Know that this drug may cause thrombocytopenia, hepatotoxicity, arrhythmias, and hypotension.
digoxin (Lanoxin)	This digitalis glycoside has positive inotropic, negative chronotropic, and negative dromotropic effects.	• Heart failure • Atrial fibrillation • Atrial flutter • Atrial tachycardia	• Withhold drug and notify the doctor if patient's apical pulse is less than 60 beats/minute. • Monitor electrolyte status, serum digoxin level, and intake and output. • Know that this drug may cause heart block, hypotension, arrhythmias, and blurred vision.
Antianginal drugs			
calcium channel blockers: diltiazem hydrochloride (Cardizem), nifedipine (Procardia), verapamil hydrochloride (Isoptin)	These drugs produce coronary vascular smooth-muscle relaxation and slow sinoatrial (SA) and AV node conduction and dilate arteries.	• Angina • Hypertension	• Use with caution in a patient with heart failure. • Monitor electrolyte balance, ECG, blood pressure, and intake and output. • Know that these drugs may cause heart failure, arrhythmias, hypotension, and AV block.
nitroglycerin (Nitro-Bid, Nitrostat)	This coronary vasodilator decreases preload.	• Angina • Heart failure caused by an MI • To produce controlled hypotension	• Monitor blood pressure, ECG, and pulse rate. • Know that this drug may cause postural hypotension, tachycardia, and headache.

(continued)

Common drugs used in critical care *(continued)*

COMMON DRUGS	ACTION	INDICATIONS	NURSING IMPLICATIONS
Central nervous system drugs			
Analgesic and antipyretic drugs			
nonsteroidal anti-inflamma-tory drugs: ibuprofen (Motrin), indomethacin (Indocin), naproxen (Naprosyn)	These drugs produce an anti-inflammatory effect by way of inhibition of pros-taglandin activity.	• Analgesia • Fever • Rheumatoid arthritis • Acute gouty arthritis	• Assess renal, hepatic, and blood studies. • Administer with food to decrease GI upset. • Report blurred vision or tinnitus to the doc-tor immediately. • Know that the most common adverse reac-tions to these drugs include GI disturbances and hepatotoxicity.
para-aminophenol deriva-tives: acetaminophen (Tylenol)	Acetaminophen produces analgesic effect by way of inhibition of prostaglandin synthesis; its antipyretic action results from inhibi-tion of hypothalamic heat regulation center.	• Pain • Fever	• Monitor liver function test results. • Know that this drug may cause hepatotoxic-ity and anemia.
salicylates: acetylsalicylic acid (aspirin)	Aspirin produces analgesic and anti-inflammatory ef-fects by way of inhibition of prostaglandin synthesis; its antipyretic effect results from stimulation of the hypothalamus, which leads to vasodilation and in-creased diaphoresis. It also inhibits platelet aggrega-tion.	• Pain • Fever • Thromboembolic disor-ders • Transient ischemic at-tacks • Post-MI	• Report tinnitus to the doctor immediately. • Monitor liver function test results. • Know that this drug may cause GI bleeding, thrombocytopenia, and bruising. • Administer with food to decrease GI symp-toms.
Opioid agonists			
codeine, fentanyl citrate (Sublimaze), hydromor-phone hydrochloride (Dilaudid), meperidine (Demerol), morphine sulfate (Duramorph PF), oxycodone hydrochloride (Percodan, Percocet), sufentanil citrate (Sufenta)	These drugs reduce pain by depressing nerve im-pulse transmission in the spinal cord level by way of interaction with opioid re-ceptors.	• Severe pain • Antitussive therapy (co-deine, hydromorphone hy-drochloride) • Preanesthesia and pri-mary anesthesia (fentanyl citrate, sufentanil citrate)	• Monitor for CNS changes and changes in respiratory or cardiovascular function. • Evaluate pain level, using a quantitative scale. • Know that these drugs may cause respira-tory depression, drowsiness, bradycardia, change in blood pressure, and constipation.

Common drugs used in critical care *(continued)*

COMMON DRUGS	ACTION	INDICATIONS	NURSING IMPLICATIONS
Central nervous system drugs *(continued)*			
Opioid antagonists			
naloxone hydrochloride (Narcan), naltrexone hydrochloride (Trexan)	These drugs occupy opioid receptor sites and displace narcotic drug molecules.	• Narcotic drug overdose • Reversal of narcotic-induced respiratory depression • Sedation	• Monitor respiratory and cardiovascular status closely after drug administration because of its short half-life. • Know that these drugs may cause nausea, vomiting, hypertension, and tachycardia.
Anticonvulsants			
barbiturates: phenobarbital (Luminal)	Barbiturates limit seizure activity by increasing the threshold for motor cortex stimuli.	• Status epilepticus • Epilepsy • Partial, generalized tonic clonic, and febrile seizures	• Evaluate for respiratory depression and blood dyscrasias. • Monitor liver function test results. • Know that this drug may cause drowsiness, nausea, and vomiting. When this drug is administered I.V., it also may cause laryngospasm, respiratory depression, and hypotension.
benzodiazepines: diazepam (Valium)	Its anticonvulsant effect may be secondary to increasing availability of the inhibitory neurotransmitter gamma-aminobutyric acid to neurons in the brain.	• Acute status epilepticus • Sedation • Confusion	• Monitor cardiac and respiratory status and liver function test results. • Know that this drug may cause cardiorespiratory depression.
hydantoins: phenytoin (Dilantin)	This hydantoin acts in the motor cortex to stabilize the nerve cells against hyperexcitability and inhibit seizure activity.	• Complex, partial, and generalized tonic-clonic seizures • Status epilepticus	• Monitor serum drug level, blood studies, and pulmonary and cardiovascular status. • Administer drug in normal saline solution at a rate of no more than 50 mg/minute. • Know that this drug may cause blood dyscrasias, hypotension, ventricular fibrillation, nausea, and vomiting.
magnesium sulfate	This drug controls seizures by blocking their transmission.	• Preeclampsia and eclampsia • Hypomagnesemic seizures • Paroxysmal atrial tachycardia • Ventricular arrhythmias	• Carefully monitor cardiovascular and pulmonary status and serum magnesium level. • Watch for depressed reflexes. • Know that this drug may cause hypotension, heart block, decreased cardiac function, and paralysis.

(continued)

Common drugs used in critical care *(continued)*

COMMON DRUGS	ACTION	INDICATIONS	NURSING IMPLICATIONS
Central nervous system drugs *(continued)*			
Psychotherapeutic drugs			
haloperidol (Haldol)	It blocks dopamine receptor sites.	• Psychotic disorders • Sedation	• Assess therapeutic response, level of consciousness, and cardiovascular status. • Know that this drug may cause extrapyramidal symptoms, hypotension, and tardive dyskinesia.
Anxiolytic, sedative, and hypnotic drugs			
barbiturates: pentobarbital sodium (Nembutal Sodium), phenobarbital (Luminal), secobarbital sodium (Seconal Sodium)	These drugs depress activity in the reticular activating system, which is located in the brain stem.	• Insomnia • Sedation • Preoperative medication • Increased intracranial pressure	• Use with caution in a patient with hypotension. • Monitor blood studies as well as cardiovascular, pulmonary, and neurologic status closely; immediately report any changes to the doctor. • Know that these drugs may cause altered level of consciousness, respiratory depression, and blood dyscrasias.
benzodiazepines: diazepam (Valium), lorazepam (Ativan), midazolam (Versed)	Benzodiazepines depress subcortical levels in the CNS; they may act on the limbic system and reticular formation.	• Sedation • Induction of general anesthesia • Hypnosis • Reduction of anxiety	• Use with caution in a patient with chronic obstructive pulmonary disease or chronic renal failure. • Monitor pulmonary and cardiovascular status; assess for therapeutic response. • Know that these drugs may cause bronchospasm, nausea, vomiting, and hypotension.
Cytoprotective drugs			
amifostine (Ethyol)	This drug protects normal tissues from cisplatin toxicity by binding to cisplatin metabolites and free radicals.	• Renal toxicity in patients who are receiving cisplatin for malignancies, including ovarian cancer.	• This drug must be diluted with normal saline solution before administration. • Infuse over 15 minutes or less. • If the patient develops severe hypotension (the major adverse effect), the medication should be stopped and the blood pressure stabilized with positioning and a fluid bolus. • Know that this medication also may cause loss of consciousness, somnolence, nausea, vomiting, hiccups, and hypocalcemia.

Common drugs used in critical care *(continued)*

COMMON DRUGS	ACTION	INDICATIONS	NURSING IMPLICATIONS
Electrolyte replacement drugs			
calcium chloride	It replaces calcium (the major cation in extracellular fluid [ECF]), which is necessary for normal maintenance of nervous, muscular, skeletal, and cardiac contractility; coagulation of blood; maintenance of enzymatic reactions; and endocrine and exocrine function.	• Acute hypocalcemia • Magnesium intoxication • Strengthening of myocardial tissue after defibrillation • Cardiac resuscitation (for positive inotropic effect)	• Infuse drug slowly, according to institutional protocol, to avoid phlebitis and necrosis. • Infuse into a central I.V. line only. • Monitor ECG (especially Q and T waves), therapeutic response, and signs and symptoms of hypercalcemia. • Know that this drug may cause arrhythmias and hypercalcemia (with signs and symptoms including drowsiness, lethargy, muscle weakness, cardiac arrest, and arrhythmias).
magnesium sulfate	This drug replaces magnesium (a common cation in intracellular fluid [ICF]); it reduces SA node conduction time in the myocardium and decreases corticotropin in the motor nerve terminals.	• Hypomagnesemia secondary to malabsorption syndrome, chronic diarrhea, prolonged diuretic therapy, or nasogastric tube suctioning • Seizures caused by hypomagnesemia	• Infuse at a rate no more than 150 mg/minute. • Monitor ECG and serum magnesium level (for hypermagnesemia). • Know that this drug may cause hypotension, decreased cardiac function, heart block, and depressed reflexes or paralysis.
potassium chloride (Kaochlor)	This drug replaces potassium (a major cation in the ICF), which is necessary for adequate transmission of nerve impulses and cardiac contraction.	• Prevention of hypokalemia and its life-threatening sequelae • Reduction of toxic effects resulting from digitalis glycoside therapy	• Know that this drug may cause hyperkalemia (with signs and symptoms including listlessness, confusion, and paralysis), phlebitis, ECG changes, heart block, and cardiac arrest. • To prevent phlebitis, administer drug in a central I.V. line at a rate no more than 20 mEq/50 ml/hour. • Monitor the patient's ECG.
3% sodium chloride solution, 5% sodium chloride solution	These solutions replace sodium (the major cation in ECF), which is necessary to maintain osmotic pressure, acid-base balance, and water balance.	• Excessive GI losses, such as from perspiration or water intoxication • Hyponatremia	• Use with caution in a patient with renal or hepatic dysfunction. • Correct sodium imbalance slowly. • Assess for changes in level of consciousness and balanced intake and output, and monitor electrolyte status. • Know that these solutions may cause hypernatremia with sequelae as well as heart failure.

(continued)

Common drugs used in critical care *(continued)*

COMMON DRUGS	ACTION	INDICATIONS	NURSING IMPLICATIONS
Gastrointestinal system drugs			
antacids: aluminum hydroxide (Amphojel), aluminum hydroxide and magnesium hydroxide (Maalox), aluminum-magnesium complex and simethicone (Riopan)	Antacids neutralize approximately 90% of gastric acid, thus increasing the pH and decreasing the amount of pepsin.	• Esophageal reflux • Acid indigestion • Heartburn • Dyspepsia • Severe stress in critically ill patients	• Monitor electrolyte status. • Know that these drugs may cause diarrhea, constipation, hyperaluminemia, hypermagnesemia, and hypophosphatemia. • Administer stool softeners if constipation occurs.
antiulcer drugs (histamine-2 [H_2]-receptor antagonists): cimetidine (Tagamet), famotidine (Pepcid), ranitidine hydrochloride (Zantac)	These drugs inhibit histamine at H_2-receptor sites in the parietal cells, thus inhibiting gastric acid secretion.	• Gastric or duodenal ulcer • Hypersecretory conditions • Stress ulcer	• Monitor intake and output, kidney and liver function, and gastric pH. • Know that these drugs may cause altered level of consciousness, hepatotoxicity, and blood dyscrasias.
sucralfate (Carafate)	This antiulcer drug forms a complex that adheres to the ulcer site and protects it from gastric acid, pepsin, and bile erosion.	• Duodenal ulcer	• Monitor gastric pH. • Know that this drug may cause drowsiness, nausea, vomiting, and pruritus. • Teach the patient (and family) that the patient should avoid caffeine, alcohol, and spicy foods.
Smooth-muscle relaxants			
bronchodilators: aminophylline (Aminophyllin, Phyllocontin)	These drugs relax the smooth muscle of the respiratory system by blocking phosphodiesterase, which increases cyclic adenosine monophosphate production.	• Bronchial asthma • Bronchospasm	• Monitor serum drug levels, ECG, and intake and output. • Assess for signs of drug toxicity. • Know that these drugs may cause anxiety, restlessness, palpitations, sinus tachycardia, hypotension, tachypnea, nausea, and vomiting.
Immunosuppressant drugs			
mycophenolate mofetil (CellCept)	Although its exact mechanism is unknown, the drug generally inhibits immune-mediated inflammatory responses.	• Prevention of organ transplant rejection in patients with allogenic kidney transplants	• If possible, administer the drug on an empty stomach with a full glass of water. • Assess the patient for signs of infection, bleeding, or bruising. • Monitor the transplanted organ for rejection. • Have the patient avoid contact with people who have an infection. • Know that this medication may cause tremor, headaches, diarrhea, hypertension, nausea, and low urine output.

Common drugs used in critical care *(continued)*

COMMON DRUGS	ACTION	INDICATIONS	NURSING IMPLICATIONS
Immunosuppressant drugs *(continued)*			
tacrolimus (FK506, Prograf)	This drug suppresses cell-mediated reactions and some types of humoral immunity.	• Prevention of organ rejection in patients receiving allogenic liver transplants.	• Dilute the drug with normal saline solution or dextrose 5% in water before using. • Do not store this drug in polyvinyl chloride container. • Do not use this medication simultaneously with cyclosporine. Use it only with steroids. • Assess the patient for signs of infection, bleeding, or bruising. • Monitor the transplanted organ for rejection. • Have the patient avoid contact with people who have an infection. • Know that this medication may cause tremor, headaches, diarrhea, hypertension, nausea, and low urine output.

Appendix B: ABG practice test

7.35-7.45

pH

PaO2 80-100

PaCO2 35-45

HCO3 22-26

Are you an expert at analyzing abnormal arterial blood gas (ABG) values and identifying their clinical significance? Take this short test to find out.

Keeping in mind the normal ABG values (pH, 7.35 to 7.45; PaO_2, 80 to 100 mm Hg; $PaCO_2$, 35 to 45 mm Hg; HCO_3^-, 22 to 26 mEq/L), analyze the following values and write your interpretation in the space to the right. Correct answers appear after the test.

	pH	PaO_2 (mm Hg)	$PaCO_2$ (mm Hg)	HCO_3^- (mEq/L)	Interpretation
1.	7.31	78	49	25	Resp acidosis
2.	7.39	49	41	25	Severe hypoxia
3.	7.30	109	50	22	Resp acidosis c̄ hyperoxia
4.	7.16	52	75	24	Resp acidosis c̄ mod hypoxia
5.	7.41	62	27	17	Comp Resp Alk
6.	7.42	67	55	36	
7.	7.36	43	22	10	
8.	7.65	354	25	36	
9.	7.39	80	39	24	
10.	7.44	63	33	22	
11.	7.40	71	37	23	
12.	7.13	111	22	7	
13.	7.44	61	36	24	
14.	7.47	62	32	23	
15.	7.55	106	32	28	
16.	7.15	46	114	7	
17.	7.11	88	40	17	
18.	7.44	99	60	36	
19.	7.38	44	22	14	
20.	7.6	123	21	26	

ABG practice test *(continued)*

Answers
1. Respiratory acidosis
2. Severe hypoxia
3. Respiratory acidosis with hyperoxia
4. Respiratory acidosis with moderate hypoxia
5. Compensated respiratory alkalosis with mild hypoxia
6. Compensated metabolic alkalosis with mild hypoxia
7. Compensated metabolic acidosis with severe hypoxia
8. Combined metabolic and respiratory alkalosis with hyperoxia
9. Normal
10. Respiratory alkalosis with mild hypoxia
11. Mild hypoxia
12. Metabolic acidosis with hyperoxia
13. Mild hypoxia
14. Respiratory alkalosis with mild hypoxia
15. Combined respiratory and metabolic alkalosis with hyperoxia
16. Combined respiratory and metabolic alkalosis with severe hypoxia
17. Metabolic acidosis
18. Compensated metabolic alkalosis
19. Compensated metabolic acidosis with severe hypoxia
20. Respiratory alkalosis with hyperoxia

Posttest #1

After you complete the posttest, or after the 50-minute time limit expires, check your responses against the correct answers and rationales provided on pages 274 to 281.

Instructions

This posttest has been designed to evaluate your readiness to take the certification examination for critical care nursing. Similar in form and content to the actual examination, the posttest consists of 50 questions based on brief clinical situations. The questions will help sharpen your test-taking skills while assessing your knowledge of critical care nursing theory and practice.

You will have 50 minutes to complete the posttest. To improve your chances for performing well, consider these suggestions:

• Read each clinical situation closely. Weigh the four options carefully, and then select the option that best answers the question. (*Note:* In this posttest, options are lettered A, B, C, and D to aid in later identification of correct answers and rationales. These letters do not appear on the certification examination.)

• Completely darken the circle in front of the answer that you select, using a #2 pencil. (You must use a #2 pencil when taking the certification examination.) Do not use check marks, Xs, or lines.

• If you decide to change your answer, erase the old answer completely. (The certification examination is scored electronically; an incomplete erasure may cause both answers to be scored, in which case you will not receive credit for answering the question.)

• If you have difficulty understanding a question or are unsure of the answer, place a small mark next to the question number and, if time permits, return to it later. If you have no idea of the correct answer, make an educated guess. (Only correct answers are counted in scoring the certification examination, so guessing is preferable to leaving a question unanswered.)

After you complete the posttest, or after the 50-minute time limit expires, check your responses against the correct answers and rationales provided on pages 274 to 281.

Now, select a quiet room where you will be undisturbed, set a timer for 50 minutes, and begin.

Questions

1. A patient is admitted to the surgical intensive care unit (ICU) with a suspected bowel obstruction. In performing the initial assessment, the nurse knows that auscultation of the abdomen:

   ○ **A.** Should be performed after palpation

   ○ **B.** Is best done with the bell of the stethoscope

   ○ **C.** Should reveal hyperactive sounds above the obstruction and absent sounds below the obstruction

   ○ **D.** Should be performed after percussion

2. A 36-year-old man who has had hypertension for 4 years was brought by family members to the emergency department. The patient complains of chest pain that is unrelieved by nitroglycerin. He states that he has had the pain for 3 hours and rates the pain as an 8 on a scale of 1 to 10. His vital signs are blood pressure 178/98 mm Hg, heart rate 116 beats minute, respiratory rate 26 breaths/minute, and temperature 98.9° F (37.1° C). A 12-lead ECG shows an elevated ST segment. The medical diagnosis is myocardial infarction (MI). The doctor orders Benadryl 25 mg I.V., nitroglycerin I.V. infusion titrated to a systolic blood pressure of 90 mm Hg and pain relief, lidocaine bolus of 100 mg I.V. followed by a lidocaine I.V. infusion of 1 mg/minute, streptokinase 1.5 million IU I.V. to run over 1 hour followed by a heparin I.V. infusion to run at 1,000 U/hour, and morphine sulfate 2 to 4 mg slow I.V. push every 2 to 4 hours as needed for chest pain. Which of the following indicates that the streptokinase therapy is effective?

   ○ **A.** Prothrombin time–partial thromboplastin time ratio (PT/PTT) 2.5 times greater than normal

   ○ **B.** Relief of chest pain

   ○ **C.** Few premature ventricular contractions and a return of the ST segment to normal

   ○ **D.** Blood pressure 120/85 mm Hg and heart rate 86 beats/minute

3. During an initial assessment, the nurse notices that the patient's arterial systolic blood pressure decreases by 14 mm Hg on inspiration. When documenting this change, the nurse should note this drop as:

   ○ **A.** Pulsus magnus

   ○ **B.** Pulsus alternans

   ○ **C.** Pulsus parvus

   ○ **D.** Pulsus paradoxus

4. A patient is admitted to the emergency department. He is unconscious, and the nurse suspects an upper airway obstruction. What is the best initial action for the nurse to take?

   ○ **A.** Perform deep tracheal suctioning

   ○ **B.** Begin mechanical ventilation

   ○ **C.** Tilt the patient's head and do a chin lift

   ○ **D.** Perform 6 to 10 upward abdominal thrusts

5. A 67-year-old woman is admitted to the ICU in a severely obtunded state. She withdraws from painful stimuli and exhibits random movement of all extremities. The admitting laboratory values are potassium 4.6 mEq/L, sodium 135 mEq/L, hematocrit 46%, blood urea nitrogen (BUN)-creatinine ratio 46:2.1, and plasma glucose 1,099 mg/dl. Arterial blood gas (ABG) values include pH 7.31, partial pressure of oxygen (Pao$_2$) 92 mm Hg, partial pressure of arterial carbon dioxide (Paco$_2$) 30 mm Hg, and HCO$_3^-$ 20 mEq/L. A medical diagnosis of hyperosmolar hyperglycemic nonketotic syndrome (HHNS) is made. Which underlying diagnosis places the patient at greatest risk for developing HHNS?

○ **A.** Insulin-dependent (type I) diabetes mellitus

○ **B.** Non-insulin-dependent (type II) diabetes mellitus

○ **C.** Long-term exogenous corticosteroid use

○ **D.** Chronic renal failure

6. A female patient is placed on oxygen delivered by way of nasal cannula at a rate of 5 L/minute with orders for repeat ABG sampling and serum glucose and electrolyte measurements in 1 hour. Urine output has dropped to 30 ml for the past hour, and the patient's current blood pressure is 94/48 mm Hg. Which of the following interventions should the nurse plan for this patient?

○ **A.** Potent diuretic therapy to increase urine flow

○ **B.** Administration of large volumes of I.V. hypertonic solutions to increase urine flow

○ **C.** Administration of large volumes of I.V. isotonic solutions, hypotonic solutions, or plasma expanders to increase circulating volume

○ **D.** Administration of large volumes of hypotonic solutions to reverse hyperosmolality

7. A 66-year-old woman is transferred to the ICU from the surgery unit after developing disseminated intravascular coagulation (DIC). The nurse develops a plan of care, knowing that the care of a patient with a bleeding disorder usually includes:

○ **A.** Close monitoring of body temperature

○ **B.** Ambulation twice daily

○ **C.** Strict bed rest

○ **D.** Avoidance of blood products that may cause reactions

8. A 55-year-old man with chest pain is admitted to the emergency department. On the 12-lead ECG, the emergency department nurse notes ST-segment elevation and large Q waves in leads II, III, and aV_F and ST-segment depression in leads I and aV_L. What is the diagnosis?

   ○ **A.** Attack of angina

   ○ **B.** Normal ECG

   ○ **C.** Inferior wall MI

   ○ **D.** Subendocardial MI

9. A woman is admitted to the ICU with a diagnosis of DIC after a serious automobile accident. Which nursing diagnosis would have the highest priority for this patient?

   ○ **A.** Impaired skin integrity related to immobility

   ○ **B.** Anxiety related to fear of dying

   ○ **C.** Fluid volume deficit related to excessive bleeding

   ○ **D.** Impaired gas exchange related to bleeding in the lungs

10. A 38-year-old man is admitted to the ICU with a diagnosis of acute pancreatitis. When assessing his condition, the nurse notes that he has a positive Trousseau's sign. This sign is associated with what condition?

    ○ **A.** Hyperglycemia

    ○ **B.** Hypoglycemia

    ○ **C.** Hypercalcemia

    ○ **D.** Hypocalcemia

11. A woman is admitted to the ICU with a diagnosis of hepatic coma. She is lethargic and responds only to painful stimuli. Which therapy would most likely be used to lower her serum ammonia level?

    ○ **A.** Provide a high-protein diet and increase fluid intake

    ○ **B.** Administer lactulose and neomycin

    ○ **C.** Administer opioid analgesics and sedatives

    ○ **D.** Administer digoxin (Lanoxin) and furosemide (Lasix)

12. A patient is diagnosed with acute transmural MI. While analyzing the patient's ECG strip, the nurse would find that the ST segment is:

    ○ **A.** Isoelectric

    ○ **B.** Elevated

    ○ **C.** Prolonged

    ○ **D.** Depressed

13. A patient's ECG pattern changed from sinus rhythm, rate 80, to junctional escape rhythm, rate 46. Of the following medications available to the nurse, which would be the most appropriate to use to correct this pattern change?

○ **A.** Digoxin (Lanoxin) 0.25 mg I.V.

○ **B.** Atropine sulfate 1 mg I.V.

○ **C.** Lidocaine 100 mg I.V.

○ **D.** Verapamil 60 mg P.O.

14. A 78-year-old man with a diagnosis of dementia who has just undergone lung resection is admitted to the surgical ICU. He is intubated, connected to a mechanical ventilator, and agitated. His vital signs are blood pressure 158/96 mm Hg, heart rate 135 beats/minute, respiratory rate 40 breaths/minute, and temperature 97.8° F (36.5° C). The ventilator settings are fraction of inspired oxygen (FIO_2) 0.40, synchronized intermittent mandatory ventilation 8, and tidal volume 800 ml. Other assessment data include pH 7.5, $PaCO_2$ 30 mm Hg, PaO_2 80 mm Hg, HCO_3^- 24 mEq/L, and arterial oxygen saturation (SaO_2) 94%. Vecuronium, a nondepolarizing neuromuscular blocker, is prescribed to induce skeletal muscle relaxation during ventilation and to decrease oxygen consumption. What other medication would the nurse expect to administer in conjunction with vecuronium?

○ **A.** Adenosine

○ **B.** Neostigmine

○ **C.** Diazepam

○ **D.** Furosemide

15. A patient is admitted with actively bleeding duodenal ulcers. What is the most important goal of treatment for this condition?

○ **A.** Stabilizing the patient to prepare for surgery as soon as possible

○ **B.** Administering I.V. vasopressin to decrease blood flow to the area

○ **C.** Replacing fluid volume loss to prevent shock

○ **D.** Administering I.V. histamine inhibitors to decrease the acid level

16. A 22-year-old man knocked a pot of hot water off the kitchen table and burned his abdomen and legs. He calls the hospital hot line. What should the nurse advise this patient to do first?

○ **A.** Take acetaminophen to relieve the pain

○ **B.** Note the extent and depth of the burn

○ **C.** Wet the burned area with cold water

○ **D.** Immediately go to the emergency department

17. A rhythm strip from a patient's ECG shows the following pattern:

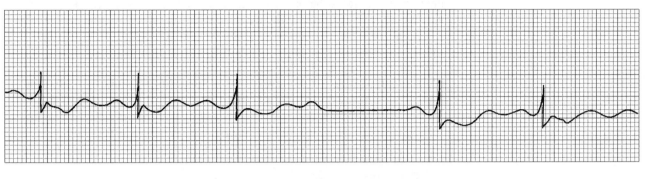

How should the nurse interpret this pattern?

- ○ **A.** Sinus bradycardia
- ○ **B.** Junctional escape rhythm
- ○ **C.** Second-degree atrioventricular (AV) block, Mobitz type II
- ○ **D.** Ventricular escape rhythm

18. A man is admitted to the ICU with acute MI. Which nursing goal would have the highest priority in planning the patient's care?

- ○ **A.** Maintain normal fluid and electrolyte balance
- ○ **B.** Maintain adequate nutrition
- ○ **C.** Prevent invasive infections
- ○ **D.** Provide physical and psychological rest

19. A patient with DIC has a severe reaction to a unit of packed cells and develops a humoral immunity. The nurse knows that humoral immunity:

- ○ **A.** Is produced by T-cell activity
- ○ **B.** Involves immunoglobulins
- ○ **C.** Only occurs in anaphylactic reactions
- ○ **D.** Involves the thymus

20. A man attending a stressful business meeting complains of severe substernal chest pain. He rates the pain as a 12 on a scale of 1 to 10. After his third sublingual nitroglycerin tablet, the man states that his pain has decreased to a 3. Vital signs are blood pressure 146/90 mm Hg, heart rate 113 beats/minute, respiratory rate 28 breaths/minute, and temperature 98.6° F (37° C). The patient is admitted to the cardiac care unit to rule out MI. Orders include creatine kinase (CK) level every 6 hours for 24 hours, nitroglycerin I.V. infusion titrated for relief of pain, Colace 100 mg/day, oxygen at 2 L by way of nasal cannula, and one enteric-coated aspirin every day. The monitoring of which vital sign should receive the highest priority?

○ **A.** Blood pressure

○ **B.** Heart rate

○ **C.** Respiratory rate

○ **D.** Temperature

21. A man who is having continuous, seizurelike movements is brought to the emergency department by the police. The patient has no identification, and his history is unknown. Which medication should the nurse administer first?

○ **A.** Naloxone

○ **B.** Sodium bicarbonate

○ **C.** Glucose

○ **D.** Diazepam

22. A patient in the ICU is intubated and connected to a mechanical ventilator. She becomes extremely anxious, and the pressure alarm sounds with each inspiration. What is the best nursing intervention for this situation?

○ **A.** Increase the tidal volume

○ **B.** Increase the oxygen concentration

○ **C.** Disconnect the ventilator and manually ventilate the patient using a ventilator bag for a few breaths

○ **D.** Administer the prescribed diazepam or morphine sulfate as needed

23. A patient is admitted to the ICU with a diagnosis of acute upper GI bleeding. Which nursing diagnosis would have the highest priority?

○ **A.** Fluid volume deficit related to bleeding

○ **B.** Impaired tissue integrity related to mucosal damage

○ **C.** Sensory or perceptual alterations related to increasedblood ammonia levels

○ **D.** Anxiety related to critical illness

24. Which laboratory values are most consistent with a medical diagnosis of HHNS?

   ○ **A.** Glucose 600 mg/dl, plasma osmolality 300 mOsm/kg, serum potassium 4.2 mEq/L

   ○ **B.** Glucose 800 mg/dl, plasma osmolality 365 mOsm/kg, pH 7.3

   ○ **C.** Glucose 450 mg/dl, pH 7.2, potassium 5.2 mEq/L

   ○ **D.** Glucose 600 mg/dl, pH 7.2, anion gap 16

25. A patient in the ICU has just undergone surgery to remove a large brain tumor. He is attached to an intracranial pressure (ICP) monitoring system using a subarachnoid screw. What is the most important nursing responsibility when caring for this patient?

   ○ **A.** Periodically obtain samples of cerebrospinal fluid

   ○ **B.** Keep the transducer below the level of the foramen of Monro

   ○ **C.** Open the system to air to zero-balance it

   ○ **D.** Use a continuous low-flow flush device to maintain patency

26. A 50-year-old woman began having chest pains at midnight. It is now 6 a.m., and she is in the emergency department having a blood sample drawn to measure enzyme levels. Which of the following laboratory values would be elevated if the patient had had an MI?

   ○ **A.** CK

   ○ **B.** Lactate dehydrogenase (LD)

   ○ **C.** Aspartate aminotransferase (AST)

   ○ **D.** Alanine aminotransferase (ALT)

27. A 47-year-old woman is admitted to the ICU with a diagnosis of syndrome of inappropriate antidiuretic hormone (SIADH) after treatment for oat cell adenocarcinoma of the lung. What is the most likely reason for the onset of SIADH in this patient?

   ○ **A.** Ectopic secretion of antidiuretic hormone (ADH) by the tumor cells

   ○ **B.** Ingestion of large amounts of water after chemotherapy

   ○ **C.** Inappropriate secretion of ADH by the posterior pituitary gland secondary to the prolonged nausea and vomiting caused by chemotherapy

   ○ **D.** Diminished ADH secretion secondary to brain metastasis

28. Laboratory values for a patient with SIADH would most likely reflect which of the following?

○ **A.** Elevated serum sodium level, decreased urine osmolality, and elevated plasma osmolality

○ **B.** Decreased serum sodium level, decreased urine sodium level, and elevated plasma osmolality

○ **C.** Decreased serum sodium level, elevated urine sodium level, and elevated urine osmolality

○ **D.** Elevated serum sodium level, elevated urine sodium level, and elevated urine specific gravity

29. A patient with DIC is receiving I.V. albumin. The nurse knows that albumin:

○ **A.** Is isotonic

○ **B.** Decreases the intravascular volume

○ **C.** Increases the interstitial volume

○ **D.** Increases the intravascular volume

30. A 34-year-old man is admitted to the ICU with severe respiratory difficulty and a diagnosis of *Pneumocystis carinii* pneumonia secondary to AIDS. Which of the following is the most important factor in planning the patient's care?

○ **A.** Pacing nursing care to avoid patient fatigue

○ **B.** Placing an "HIV positive" sign on the door so that laboratory and nursing personnel take appropriate precautions when handling blood and body fluids

○ **C.** Ensuring that the patient wears a mask and gloves outside the room to prevent the spread of infection

○ **D.** Restricting visitors to the immediate family to prevent contamination

31. A patient is admitted to the ICU with a blood pressure of 76/38 and a diagnosis of septic shock. Which assessment finding would best confirm this diagnosis?

○ **A.** Hot, dry skin with poor skin turgor

○ **B.** ABG analysis revealing metabolic alkalosis

○ **C.** Temperature of 105° F (40.6° C) and a pulse rate of 122 beats/minute

○ **D.** Urine output of 30 ml/hour and central venous pressure of 8 cm H_2O

32. A patient with head trauma is admitted to the ICU for observation and exhibits the following signs: decreased level of consciousness, altered respiratory pattern with frequent yawns, small but reactive pupils, and positive bilateral Babinski's reflex. Shortly after admission, Cheyne-Stokes respirations, decorticate posturing, and coma occur. What is the most likely cause of this deterioration?

  ○ **A.** Uncal herniation

  ○ **B.** Central herniation

  ○ **C.** Transcranial herniation

  ○ **D.** Nucleus pulposus herniation

33. For a patient with an acute, uncomplicated MI, the nurse should question which of the following doctor's orders?

  ○ **A.** Morphine 5 mg I.V. push every 2 hours p.r.n. for chest pain

  ○ **B.** Isoproterenol (Isuprel) infusion at 20 mcg/minute

  ○ **C.** Heparin 5,000 units S.C. every 12 hours

  ○ **D.** Diltiazem (Cardizem) 60 mg P.O. every 8 hours

34. A 53-year-old woman with a history of coronary artery disease and alcohol abuse is in the ICU with a diagnosis of bleeding esophageal varices. Her vital signs are blood pressure 105/60 mm Hg, heart rate 130 beats/minute, respiratory rate 28 breaths/minute, and temperature 98° F (36.6° C). Significant laboratory values are hemoglobin 8 g/dl and hematocrit 26%. Burgundy-colored aspirate appears in the nasogastric (NG) tube. The patient is receiving cimetidine I.V. at a rate of 42 ml/hour and dextrose 5% in water in combination with normal saline solution and 20 mEq potassium chloride I.V. at a rate of 150 ml/hour. After 1 hour, the nurse notices that NG tube drainage has changed from burgundy to bright red, the blood pressure has decreased to 90/50 mm Hg, and the heart rate is 142 beats/minute. The doctor is notified and gives a verbal order to start avasopressin infusion at 0.3 U/minute. After initiating the infusion, the nurse instructs the patient to notify the nurse immediately if she experiences which of the following?

  ○ **A.** Increase in urinary urgency

  ○ **B.** Numbness or tingling

  ○ **C.** Metallic taste in the mouth

  ○ **D.** Chest pain

35. A patient experiencing transient confusion and drowsiness is scheduled for a lumbar puncture. Knowing that the spinal subarachnoid space is continuous with the cerebral subarachnoid space, the nurse discusses her concern with the doctor about performing lumbar puncture when the patient's level of consciousness changes. In what circumstances is lumbar puncture contraindicated?

○ **A.** If the patient's blood pressure is 100/60 mm Hg

○ **B.** If the patient's family reports that the patient recently had a severe viral cold

○ **C.** If the patient shows signs of increasing ICP

○ **D.** All of the above

36. A 30-year-old pregnant woman who is admitted to the emergency department has a history of sudden onset of severe headaches followed by seizures. Bruits are heard over the patient's carotid arteries and eyeballs. Nuchal rigidity is present. What is the most likely diagnosis and what test can be used to confirm this diagnosis?

○ **A.** Guillain-Barré syndrome and electromyography

○ **B.** Meningitis and lumbar puncture

○ **C.** Autonomic dysreflexia and spinal series

○ **D.** Arteriovenous malformation and computed tomography (CT) scan

37. An 84-year-old man is diagnosed with septic shock. Aggressive treatment is started in the ICU. Which is the most important action for the nurse to take during this therapy?

○ **A.** Place the patient in the shock position to increase blood pressure

○ **B.** Keep the patient on strict bed rest

○ **C.** Control the patient's temperature by placing him on a hypothermia blanket

○ **D.** Monitor the patient's vital signs and urine output every 4 hours for changes

38. A 24-year-old man has accidentally ingested about 200 ml of a lye-based liquid drain cleaner. Which of the following should the nurse be prepared to administer when the patient arrives at the emergency department?

○ **A.** A cathartic, to promote elimination of the caustic substance

○ **B.** 30 ml of ipecac syrup, followed by 240 ml of water, to induce vomiting

○ **C.** 150 ml of milk or water, to dilute the caustic substance

○ **D.** 75 g of activated charcoal, to absorb the ingested chemical

39. A 29-year-old man is brought to the emergency department by emergency medical service personnel after he was found sitting in his car in an enclosed garage with the motor running. He is unresponsive and hypotensive, and his skin is bright red. Which of the following nursing diagnoses is of the highest priority for this patient?

○ **A.** Ineffective individual coping related to depression

○ **B.** Altered tissue perfusion related to decreased cardiac output

○ **C.** Altered cerebral tissue perfusion related to depressed neurologic functioning

○ **D.** Ineffective breathing pattern related to suppressed respirations

40. A patient with burns on the face and neck is at risk for airway obstruction. Which of the following would be most indicative of a potential airway obstruction?

○ **A.** Singed nasal hairs

○ **B.** Neck and face pain

○ **C.** PaO_2 of 80 mm Hg

○ **D.** Coughing up large amounts of thick, white sputum

41. A 63-year-old man is admitted to the ICU with a diagnosis of a dissecting thoracic aneurysm. His vital signs are blood pressure 180/110 mm Hg, heart rate 110 beats/minute, respiratory rate 12 breaths/minute, and temperature 99° F (37.2° C). The patient is anxious, and several family members are present. What medications will most likely be ordered to lower the patient's blood pressure and decrease his anxiety level?

○ **A.** Meperidine (Demerol) and propranolol (Inderal)

○ **B.** Midazolam (Versed) and nifedipine (Procardia)

○ **C.** Morphine and digoxin (Lanoxin)

○ **D.** Lorazepam (Ativan) and nitroprusside sodium

42. A 50-year-old woman comes to the emergency department complaining of "fluttering" in her chest, dyspnea, lethargy, and syncope. She is barrel-chested, has a history of schizophrenia, and smokes two packs of cigarettes a day. Her vital signs are blood pressure 99/50 mm Hg, heart rate 220 beats/minute, respiratory rate 38 breaths/minute, and temperature 98.6° F (37° C). An ECG shows that she is experiencing atrial fibrillation with a rapid ventricular response. Verapamil 2.5 mg I.V. is administered twice. To determine the desired therapeutic response, the nurse should watch for which of the following?

○ **A.** Decrease in blood pressure

○ **B.** Decrease in respiratory rate

○ **C.** Decrease in hallucinations

○ **D.** Decrease in heart rate

43. A patient with a closed head injury begins to show a decreased level of consciousness and increased ICP. His arms extend and adduct, his wrists are hyperpronated, and his lower extremities extend stiffly, with the feet in plantar flexion. His ABG values show a PaO_2 of 90 mm Hg and a $PaCO_2$ of 50 mm Hg. He is on a ventilator with a tidal volume of 900 ml, FIO_2 0.40, and respiratory rate 14 breaths/minute. What type of posturing is the patient displaying and what can be done to correct this?

○ **A.** Opisthotonic posturing, increase tidal volume

○ **B.** Decorticate posturing, increase FIO_2

○ **C.** Decerebrate posturing, increase ventilation rate

○ **D.** Temporary posturing, no changes necessary

44. A patient has suffered deep partial-thickness and full-thickness burns over 35% of his body. In what ambient environment would the patient be most comfortable?

○ **A.** Room temperature is lower than skin surface temperature and humidity at 25% or lower

○ **B.** Room temperature is lower than skin surface temperature and humidity at 50% or higher

○ **C.** Room temperature is slightly higher than skin surface temperature and humidity at 25% or lower

○ **D.** Room temperature is slightly higher than skin surface temperature and humidity at 40% to 50%

45. A patient with myasthenia gravis arrives in the emergency department. Based on the presenting symptoms, she appears to be in cholinergic crisis. The administration of which drug and which response to the drug would confirm the diagnosis?

○ **A.** Edrophonium chloride (Tensilon); worsening of symptoms

○ **B.** Ambenonium chloride (Mytelase); worsening of symptoms

○ **C.** Edrophonium chloride; improvement of symptoms

○ **D.** Ambenonium chloride; improvement of symptoms

46. A patient with chronic bronchitis requires tracheobronchial suctioning. Which of the following nursing actions would best help prevent the potential complications of this procedure?

○ **A.** Hyperoxygenate the patient with 100% oxygen

○ **B.** Keep the patient in a supine position

○ **C.** Insert the suction catheter no further than 12 cm

○ **D.** Give an I.V. bolus dose of lidocaine to prevent ventricular ectopic beats

47. A patient is in the emergency department. The following ABG values have been obtained: pH 7.36, PaO_2 88 mm Hg, $PaCO_2$ 62 mm Hg, and HCO_3^- 35 mEq/L. Which condition is reflected by these values?

○ **A.** Respiratory acidosis

○ **B.** Compensated respiratory acidosis

○ **C.** Metabolic alkalosis

○ **D.** Compensated metabolic alkalosis

48. A 35-year-old man with bacterial meningitis is at risk for increasing ICP. Which measure is appropriate for preventing increased ICP?

○ **A.** Encouraging the patient to avoid straining or performing maneuvers similar to the Vasalva maneuver

○ **B.** Avoiding hyperoxygenation before and after suctioning by limiting suctioning to 5 to 10 seconds each time

○ **C.** Keeping the head of the bed flat

○ **D.** Encouraging hyperextension or hyperflexion of the neck and extremities

49. A patient suffered deep partial-thickness and full-thickness burns over 40% of his body approximately 12 hours ago. Urine output is 22 ml/hour and the hematocrit is 50%. ABG values show pH 7.32, PaO_2 95 mm Hg, $PaCO_2$ 35 mm Hg, and HCO_3^- 18 mEq/L. Based on these data, the nurse would assume that the patient:

○ **A.** Is dehydrated, developing renal failure, and in metabolic acidosis

○ **B.** Is in the early stages of heart failure caused by overhydration

○ **C.** Is adequately hydrated but in acute renal failure and respiratory acidosis

○ **D.** Has developed a polycythemia as his body attempts to compensate for metabolic acidosis and renal failure

50. After an insulin infusion is initiated, serial fingerstick blood glucose tests reveal a progressive decrease in the patient's serum glucose level. At which of the following plasma glucose levels will the nurse most likely begin adding dextrose to the maintenance I.V. infusion?

○ **A.** 250 mg/dl

○ **B.** 200 mg/dl

○ **C.** 150 mg/dl

○ **D.** 100 mg/dl

Answers and rationales

1. Answer: C

In a patient with bowel obstruction, bowel sounds typically are hyperactive above the obstruction and absent below the obstruction. Palpation and percussion tend to increase bowel sounds. The diaphragm, not the bell, of the stethoscope is best for hearing high-pitched bowel sounds.

2. Answer: C

As the clot dissolves and the myocardium is perfused, a few arrhythmias may occur; these are known as reperfusion anomalies. After these initial events, the ST segment slowly returns to baseline value or within normal limits as a result of the decreased pain and increased oxygen levels. Heparin therapy, not streptokinase therapy, will increase the PT/PTT to 2 to 2.5 times greater than normal. Although chest pain may be relieved by streptokinase, pain relief also may result from administration of nitroglycerin or morphine sulfate. Vital signs are not used to evaluate the effectiveness of streptokinase therapy.

3. Answer: D

A small decrease in systolic blood pressure normally occurs during inspiration, but decreases greater than 10 mm Hg are abnormal. Pulsus paradoxus (paradoxical pulse) is the correct term for describing this decrease in systolic blood pressure. Pulsus magnus refers to a large or strong pulse. Pulsus alternans describes an alternating strong and weak heartbeat. Pulsus parvus is a small or weak pulse.

4. Answer: C

The most common cause of airway obstruction in an unconscious person is the tongue blocking the airway. Opening the airway by tilting the patient's head will relieve the obstruction. Deep tracheal suctioning is unnecessary unless some blockage is present. Mechanical ventilation should be used only if the patient is not breathing after the airway is opened. Upward abdominal thrusts are performed only if an obstruction is present in the airway.

5. Answer: B

Patients with non-insulin-dependent diabetes mellitus are most at risk for developing HHNS because low levels of circulating endogenous insulin are thought to inhibit glycogenolysis and gluconeogenesis in the liver. Patients with insulin-dependent diabetes mellitus tend to develop diabetic ketoacidosis. Long-term exogenous corticosteroid use can lead to the development of insulin-dependent diabetes. Chronic renal failure is not indicated by the laboratory values reported for this patient.

6. Answer: C

Isotonic solutions (such as normal saline solution) are administered initially. As fluid volume approaches normal, hypotonic fluids (such as half-normal saline solution or 0.225% sodium chloride solution) are administered until blood pressure and serum electrolyte and glucose values approach normal. Plasma expanders may be required in the presence of hypovolemic shock. Diuretic therapy would be detrimental to this patient because her urine output has dropped due to severe osmotic diuresis. Serum osmolality should be increased, not decreased.

7. Answer: C

Bed rest is important to prevent further injury and, possibly, bleeding. Body temperature is not a critical consideration. Ambulation should be avoided until the patient is stable. Blood products commonly are used to treat DIC.

8. Answer: C

The ECG changes noted by the emergency department nurse clearly are not normal. They are classic signs of an inferior (diaphragmatic) MI. Attacks of angina typically do not cause ECG changes. A subendocardial MI is a type of MI, not a location.

9. Answer: D

Problems related to breathing always receive highest priority. Fluid volume deficit related to excessive bleeding is a close second in terms of priority. The other options are of lower priority in the care of this patient.

10. Answer: D
The carpal spasm caused by compressing the upper arm is an indication of a low calcium level. Trousseau's sign is not an indication of hyperglycemia, hypoglycemia, or hypercalcemia.

11. Answer: B
Neomycin kills bacteria in the intestine to diminish protein breakdown, whereas lactulose eliminates protein from the GI tract. Appropriate therapy for this patient includes a low-protein diet and fluid restrictions. Opioid analgesics and sedatives are inappropriate for a patient who is lethargic. Digoxin and furosemide are prescribed for heart failure, not hepatic coma.

12. Answer: B
The ECG of a patient with transmural MI most often shows an elevated ST segment. An isoelectric ST segment is the normal configuration. A prolonged ST segment indicates hypocalcemia. A depressed ST segment is a sign of angina, right ventricular hypertrophy, or digoxin toxicity.

13. Answer: B
Atropine is used for most slow arrhythmias. It blocks the parasympathetic system and directly increases the rate of the AV node and the atria and indirectly increases the rate of the ventricles. Digoxin slows the rate and increases the force of contraction. Lidocaine is used exclusively for ventricular arrhythmias. Verapamil is used to slow atrial arrhythmias.

14. Answer: C
Because skeletal muscle relaxants do not inhibit the patient's awareness, a sedative or anxiolytic agent such as diazepam also would be administered. Adenosine is used to treat supraventricular tachycardia, neostigmine is used to treat myasthenia gravis or overdose of a nondepolarizing blocking agent, and furosemide is used to induce diuresis.

15. Answer: C
The best way to stabilize the patient is to maintain fluid volume, blood pressure, and pulse rate. Preparing for surgery may not be necessary because many patients stop bleeding on their own. Administering I.V. vasopressin would be an ineffective treatment. Administering I.V. histamine inhibitors is a long-term treatment after recovery from active bleeding.

16. Answer: C
Wetting the burned area with cold water stops the burning process and helps relieve the pain. The other options are of lesser priority.

17. Answer: C
An ECG pattern of two P waves for each QRS complex and a PR interval that is uniform across the strip indicates second-degree AV block, Mobitz type II. The pattern for sinus bradycardia is one P wave for each QRS complex. Junctional escape rhythm would not have P waves or P waves after the QRS complex. The QRS complexes on this strip are too narrow for a ventricular escape rhythm.

18. Answer: D
Resting the heart is a major goal of treatment after an acute MI. The other options all have lower priorities.

19. Answer: B
B lymphocytes initiate the development of immunoglobulins and the antigens. Only helper T cells play a small role in the development of humoral immunity, which usually occurs in conjunction with hemolytic, not anaphylactic, reactions. The bone marrow and lymph cells, not the thymus, are involved in humoral immunity.

20. Answer: A
Hypotension is one of the most common adverse effects of nitroglycerin. Although the heart rate may be increased, it usually acts as a compensatory mechanism for the hypotension. Respiratory rate and temperature generally are not affected.

21. Answer: C
Hypoglycemia is a common cause of seizurelike movements. It is easily corrected but can be fatal if left untreated. Given the situation, the nurse could safely administer glucose. Naloxone is inappropriate because the patient's condition is not consistent with an opioid overdose. Sodium bicarbonate is inappropriate because there is no evidence of acidosis. Diazepam would be appropriate after glucose has been administered.

22. Answer: C
Disconnecting the ventilator and manually ventilating the patient enables the nurse to evaluate whether the endotracheal tube or the patient's airway is blocked. Increasing the tidal volume may cause pneumothorax. Increasing the oxygen concentration or administering prescribed medications will not help the underlying problem.

23. Answer: A
According to Maslow's hierarchy of needs, a fluid volume deficit has the highest priority.

24. Answer: B
In HHNS, the glucose level usually is higher than that seen in diabetic ketoacidosis. Plasma osmolality greater than 350 mOsm/kg is the most significant finding in HHNS. Because ketoacidosis does not occur in HHNS, pH should be normal or slightly decreased.

25. Answer: C
This type of monitoring system needs to be balanced against atmospheric pressure, usually every 8 hours. Cerebrospinal fluid cannot be obtained through this device. The transducer should be level. A flush device should never be used with an ICP monitoring system.

26. Answer: A
In a patient with MI, the CK level begins to rise within 2 to 6 hours after the MI occurs and peaks at 24 hours. The LD level begins to rise within 6 to 12 hours after the MI and peaks at 48 to 72 hours. AST begins to rise within 6 to 8 hours and peaks at 24 to 48 hours. ALT does not increase with cardiac damage.

27. Answer: A
Ectopic production of ADH is the most common cause of SIADH. There is no evidence that excessive fluid intake or dehydration contributes to the inappropriate release of ADH by the posterior pituitary gland. SIADH is associated with increased, not decreased, levels of ADH.

28. Answer: C
Hyponatremia, elevated urine sodium level, and elevated urine osmolality are consistent with the clinical findings of SIADH. Elevated serum sodium level, decreased urine osmolality, and elevated plasma osmolality are indicative of diabetes insipidus.

29. Answer: D
Albumin consists of large protein molecules that help draw and hold fluid in the vascular system. Albumin is hypertonic and helps to decrease fluid volume in the tissues.

30. Answer: A
The patient's generalized weakened condition can lead to severe dyspnea even with minimal activity. An "HIV positive" sign is not necessary and would be an invasion of privacy. The patient need not wear mask and gloves nor must visitors be restricted to immediate family because HIV is not spread through airborne organisms or casual contact.

31. Answer: C
In response to an infection, body temperature rises and pulse rate increases. In a patient in septic shock, the skin is cold and diaphoretic. Arterial blood gas analysis would reveal metabolic acidosis caused by lactic acid buildup. A urine output of 30 ml/hour and a central venous pressure of 8 cm H_2O are normal parameters; in septic shock, urine output is likely to be lower and central venous pressure is likely to be decreased.

32. Answer: B
Central herniation causes bilateral rostral-caudal deterioration. Uncal herniation causes unilateral signs. Transcranial herniation is related to herniation of cerebral tissue through the skull. Nucleus pulposus herniation involves the spinal canal and spinal cord.

33. Answer: B
Isoproterenol is a powerful cardiac stimulant used for heart blocks and heart failure. In uncomplicated MI, it is not needed and would increase the workload of the heart. Morphine typically is prescribed for pain relief. Heparin is administered to prevent clots while the patient is on bed rest. Diltiazem reduces the workload of the heart.

34. Answer: D
Caution must be used when administering vasopressin to patients with coronary disease because of the drug's constrictive effects on the coronary arteries. Vasopressin causes urine retention and reabsorption by the kidneys. Although numbness and tingling may be experienced in the extremities, chest pain is a more ominous sign. Vasopressin usually does not cause a metallic taste in the mouth.

35. Answer: C
A decreasing level of consciousness is possibly a sign of increasing ICP. If a lumbar puncture is performed in the presence of increased ICP, brain stem herniation may occur. As the lumbar puncture needle enters the spinal subarachnoid space, pressure is released and the brain stem is forced down through the foramen magnum. A blood pressure of 100/60 is normal and does not preclude lumbar puncture. A viral infection may precipitate sterile meningitis but is not a contraindication for lumbar puncture.

36. Answer: D
The presence of bruits over the eyes with nuchal rigidity suggests a leaking arteriovenous malformation, which can be confirmed with a CT scan. Most arteriovenous malformations are present at birth but are asymptomatic until the third decade of life. The likelihood of hemorrhage is increased during pregnancy. Seizures and headaches are common presenting symptoms. Guillain-Barré syndrome is a neuromuscular demyelination disease characterized by progressive ascending paralysis. Although nuchal rigidity, headache, and seizures are signs and symptoms of meningitis, this disease does not cause bruits. Autonomic dysreflexia is a syndrome associated with spinal cord injuries below the level of T6 and is characterized by loss of sympathetic inhibition.

37. Answer: B
Bed rest reduces the energy and oxygen demands on the circulatory system. The shock position may be unnecessary or contraindicated. Hypothermia blankets may be unnecessary because body temperature commonly is normal in early septic shock. Vital signs should be checked every 15 minutes and urine output, every hour.

38. Answer: C
If the patient is alert and able to swallow, he should drink milk or water to dilute the caustic substance. The use of ipecac syrup is not advisable because caustic and corrosive substances should not be vomited to prevent further damage to the esophagus. Activated charcoal and a cathartic are not effective in decreasing the caustic properties of the ingested chemical.

39. Answer: D
Respiratory diagnoses are always of the highest priority.

40. Answer: A
Singed nasal hairs indicate that the patient has inhaled hot toxic gases or flames that may cause respiratory problems. A patient can have facial burns without airway damage. A PaO_2 of 80 mm Hg is a normal laboratory value. White sputum is normal; black sputum would indicate possible respiratory problems.

41. Answer: D
Lorazepam is used to decrease anxiety. Nitroprusside sodium is used to quickly lower the blood pressure in an attempt to prevent rupture of the aneurysm. The other drugs do not effectively lower the patient's blood pressure or decrease anxiety.

42. Answer: D
The priority for this patient is to slow the heart rate. Verapamil interrupts the re-entry pathway to effectively decrease the heart rate. Verapamil also may decrease the blood pressure, which, in this case, is an undesirable effect because of the patient's already low blood pressure. Although the respiratory rate may decrease, it is not the priority in this case. Verapamil has no effect on hallucinations.

43. Answer: C
Decerebrate posturing, or abnormal extension, is an ominous sign, indicating rostral-caudal deterioration. A $PaCO_2$ of 50 mm Hg is slightly high but can be lowered by increasing the rate of ventilation. A decreasing $PaCO_2$ causes cerebral vessels to constrict, thereby decreasing ICP. Opisthotonic posturing is characterized by rigid spinal hyperextension. It is seen in tetanus and some acute cases of meningitis and is indicative of meningeal irritation. A tidal volume of 900 ml is normal for an adult. Decorticate posturing, or abnormal flexion, is characterized by rigid flexion of the arms and extension of the legs. Decorticate posturing commonly precedes decerebrate posturing in cases of neurologic deterioration. An FIO_2 of 0.40 is normal.

44. Answer: D
Patients with burns over a large area of the body lose heat and moisture through the open wounds. An environment in which the temperature is slightly higher than the skin surface temperature with the humidity at 40% to 50% helps prevent heat and fluid loss.

45. Answer: A
Edrophonium chloride is a short-acting anticholinesterase agent. It is the drug of choice for differentiating between the two types of crisis in a patient with myasthenia gravis. Administration of edrophonium chloride to a patient in myasthenic crisis resulting from inadequate anticholinesterase would improve the symptoms. Ambenonium chloride is a long-acting anticholinesterase agent. Administration of ambenonium chloride to a patient who has been overmedicated with anticholinesterase drugs would intensify or worsen the symptoms.

46. Answer: A
Hypoxia is one of the most common complications of tracheobronchial suctioning and can cause arrhythmias and changes in heart rate. An upright position is best for suctioning. The catheter must be inserted approximately 20 cm. Ventricular ectopic beats that occur during suctioning are best treated by reoxygenating the patient.

47. Answer: B
The pH is in the normal range, but the $PaCO_2$ value indicates acidosis.

48. Answer: A
Maneuvers that are similar to the Valsalva maneuver increase central venous and central thoracic pressures, thereby hindering outflow of venous return from the cerebral vessels and possibly causing increased ICP. Hypercapnia and hypoxemia cause vasodilation, which increases ICP. Lengthy suctioning times can cause a sympathetic response of increased heart rate and blood pressure, leading to increased cerebral blood flow and cerebral edema. Keeping the head of the bed elevated 15 to 30 degrees and avoiding hyperextension or hyperflexion of the neck and extremities facilitate drainage of blood and CSF from the head and decrease impedance.

49. Answer: A
The elevated hematocrit indicates insufficient fluids, the low urine output is an early sign of renal failure, and the ABG values indicate metabolic acidosis. A patient with heart failure would have edema and crackles on auscultation of lungs. A patient who is adequately hydrated would have a hematocrit lower than 50%. Polycythemia takes longer than 12 hours to develop.

50. Answer: A
Dextrose is added to the I.V. infusion at a glucose level of 250 mg/dl to prevent hypoglycemia and to accelerate the resolution of ketone bodies by decreasing lipolysis. The other values listed are too low and increase the risk of hypoglycemia.

Analyzing the posttest

Total the number of *incorrect* responses to posttest #1. A score of 1 to 9 indicates that you have an excellent knowledge base and that you are well prepared for the certification examination; a score of 10 to 14 indicates adequate preparation, although more study or improvement in test-taking skills is recommended; a score of 15 or more indicates the need for intensive study before taking the certification examination.

For a more detailed analysis of your performance, complete the self-diagnostic profile worksheet below.

Self-diagnostic profile for posttest #1

In the top row of boxes, record the number of each question you answered incorrectly. Then, beneath each question number, check the box that corresponds to the reason you answered the question incorrectly. Finally, tabulate the number of check marks on each line in the right-hand column marked "Totals." You now have an individualized profile of weak areas that require further study or improvement in test-taking ability before you take the Critical Care Nursing Certification Examination.

QUESTION NUMBER																					TOTALS
Test-taking skills																					
1. Misread question																					
2. Missed important point																					
3. Forgot fact or concept																					
4. Applied wrong fact or concept																					
5. Drew wrong conclusion																					
6. Incorrectly evaluated distractors																					
7. Mistakenly filled in wrong circle																					
8. Read into question																					
9. Guessed wrong																					
10. Misunderstood question																					

Posttest #2

Instructions

This posttest has been designed to evaluate your readiness to take the certification examination for critical care nursing. Similar in form and content to the actual examination, the posttest consists of 50 questions based on brief clinical situations. The questions will help sharpen your test-taking skills while assessing your knowledge of critical care nursing theory and practice.

You will have 50 minutes to complete the posttest. To improve your chances for performing well, consider these suggestions:

• Read each clinical situation closely. Weigh the four options carefully, and then select the option that best answers the question. (*Note:* In this posttest, options are lettered A, B, C, and D to aid in later identification of correct answers and rationales. These letters do not appear on the certification examination.)
• Completely darken the circle in front of the answer that you select, using a #2 pencil. (You must use a #2 pencil when taking the certification examination.) Do not use check marks, Xs, or lines.
• If you decide to change your answer, erase the old answer completely. (The certification examination is scored electronically; an incomplete erasure may cause both answers to be scored, in which case you will not receive credit for answering the question.)
• If you have difficulty understanding a question or are unsure of the answer, place a small mark next to the question number and, if time permits, return to it later. If you have no idea of the correct answer, make an educated guess. (Only correct answers are counted in scoring the certification examination, so guessing is preferable to leaving a question unanswered.)

After you complete the posttest, or after the 50-minute time limit expires, check your responses against the correct answers and rationales provided on pages 297 to 305.

Now, select a quiet room where you will be undisturbed, set a timer for 50 minutes, and begin.

Questions

1. The nurse is preparing to discharge a 75-year-old patient who has experienced a myocardial infarction (MI). Which of the following evaluation outcomes would be inappropriate for this patient?

   ○ **A.** The patient will be free of arrhythmias

   ○ **B.** The patient will have no signs of infection at the invasive line sites

   ○ **C.** The patient will gain no more than 4 lb a week

   ○ **D.** The patient will remain alert and oriented

2. A 46-year-old teacher with advanced cirrhosis is being examined by the emergency department nurse. What can the nurse expect to find when palpating the patient's liver?

○ **A.** Rebound tenderness

○ **B.** Enlarged, soft, painful mass

○ **C.** Enlarged, hard, painless mass

○ **D.** Enlarged, soft mass

3. A 21-year-old man is admitted to the intensive care unit (ICU) after suffering a traumatic injury to the left side of his neck. The patient has flaccid paralysis of the upper and lower extremities on the left side but retains the sensations of pain and temperature on the left side. He has some movement of his upper and lower extremities on the right side but no sensations of pain or temperature on the right side. What type of spinal cord injury should the nurse suspect when doing an assessment?

○ **A.** Posterior spinal cord injury associated with hyperextension

○ **B.** Central spinal cord compression

○ **C.** Brown-Séquard syndrome associated with intervertebral disk rupture

○ **D.** Anterior spinal cord injury associated with dislocation

4. A 21-year-old man is admitted to the ICU complaining of polydipsia, polyuria, nocturia, and weight loss. He reports that he has been voiding large amounts of clear, colorless urine about 20 times a day. His vital signs are blood pressure 96/48 mm Hg, heart rate 124 beats/minute, and respiratory rate 22 breaths/minute. His laboratory test values are potassium 4.1 mEq/L, sodium 146 mEq/L, serum osmolality 306 mOsm/kg, serum glucose 122 mg/dl, urine specific gravity 1.004, hemoglobin 13.2 g/dl, and hematocrit 48%. Based on the clinical evidence, what is the most likely medical diagnosis?

○ **A.** Diabetic ketoacidosis (DKA)

○ **B.** Hyperosmolar hyperglycemic nonketotic syndrome (HHNS)

○ **C.** Syndrome of inappropriate antidiuretic hormone (SIADH)

○ **D.** Diabetes insipidus

5. A patient is admitted with a diagnosis of diabetes insipidus. Which nursing interventions should be planned for this patient?

○ **A.** Administration of vasopressin, administration of I.V. hypertonic sodium chloride solution, and measurement of hourly intake and output

○ **B.** Administration of insulin, administration of I.V. normal saline solution, and measurement of hourly intake and output

○ **C.** Administration of vasopressin, administration of I.V. and oral fluid replacements, and measurement of hourly intake and output

○ **D.** Administration of furosemide, administration of I.V. hypertonic sodium chloride solution, and measurement of hourly intake and output

6. A woman has been admitted with acute upper GI bleeding. She is receiving I.V. aqueous vasopressin (Pitressin) at a rate of 0.4 U/minute. Which other medication would be used concurrently with vasopressin?

○ **A.** I.V. dopamine infusion

○ **B.** I.V. nitroglycerin infusion

○ **C.** I.M. vitamin K

○ **D.** I.V. lidocaine infusion

7. A patient is admitted to the ICU with heart failure. He is 5′ 4″ tall, weighs 125 lb, and has a cardiac output of 6 L/minute. What is the correct cardiac index for this patient?

○ **A.** 4.4 L/minute/m²

○ **B.** 4.0 L/minute/m²

○ **C.** 3.8 L/minute/m²

○ **D.** 2.8 L/minute/m²

8. A patient with severe head trauma is monitored for Cushing's triad, which results when pressure is exerted on the brain stem by intracranial hypertension or a herniation syndrome. What are the three signs of Cushing's triad?

✗ **A.** Increased blood pressure with widening pulse pressure, bradycardia, and abnormal respiratory pattern

○ **B.** Hypertension, seizures, and cluster breathing pattern

○ **C.** Pinpoint pupils, unilateral paresthesias, and Wernicke's aphasia

○ **D.** Contralateral loss of vision in the same side of each eye, diplopia, and loss of contralateral sensation

9. A 62-year-old man has been in the ICU for 2 weeks after an acute MI. His activity level has been increased to include bathroom privileges. While in the bathroom, he calls out that he does not feel well. Simultaneously, the monitor technicians report a decrease in heart rate. The nurse finds the patient unresponsive and slumped against the wall. After lowering him to the floor and calling for help, the nurse notes the following vital signs: blood pressure 60/36 mm Hg, heart rate 38 beats/minute, and respiratory rate 12 breaths/minute. The doctor orders 1 mg atropine by I.V. push to be administered immediately. What is the minimum time the nurse should allow before suggesting that the dose be repeated?

○ **A.** 1 to 2 minutes

○ **B.** 3 to 5 minutes

○ **C.** 15 to 30 minutes

○ **D.** 1 to 2 hours

10. The nurse is educating a patient about the consequences of chronic cirrhosis of the liver caused by hepatitis. The nurse knows that her teaching is successful if the patient states that which of the following is caused by the disease?

○ **A.** Gynecomastia

○ **B.** Peptic ulcers

○ **C.** Thrombotic events

○ **D.** Increased osmotic pressure

11. Which of the following is an appropriate treatment for a patient with pancreatitis?

○ **A.** Codeine to control the pain

○ **B.** Anticholinergic or antienzyme agents to suppress pancreatic function

○ **C.** Antibiotics to prevent abscess formation

○ **D.** Place patient on nothing-by-mouth status during the acute phase and a low-fat diet during the recovery phase

12. The nurse has noticed that a patient's electrocardiogram (ECG) pattern has changed. There are now erratic, undulating waveforms in place of identifiable QRS complexes. What does this change in pattern indicate?

○ **A.** Atrial fibrillation

○ **B.** Junctional tachycardia

○ **C.** Ventricular fibrillation

○ **D.** Agonal rhythm

13. A 19-year-old patient with insulin-dependent (type I) diabetes is admitted to the emergency department complaining of nausea, vomiting, abdominal cramping, and fever. Her blood pressure is 132/74 mm Hg, heart rate 118 beats/minute, and respiratory rate 32 breaths/minute. Her breath has a fruity odor, and she appears lethargic and has slurred speech. A diagnosis of DKA is made. Which of the following admission laboratory values would the nurse expect to find for this patient?
(1) pH less than 7.3
(2) Serum osmolality greater than 350 mOsm/kg
(3) Serum potassium less than 3.5 mEq/L
(4) Acetone present in serum and urine

- ○ **A.** 2 and 3
- ○ **B.** 1 and 3
- ○ **C.** 1 and 4
- ○ **D.** 2 and 4

14. The nurse is caring for a patient who had a heart transplantation 2 weeks ago. Which of the following signs would indicate that the patient is experiencing a rejection episode?

- ○ **A.** Chest pain and low blood pressure
- ○ **B.** Abnormally low temperature and renal failure
- ○ **C.** Dizziness and weakness
- ○ **D.** Bounding pulses and flushed skin

15. A 56-year-old man is scheduled for bypass surgery. His critical care nurse notes that his platelet count is 28,000/mm³. Which of the following is the best course of action for the nurse to take?

- ○ **A.** Complete the preoperative checklist and administer the preoperative medication as prescribed.
- ○ **B.** Call the laboratory to have the complete blood count redone.
- ○ **C.** Delay preoperative preparations and call the doctor.
- ○ **D.** Check the patient's blood pressure, heart rate, and respiratory status.

16. A 68-year-old man is admitted with an acute MI. A thermodilution catheter and arterial line are in place. The nurse notes the following readings during the past hour: mean arterial pressure 106 mm Hg, diastolic blood pressure 90 mm Hg, systolic blood pressure 140 mm Hg, cardiac output 5.2 L/minute, mean pulmonary artery pressure 20 mm Hg, and mean right arterial pressure 16 mm Hg. What is the patient's systemic vascular resistance (SVR)?

   ○ **A.** 1,730 dynes/second/cm^2

   ○ **B.** 1,384 dynes/second/cm^2

   ○ **C.** 1,323 dynes/second/cm^2

   ○ **D.** 1,138 dynes/second/cm^2

17. A patient has just been intubated. The nurse auscultates his lungs soon after intubation and notes normal breath sounds on the right side and diminished breath sounds on the left side. What is the best action for the nurse to take?

   ○ **A.** Increase the tidal volume on the ventilator.

   ○ **B.** Pull the endotracheal tube back 1".

   ○ **C.** Suction the patient to remove the mucus plug.

   ○ **D.** Leave the tube alone because this is a normal finding.

18. A patient is admitted with a diagnosis of hepatocellular damage. In reviewing his laboratory values, the nurse would consider which of the following most relevant to his diagnosis?

   ○ **A.** Prothrombin time (PT) and partial thromboplastin time (PTT)

   ○ **B.** Alkaline phosphatase level

   ○ **C.** Alanine aminotransferase and aspartate aminotransferase levels

   ○ **D.** Amylase level

19. A 20-year-old college student develops toxic shock syndrome. Assuming that all of the following are appropriate, which nursing diagnosis has the highest priority for this patient?

   ○ **A.** Knowledge deficit related to use of tampons

   ○ **B.** Altered cerebral perfusion related to low cardiac output

   ○ **C.** Infection related to streptococcal organisms

   ○ **D.** Impaired gas exchange related to depressed respirations

20. A 44-year-old man is admitted to the ICU. He attempted suicide by ingesting approximately 30 tablets of clorazepate dipotassium (each tablet contains 7.5 mg). What are the toxic effects of this drug?

   ○ **A.** Tachycardia and cerebral hemorrhage

   ○ **B.** Respiratory depression and hypotension

   ○ **C.** Complete heart block and paralytic ileus

   ○ **D.** Liver failure and GI bleeding

21. A patient is receiving nitroglycerin by I.V. infusion. The nurse notes that the nitroglycerin is mixed in a glass I.V. bottle of dextrose 5% in water (D_5W) and being administered through normal I.V. tubing using an infusion pump. The nitroglycerin is being administered at a rate of 20 mcg/minute. What should be the nurse's first action?

   ○ **A.** Decrease the rate of the infusion

   ○ **B.** Change the dilution solution to normal saline solution because the medication will precipitate in D_5W

   ○ **C.** Change the normal I.V. tubing to nonabsorbent tubing

   ○ **D.** Remove the infusion pump because it will cause the medication to crystallize

22. A patient has been taking quinidine for an arrhythmia. Which of the following would indicate that the patient is experiencing quinidine toxicity?

   ○ **A.** Frequent diarrhea

   ○ **B.** Slow, irregular pulse rhythm

   ○ **C.** Tinnitus and rash

   ○ **D.** Widening QRS complex

23. A 22-year-old woman is brought to the emergency department by her mother, who states that her daughter has just ingested 50 iron tablets. Treatment is started. The nurse knows that activated charcoal should:

   ○ **A.** Be administered after ipecac syrup has been administered and after vomiting has stopped

   ○ **B.** Be administered first to help absorb the iron

   ○ **C.** Not be administered to patients who have ingested iron

   ○ **D.** Be mixed with ipecac syrup and water to increase its effectiveness

24. A 33-year-old firefighter is admitted to the emergency department with burns on his face and neck; he had been fighting a fire at a plastics factory. During her assessment, the nurse would give highest priority to which of the following actions?

○ **A.** Noting signs of increased intracranial pressure (ICP)

○ **B.** Obtaining an accurate weight

○ **C.** Assessing psychological status

○ **D.** Assessing changes in the circumference of the neck

25. A 31-year-old woman is admitted to the ICU after a motor vehicle accident during which she sustained a head injury. She is lethargic but responsive to tactile stimulation. Several hours later, her level of consciousness deteriorates, and she cannot be aroused. Her vital signs are blood pressure 108/55 mm Hg, heart rate 45 beats/minute, respiratory rate 8 breaths/minute, and temperature 101.5° F (38.6° C). Other assessment data include pH 7.31, $PaCO_2$ 70 mm Hg, PaO_2 75 mm Hg, HCO_3^- 26 mEq/L, SaO_2 88%, and ICP 20 mm Hg. The doctor intubates the patient to correct the respiratory acidosis. The patient also receives 75 ml of a 20% solution of mannitol. The nurse knows that the patient is responding to the mannitol when which of the following occurs?

○ **A.** The patient spontaneously opens her eyes

○ **B.** The patient experiences diuresis

○ **C.** The patient has a decreased heart rate

○ **D.** The patient has diarrhea

26. In monitoring a patient for adverse reactions to vasopressin therapy, the nurse should check for which of the following signs and symptoms?

○ **A.** Headache, decreased level of consciousness, decreased urine output, nausea, and vomiting

○ **B.** Pallor, diaphoresis, tremor, and seizures

○ **C.** Hemoconcentration, increased urine output, and complaints of thirst

○ **D.** Hyperglycemia, hyperkalemia, and increased urine output

27. A patient is admitted to the ICU with a temperature of 105.6° F (40.9° C). In reviewing the laboratory data, the nurse notices a leukocyte shift to the left, evidenced by an increased number of immature neutrophils. This is an indication of which condition?

○ **A.** Anemia

○ **B.** Thrombocytopenia

○ **C.** Acute infection

○ **D.** Leukemia

28. A patient was burned on the face, head, and neck while trying to light a barbecue grill. Which of the following measures would be most effective in preventing pulmonary congestion for this patient?

- ○ **A.** Encourage the patient to increase his oral fluid intake
- ○ **B.** Administer high-flow oxygen therapy
- ○ **C.** Encourage the patient to cough
- ○ **D.** Use tracheal suctioning to remove burn residue

29. In developing a plan of care for a patient with a severe burn, the nurse establishes a goal to monitor for bleeding to detect stress ulcers. To achieve this goal, the nurse also should monitor for:

- ○ **A.** Renal failure
- ○ **B.** Hepatic failure
- ○ **C.** Disseminated intravascular coagulation
- ○ **D.** Increased ICP

30. A 44-year-old man suffered an MI 2 days ago. He tells the nurse that he is having trouble sleeping because of all the beeps and buzzes he hears whenever he moves. Which of the following actions would be best for the nurse to take?

- ○ **A.** Close the patient's door so that the noise is blocked out
- ○ **B.** Tell the patient not to worry about the noises because they are not that important
- ○ **C.** Take the patient to the nurses' station and show him what the alarms indicate and how they work
- ○ **D.** Turn the alarms off or turn the volume down so that he cannot hear them

31. A patient arrives in the emergency department after having been burned with boiling water over the lower anterior trunk and the anterior thigh to the knee. Which of the following would the nurse expect to find during the assessment?

- ○ **A.** Third-degree burns over 20% of the body
- ○ **B.** Fourth-degree burns over 12% of the body
- ○ **C.** Second-degree burns over 33% of the body
- ○ **D.** Second-degree burns over 22% of the body

32. A patient with diabetes mellitus was discharged from the hospital 3 months ago. Which of the following laboratory data would indicate that the patient complied with the ICU nurse's instructions about postdischarge care?

    ○ **A.** Fasting serum glucose 125 mg/dl

    ○ **B.** Glycosylated hemoglobin (Hb A_{1C}) 6%

    ○ **C.** Serum potassium 4.2 mEq/L

    ○ **D.** Arterial pH 7.38

33. A 60-year-old man underwent heart transplantation 7 days ago. He is to be transferred out of the ICU tomorrow. The nurse will know that her teaching about posttransplantation care has been successful when the patient states:

    ○ **A.** "I can stop taking these immunosuppressant medications after I feel better."

    ○ **B.** "I need to avoid crowds and people with colds."

    ○ **C.** "I can never kiss my wife again because I will get an infection."

    ○ **D.** "I will never be able to go hunting again."

34. A patient is admitted with septic shock. The following arterial blood gas values are obtained: pH 7.23, PaO_2 82 mm Hg, $PaCO_2$ 44 mm Hg, and HCO_3^- 18 mEq/L. What would be the best initial action for the nurse to take?

    ○ **A.** Administer one ampule of sodium bicarbonate by I.V. push

    ○ **B.** Intubate and hyperventilate the patient

    ○ **C.** Have the patient breathe into a paper bag

    ○ **D.** Start oxygen therapy by nasal cannula

35. A 20-year-old patient is admitted to the ICU with a severe closed head injury. He was riding a bicycle when he collided with an automobile. Intracranial monitoring shows an ICP of 23 mm Hg, and uncal herniation is occurring. During the assessment, the nurse would look for which eye signs and would expect which cranial nerves to be affected?

    ○ **A.** Hippus; cranial nerve III

    ○ **B.** Absent doll's eyes; cranial nerves III, VI, and VIII

    ○ **C.** Anisocoria; cranial nerve III

    ○ **D.** All of the above

36. A 42-year-old woman is in the early recovery period after heart transplantation. She is receiving immunosuppressant medications, including cyclosporine. Which of the following signs or symptoms are considered to be the most serious adverse reactions to this medication?

○ **A.** Gastritis and development of peptic ulcers

○ **B.** Paresthesia and headache

○ **C.** Elevated blood urea nitrogen (BUN) and serum creatinine levels

○ **D.** Decreased HCO_3^- level and hypertension

37. A patient with myasthenia gravis is in crisis and about to be admitted to the ICU. The patient has bradycardia and is complaining of blurred vision, nausea, and vomiting. What type of crisis is this patient experiencing and what drug might be needed?

○ **A.** Myasthenic crisis; atropine

○ **B.** Cholinergic crisis; atropine

○ **C.** Myasthenic crisis; neostigmine bromide (Prostigmin)

○ **D.** Cholinergic crisis; neostigmine bromide

38. A 49-year-old man is brought to the unit with a diagnosis of status epilepticus. He is having generalized tonic-clonic seizures every 5 minutes, with each seizure lasting 30 to 90 seconds. He received a total of 50 mg of diazepam before arriving at the ICU. In accordance with accepted safety precautions, the nurse should ensure that which drug is at the patient's bedside?

○ **A.** Phenobarbital

○ **B.** Flumazenil (Mazicon)

○ **C.** Naloxone (Narcan)

○ **D.** Phenytoin (Dilantin)

39. A 56-year-old man has severe, long-term lung disease related to heavy smoking. In planning his care, which of the following would the nurse rank as most important?

○ **A.** Administering prophylactic antibiotics

○ **B.** Performing a thorough psychological assessment

○ **C.** Increasing the patient's level of exercise

○ **D.** Planning large, high-protein meals to maintain the patient's energy

40. A 50-year-old man with a diagnosis of cerebral aneurysm and subarachnoid hemorrhage is admitted to the surgical ICU. The patient has progressed through the first few days without increased neurologic deficits. What intervention is important on the 7th postoperative day and why?

○ **A.** Discharge planning because 7 days is the usual length of stay for these patients.

○ **B.** Neurologic checks and assessment of level of consciousness because the incidence of vasospasm or rebleeding is highest 7 to 10 days after surgery.

○ **C.** Elevation of the head of the bed because the development of Brudzinski's sign is seen after 7 postoperative days.

○ **D.** Increasing the dose of osmotic diuretics because this action decreases transient cerebral edema.

41. A 65-year-old man is admitted to the ICU after undergoing coronary artery bypass graft. He has a history of angina, coronary artery disease, and insulin-dependent diabetes mellitus. The effects of the anesthesia have not yet reversed, and the patient's blood pressure is labile. His vital signs are systolic blood pressure 98 mm Hg (using Doppler flow probe), heart rate 135 beats/minute, respiratory rate 14 breaths/minute, and temperature 96.8° F (36° C). Other assessment data include pulmonary artery diastolic pressure 32 mm Hg, pulmonary artery wedge pressure 18 mm Hg, central venous pressure 12 mm Hg, $PaCO_2$ 45 mm Hg, and SVR 700 dynes/second/cm². The doctor orders vital signs assessment per ICU protocol, dopamine 800 mg in 500 ml D_5W titrated to keep the systolic blood pressure between 90 and 120 mm Hg, and nitroprusside sodium (Nipride) 50 mg in 250 ml D_5W. The doctor is to be notified if the systolic blood pressure is less than 90 or greater than 120 mm Hg. As the hours pass, the nurse notices that frequent increases in the dose of dopamine are required to maintain the blood pressure within the ordered parameters. At what dosage should the nurse initially notify the doctor of the amount of dopamine being administered?

○ **A.** 5 mcg/kg/minute

○ **B.** 10 mcg/kg/minute

○ **C.** 15 mcg/kg/minute

○ **D.** 20 mcg/kg/minute

42. A patient is admitted with a head injury after falling off his roof. He is now exhibiting a respiratory pattern that alternates between hyperpnea and apnea. What description should the nurse use to describe this pattern during charting?

○ **A.** Biot's respirations

○ **B.** Cheyne-Stokes respirations

○ **C.** Kussmaul's respirations

○ **D.** Intermittent apnea

43. A 29-year-old woman arrives in the emergency department exhibiting audible wheezes and complaining of dyspnea and anxiety. The doctor's diagnosis is status asthmaticus. The patient's vital signs are blood pressure 165/94 mm Hg, heart rate 120 beats/minute, respiratory rate 44 breaths/minute and labored, and temperature 97.8° F (36.5° C). Other assessment data include pH 7.32, SaO_2 87%, $PaCO_2$ 62 mm Hg, PaO_2 74 mm Hg, HCO_3^- 24 mEq/L, and hemoglobin 14.4g/dl. Auscultation reveals coarse crackles and wheezes. Inspection reveals forceful exhalation, diaphoresis, use of accessory muscles, and pale skin color. The doctor orders epinephrine 0.1 mg S.C. and an aminophylline I.V. loading dose of 5 mg/kg infused over 20 minutes followed by I.V. infusion at a rate of 0.5 mg/kg/hour. When the patient's heart rate increases to 170 beats/minute, what should the nurse do?

○ **A.** Stop the aminophylline infusion and notify the doctor.

○ **B.** Increase the aminophylline infusion and notify the doctor.

○ **C.** Teach the patient to do pursed-lip breathing.

○ **D.** Provide a quiet atmosphere to promote relaxation.

44. A patient suffered an acute head injury after a head-on automobile collision. He is displaying cerebrospinal fluid (CSF) rhinorrhea. What would be a high priority of nursing care for this patient?

○ **A.** Insertion of a nasogastric tube to eliminate swallowed CSF

○ **B.** Repacking the nasal passages every 4 hours and as needed

○ **C.** Administering prophylactic antibiotics

○ **D.** Testing the pH of the CSF every 2 hours

45. A patient suffered a major burn injury and is diagnosed with adult respiratory distress syndrome (ARDS). His nurse is formulating a plan of care to reflect ARDS and knows that the goals with the highest priority should include:

○ **A.** Improving the patient's nutritional status and decreasing his pulmonary compliance

○ **B.** Administering steroids and antibiotics to combat infection

○ **C.** Lowering the patient's blood pressure and increasing his $PaCO_2$ level

○ **D.** Maintaining adequate oxygenation and eliminating the underlying cause of ARDS

46. A 51-year-old man is admitted to the emergency department complaining of dyspnea, weakness, poor appetite, and headache. He has no drug allergies but had an MI 3 years ago and has a history of atrial fibrillation and flutter. Current medications include enteric-coated aspirin, furosemide (Lasix), quinidine, and digoxin. His vital signs are blood pressure 98/58 mm Hg, heart rate 54 beats/minute, respiratory rate 28 breaths/minute, and temperature 99.2° F (37.4° C). Emergency department personnel inserted two I.V. lines, sent admitting samples to the laboratory, and performed a 12-lead ECG that showed ST-segment depression. A report is called to ICU, and the patient will be arriving in approximately 30 minutes, after a chest X-ray is done. After preparing the patient's room, what is the first thing the nurse should do?

○ **A.** Anticipate that the patient will require additional digoxin, and ensure that the admitting orders include an order for digoxin administration

○ **B.** Anticipate that the patient may be agitated, and ensure that the admitting orders include an antianxiety medication

○ **C.** Check the patient's laboratory test results

○ **D.** Order a late dinner tray because the other patients' dinner trays have already been delivered

47. A patient is intubated with a low-pressure-cuff endotracheal tube. Which of the following measures is most important for the nurse to include in the plan of care for this patient?

○ **A.** Maintaining 30 mm Hg pressure in the cuff at all times

○ **B.** Deflating the cuff every shift for 10 minutes to prevent pressure necrosis

○ **C.** Monitoring the cuff pressure every 4 hours

○ **D.** Changing the endotracheal tube every 2 days

48. A patient is intubated and connected to a mechanical ventilator. The nurse would recognize an accumulation of secretions that alter the patient's airway resistance by which of the following responses?

○ **A.** Sudden decrease in the positive end-expiratory pressure (PEEP)

○ **B.** Gradual decrease in the inspired tidal volume

○ **C.** Increase in the amount of pressure required to deliver the selected tidal volume

○ **D.** Increase in the tidal volume without pressure changes

49. A 42-year-old woman who fell from the back of a pickup truck was admitted to the ICU with a diagnosis of basilar skull fracture. The patient has ecchymosis over the mastoid bone and around the eyes. She also has clear fluid draining from her nose and ears. What should the nurse do first?

○ **A.** Test the clear fluid for sugar

○ **B.** Test the patient for cardinal signs of vision

○ **C.** Send the clear fluid for culture

○ **D.** Raise the head of the bed

50. An 89-year-old woman suffers respiratory arrest at a nursing home. She is rushed to the emergency department, where she is breathing on her own. The nurse knows that before this patient is treated, her oxyhemoglobin dissociation curve must:

○ **A.** Be normal

○ **B.** Show a shift to the right

○ **C.** Show a shift to the left

○ **D.** Be flattened out

Answers and rationales

1. Answer: C
Rapid weight gain in a patient who has had an MI commonly is a sign of fluid retention and the development of heart failure. All the other goals are appropriate for this patient.

2. Answer: C
In advanced cirrhosis, the liver has turned into scar tissue and is hard; auscultation does not cause pain. Rebound tenderness is found in acute appendicitis. An enlarged, soft, painful mass is seen in hepatitis. An enlarged, soft mass usually indicates some type of cancer or tumor.

3. Answer: C
Brown-Séquard syndrome should be suspected because of the presence of ipsilateral loss of motor function with contralateral loss of pain and temperature sensations. The nurse can assume that laceration or hemisection of the spinal cord has occurred in this patient. The corticospinal (motor) tracts cross at the level of the medulla. Thus, the decussation is above the site of injury, which leads to

motor loss on the same side. Trauma to the left side of the spinal cord below the level of decussation results in left-sided motor deficits. However, the spinothalamic (sensory) tracts cross at the level of entry into the spinal cord. Trauma to the left side of the spinal cord results in right-sided sensory deficits.

Posterior cord injuries are rare and generally occur with hyperextension. Damage affects the posterior horns of the spinal cord; proprioception and light touch would be impaired bilaterally, but motor function would remain intact bilaterally. Anterior cord damage affects the anterior horns of the spinal cord; motor function, pain, and temperature sensations would be lost at the level of injury.

4. Answer: D

Diabetes insipidus is characterized by symptoms of dehydration, such as hemoconcentration, tachycardia, and hypotension. The glucose level is too low to consider DKA or HHNS as possible medical diagnoses, although the elevated plasma osmolality is consistent with osmotic diuresis. Syndrome of inappropriate antidiuretic hormone is characterized by low serum osmolality, high urine specific gravity, and urine output less than 30 ml/hour.

5. Answer: C

Administration of vasopressin and I.V. hypertonic sodium chloride solution is an appropriate intervention for diabetes insipidus. I.V. normal saline solution is inappropriate because the plasma sodium level already is elevated. Vasopressin administration and I.V. and oral fluid replacement is an appropriate intervention for DKA and HHNS. Furosemide and I.V. hypertonic sodium chloride solution administration are appropriate for SIADH.

6. Answer: B

Nitroglycerin counteracts the adverse vasoconstricting effects of vasopressin and helps maintain coronary perfusion. Dopamine will exacerbate the vasoconstriction. Vitamin K may be given, but it has no effect on vasopressin. Lidocaine is not indicated for GI bleeding.

7. Answer: C

The cardiac index is calculated as follows: cardiac index equals cardiac output divided by body surface area. For this patient, $6 \div 1.57 = 3.82$ L/minute/m^2.

8. Answer: A

The brain stem provides parasympathetic control to the heart and controls respiration. As the centers for autoregulation lose control and parasympathetic stimulation from the compressing medulla occurs, a hyperdynamic state ensues with hypertension and decreased heart and respiratory rates. Cluster respirations are seen in lesions of the upper medulla and may be part of Cushing's triad, but seizures are not. Pinpoint pupils are seen in medullary compression caused by parasympathetic innervation, but Wernicke's (receptive) aphasia is seen in patients with cerebrovascular accidents, not those with head trauma. Homonymous hemianopsia, double vision, and hemiparesis also are seen in patients suffering from cerebrovascular accidents.

9. Answer: B

Atropine can be repeated every 3 to 5 minutes up to a maximum total dose of 3 mg. If the total dose is more than 3 mg, atropine has a vagolytic effect and does not have a positive effect. Atropine may take up to 5 minutes to be effective. If the desired effect is not achieved within 5 to 10 minutes, atropine is not likely to work within 30 minutes. Crisis intervention should be completed within 1 to 2 hours.

10. Answer: A

An increase in breast size is a common development in patients with cirrhosis. Peptic ulcers are not associated with cirrhosis. Patients tend to bleed because of cirrhosis; the disease does not cause clot formation. Osmotic pressure is decreased by cirrhosis.

11. Answer: D

The pancreas stops producing secretions when the patient receives nothing by mouth. A low-fat diet is necessary because fat is digested poorly by patients with pancreatitis. Codeine is inappropriate because it causes spasms of the biliary tract. Anticholinergic and antienzyme agents have not proved effective in pancreatic disease. Antibiotics are unnecessary.

12. Answer: C

In ventricular fibrillation, the ventricles quiver and produce no distinct QRS complexes. In atrial fibrillation, there are no distinct P waves, but the QRS complexes are normal. In junctional tachycardia, P waves may be hidden, but the QRS complexes are normal. Agonal rhythm is marked by wide, slow, semiregular QRS complexes.

13. Answer: C

Metabolic acidosis and the presence of serum and urine ketones are indicators of ketogenesis, a hallmark of DKA. Serum osmolality greater than 350 mOsm/L H_2O is seen in HHNS but is normal or slightly elevated in patients with DKA. The serum potassium level typically is normal or elevated in DKA. A decreased potassium level on admission indicates severe potassium depletion and constitutes a medical and nursing emergency.

14. Answer: A

Most rejected organs begin to swell or enlarge, causing pain and poor functioning. Temperature would be elevated during a rejection episode. Dizziness and weakness are not associated with rejection. Rejection causes weak pulses and pale skin.

15. Answer: C

A normal platelet count is 150,000 to 400,000/mm³. Platelet counts below 30,000/mm³ place the patient at increased risk for bleeding, and most doctors would not operate on such patients. Laboratory tests could be redone only with the doctor's approval. Checking the patient's vital signs is appropriate but not of the highest priority.

16. Answer: B
Systemic vascular resistance is calculated as follows:

$$SVR = \frac{\text{mean arterial pressure} - \text{right arterial pressure}}{\text{cardiac output}} \times 80$$

SVR is the same as afterload. Normal SVR is 800 to 1,500 dynes/second/cm^2.

17. Answer: B
These findings indicate that the endotracheal tube has been inserted too far and has entered the right bronchus. Increasing the tidal volume may cause pneumothorax. The patient is not likely to have a mucus plug immediately after intubation.

18. Answer: C
Alanine aminotransferase and aspartate aminotransferase are most likely to be elevated in patients with liver disease, although other diseases also may cause increases in these laboratory values. The PT and PTT may be elevated indirectly. Alkaline phosphatase and amylase levels are elevated in pancreatic disease.

19. Answer: D
Nursing diagnoses related to the airway and breathing have the highest priority. Altered cerebral perfusion diagnoses have the next highest priority, followed by the nursing diagnoses relating to infection and knowledge deficit.

20. Answer: B
Respiratory depression and hypotension are toxic effects of clorazepate, which is a benzodiazepine. Tachycardia and cerebral hemorrhage are toxic effects of cocaine. The toxic effects of tricyclic antidepressants include complete heart block and paralytic ileus. Liver failure and GI bleeding result from aspirin toxicity.

21. Answer: C
The plastic in I.V. bags and normal I.V. tubing will absorb the nitroglycerin, thereby reducing its effectiveness. The infusion rate need not be decreased; the normal dosage range is 5 to 100 mcg/minute. Nitroglycerin can be diluted in D$_5$W or normal saline solution. An infusion pump should always be used; no crystallization problem exists with nitroglycerin administration.

22. Answer: D
Quinidine works by slowing electrical conduction through the ventricles. Quinidine toxicity often widens the QRS complex. Frequent diarrhea is an adverse effect that may occur long before toxicity occurs. Quinidine tends to increase the heart rate. Tinnitus and rash usually are not seen in quinidine toxicity.

23. Answer: A
Activated charcoal works in the intestine to absorb medications and toxic substances. It would be vomited if administered after ipecac syrup. Mixing activated charcoal with ipecac syrup and water reduces its effectiveness.

24. Answer: D
Changes in neck size indicate edema and potential airway problems. The other options have a lower priority.

25. Answer: B
Mannitol is an osmotic diuretic used to reduce cerebral edema. Diuresis will occur before a change in the level of consciousness is noted. Mannitol will increase, not decrease, the heart rate. Diarrhea is an adverse effect of the medication but does not indicate that the patient is responding to the drug.

26. Answer: A
Water intoxication, which is characterized by the signs and symptoms listed in option A, is the most serious adverse effect of exogenous antidiuretic hormone (vasopressin) therapy. Pallor, diaphoresis, tremor, and seizures are signs of severe hypoglycemia. Hemoconcentration, increased urine output, and complaints of thirst are signs and symptoms of dehydration, which would be observed if the patient did not respond to vasopressin therapy. Hyperglycemia, hyperkalemia, and increased urine output are presenting symptoms of DKA and HHNS.

27. Answer: C
A shift to the left usually indicates an acute infection. Anemia is indicated by a low blood count. Thrombocytopenia is indicated by a low platelet count. Leukemia is indicated by a shift to the right.

28. Answer: C
Coughing increases lung expansion and tends to eliminate burn residue without damaging the trachea. Increasing oral fluid intake could induce vomiting. High-flow oxygen therapy does not prevent pulmonary congestion. Suctioning may further damage the tracheal lining.

29. Answer: C
Disseminated intravascular coagulation is a generalized bleeding disorder in which microembolisms deplete clotting factors. Renal failure, hepatic failure, and increased ICP are possible complications of burns but are not related to bleeding problems.

30. Answer: C
Allowing the patient to see how the alarms work will increase the patient's understanding of the importance of the alarms and will help reduce his anxiety. The other options will not reduce the patient's anxiety level.

31. Answer: D
Boiling water usually produces second-degree burns. According to the Rule of Nines, the anterior chest makes up 18% of the body surface area and the thigh makes up 4%, for a total of 22% of the body.

32. Answer: B
Glycosylated hemoglobin measures glucose levels over 120 days (the life span of an erythrocyte). The results of this test provide the most accurate indication of long-term glucose control. A fasting serum glucose level of 125 mg/dl, although considered acceptable for a patient with insulin-dependent diabetes, reflects a one-time measurement—not a span of days—of glucose control. The other measurements, although helpful in determining clinical status, do not provide information about glucose control.

33. Answer: B
Patients who have undergone organ transplantation receive immunosuppressant medications and need to avoid crowds and people with infections. Immunosuppressant medications are needed indefinitely to prevent organ rejection. Although kissing his wife presents a small risk for infection, it should not be a problem. After an extended recovery period, the patient should be able to resume most normal activities, including hunting.

34. Answer: A
The patient has metabolic acidosis, which can be reversed by administering sodium bicarbonate. Intubation and hyperventilation are useful for respiratory acidosis. Having the patient breathe into a paper bag is an appropriate action for respiratory alkalosis. Oxygen therapy is used to treat hypoxia.

35. Answer: D
Options A, B, and C describe pathologic pupil signs indicative of brain herniation. Hippus is the term given to a pupil that constricts to light but, because of oculomotor nerve involvement, cannot sustain constriction and dilates. Absent doll's eyes is a pathologic condition in which the sensory acoustic nerve fails to accept stimuli, and both the oculomotor and acoustic nerves fail to respond. This results in a fixed midline position of the pupils when the head is turned to the side. Anisocoria refers to unequal pupil size. It may be pathologic or a normal finding. When pathologic, it signifies dysfunction of the oculomotor nerve and occurs in early brain herniation.

36. Answer: C
Elevated BUN and serum creatinine levels are indicative of nephrotoxicity, which can lead to renal failure. The other adverse reactions are of a less serious nature.

37. Answer: B
Cholinergic crisis is caused by an excess of acetylcholine, which most often results from overmedication. Atropine may be needed to increase sympathetic responses. Myasthenic crisis is characterized by tachycardia, hypertension, and an absence of GI symptoms. Treatment includes the administration of anticholinesterase agents, such as neostigmine bromide.

38. Answer: B
Flumazenil is a benzodiazepine antagonist that reverses the effects of diazepam. It should be administered if respiratory distress secondary to an overdose of diazepam is noted. Although phenobarbital can effectively control seizure activity, the nurse must be aware of the amount of medication that has already been given because this medication may further suppress respiration. Naloxone is used to reverse the effects of opioid analgesics. Phenytoin will not reverse the effects of a benzodiazepine.

39. Answer: B
Long-term lung disease has a significant psychological component, and psychological support is an essential part of the treatment and recovery process. Prophylactic antibiotics may or may not be used, depending on the underlying disease. Exercise levels should be increased in the later rehabilitative stages of treatment. Patients with lung disease respond better to small, high-calorie meals.

40. Answer: B
Neurologic checks and assessment of the level of consciousness are needed to detect a rebleeding episode. Because the bleeding has been sealed by a clot, normal fibrinolysis increases the chances for rebleeding during this period. The incidence of vasospasm is thought to be related to the breakdown of blood products in the subarachnoid space. Erythrocytes and platelets produce spasmogenic substances as they degrade.

The usual length of stay for patients with cerebral aneurysm and subarachnoid hemorrhage is much longer than 7 days. Brudzinski's sign is the involuntary flexion of the hips and knees in response to passive flexion of the neck and is a sign of meningeal irritation. Osmotic diuretics are used during the early stages of treatment and gradually tapered off.

41. Answer: B
Once the dosage of dopamine rises above 10 mcg/kg/minute, the drug has strictly alpha-stimulating effects. Prolonged use at this or higher levels can lead to temporary or permanent renal damage because of vasoconstriction of the renal vasculature. A dosage of 5 mcg/kg/minute produces a mixture of beta- and alpha-receptor stimulation and does not decrease kidney perfusion. At 20 mcg/kg/minute, renal perfusion is severely decreased, and the patient may be at risk for renal failure. Although 15 mcg/kg/minute can be administered, it should be given only under a doctor's order.

42. Answer: B
Cheyne-Stokes respirations describe this type of breathing pattern, which is often seen in patients with head injuries. Biot's respirations consists of a rapid, deep, completely irregular breathing pattern. Kussmaul's respirations are regular, deep, sighing respirations that are present in metabolic acidosis. Intermittent apnea does not fit the description.

43. Answer: A

Aminophylline commonly increases the heart rate. A rate of 170 beats/minute, however, can be harmful to the patient and must be evaluated by the doctor before the infusion is continued. Increasing the aminophylline infusion rate would exacerbate the problem. During a crisis situation, the patient would not be receptive to teaching. Although a quiet environment may be beneficial, it will not alleviate the crisis or decrease the patient's heart rate.

44. Answer: C

Patients with CSF leakage are at high risk for infection. A nasogastric tube should not be used because it may enter the brain through the tear. Packing is not needed; CSF should drain freely. Frequent testing of pH is not required.

45. Answer: D

Decreased compliance of the lungs in ARDS reduces the body's ability to oxygenate tissues. Patients are intubated and mechanically ventilated, with positive end-expiratory pressure used to maintain oxygenation. The other nursing goals have lower priority.

46. Answer: C

The nurse should check the patient's admitting laboratory test results first. Digoxin commonly is used to treat atrial arrhythmias, and approximately 20% of patients who take digoxin experience toxic effects. The signs and symptoms of digoxin toxicity include dyspnea, bradycardia, nausea, vomiting, vision disturbances, and weakness. Additional digoxin should not be administered unless a subtherapeutic level is verified by laboratory test results. The other options—relieving anxiety and ordering a meal—have lower priority.

47. Answer: C

Low-pressure cuffs are designed to prevent necrosis as long as the pressure is at or below 20 mm Hg. A pressure of 30 mm Hg is too high. Deflating the cuff is not required and can cause aspiration and respiratory problems. Changing the endotracheal tube is not necessary unless there is a problem with the tube.

48. Answer: C

Secretions block the airway, necessitating a higher pressure to obtain the same tidal volume. A sudden decrease in the PEEP required is not an indication of a blocked airway. A gradual decrease in the inspired tidal volume does not occur with a volume-cycled ventilator. Increasing the tidal volume almost always requires pressure increases.

49. Answer: A

The nurse should first test the clear fluid for sugar. If sugar is present, the fluid is CSF. Testing the cardinal signs of vision and elevating the head of the bed have lower priority. Although the fluid may be sent for culture, a sterile sample would need to be obtained, and this is not an initial intervention.

50. Answer: B
A shift to the right indicates that more oxygen is being delivered and released to the tissues, which is caused by acidosis and an elevated $PaCO_2$ level. A normal oxyhemoglobin curve would not require treatment. A shift to the left occurs with alkalosis. A flattening of the curve never occurs.

Analyzing the posttest

Total the number of *incorrect* responses to the posttest. A score of 1 to 9 indicates that you have an excellent knowledge base and that you are well prepared for the certification examination; a score of 10 to 14 indicates adequate preparation, although more study or improvement in test-taking skills is recommended; a score of 15 or more indicates the need for intensive study before taking the certification examination.

For a more detailed analysis of your performance, complete the self-diagnostic profile worksheet below.

Self-diagnostic profile for posttest #2

In the top row of boxes, record the number of each question you answered incorrectly. Then, beneath each question number, check the box that corresponds to the reason you answered the question incorrectly. Finally, tabulate the number of check marks on each line in the right-hand column marked "Totals." You now have an individualized profile of weak areas that require further study or improvement in test-taking ability before you take the Critical Care Nursing Certification Examination.

QUESTION NUMBER																			TOTALS
Test-taking skills																			
1. Misread question																			
2. Missed important point																			
3. Forgot fact or concept																			
4. Applied wrong fact or concept																			
5. Drew wrong conclusion																			
6. Incorrectly evaluated distractors																			
7. Mistakenly filled in wrong circle																			
8. Read into question																			
9. Guessed wrong																			
10. Misunderstood question																			

Selected references

American Association of Critical Care Nurses. *AACN Procedure Manual for Critical Care,* 3rd ed. Philadelphia: W.B. Saunders Co., 1993.

Conover, M.B. *Understanding Electrocardiography,* 7th ed. St. Louis: Mosby–Year Book, Inc., 1996.

Darovic, G.A., ed. *Hemodynamic Monitoring: Invasive and Noninvasive Clinical Application,* 2nd ed. Philadelphia: W.B. Saunders Co., 1995.

Des Jardins, T.R. *Cardiopulmonary Anatomy and Physiology: Essentials for Respiratory Care,* 3rd ed. Albany, N.Y.: Delmar Publishers, 1998.

Dolan, J.T. *Critical Care Nursing: Clinical Management Through the Nursing Process,* 2nd ed. Philadelphia: F.A. Davis Co., 1996.

Harthorn, J.C., et al. *Introduction to Critical Care Nursing,* 2nd ed. Philadelphia: W.B. Saunders Co., 1997.

Hudak, C.M., and Gallo, B.M. *Critical Care Nursing: A Holistic Approach,* 7th ed. Philadelphia: Lippincott-Raven Publishers, 1998.

Kinney, M., et al. *Comprehensive Cardiac Care,* 8th ed. St. Louis: Mosby–Year Book, Inc., 1995.

Metheny, N.M. *Fluid and Electrolyte Balance: Nursing Considerations,* 3rd ed. Philadelphia: Lippincott-Raven Publishers, 1996.

Roberts, S.L. *Critical Care Nursing.* East Norwalk, Conn.: Appleton & Lange, 1996.

Stillwell, S. *Mosby's Critical Care Nursing Reference,* 2nd ed. St. Louis: Mosby–Year Book, Inc., 1996.

Swearingen, P.L., and Keen, J.H. *Manual of Critical Care: Applying Nursing Diagnosis to Adult Critical Illness,* 3rd ed. St. Louis: Mosby–Year Book, Inc., 1995.

Thelan, L.A., et al. *Critical Care Nursing: Diagnosis and Management,* 2nd ed. St. Louis: Mosby–Year Book, Inc., 1994.

Index

i refers to an illustration; t refers to a table.

i refers to an illustration; t refers to a table.

i refers to an illustration; t refers to a table.

i refers to an illustration; t refers to a table.

Stroke volume, 21, 22t
Subarachnoid hemorrhage, grades of, 163
Succinylcholine chloride, 248t
Sucralfate, 256t
Sufentanil citrate, 252t
Syndrome of inappropriate secretion of antidiuretic hormone, 114-116, 267, 268, 278
Systemic vascular resistance, 22t, 288, 300
Systole, 20

T
Tacrolimus, 257t
Temperature dysfunctions, 149
Tensilon test, 172, 273, 281
Tension pneumothorax, 88
Third-degree atrioventricular block, 48-49, 49i
Thirst mechanism, 212
Thorax, 73
Thrombophlebitis, assessing for, 24-25
Thymus gland, 117, 118
Thyroid gland, 98, 99t, 100
Thyroid-stimulating hormone, 99
Thyroxine, 100
Toxic ingestions, 240-242
Toxic shock syndrome, 288, 300
Trachea, 72
Tracheobronchial suctioning, 273, 281
Tricyclic antidepressant overdose, 300
Triiodothyronine, 100
Turner's sign, 186

U
Urea, 212
Uremia, signs of, 216
Urine, formation of, 210-212
Urine tests, 217

V
Valsalva maneuver, intracranial pressure and, 273, 281
Vasopressin, 269, 279, 290, 301
Vecuronium bromide, 248t
Ventilation-perfusion mismatching, 79
Ventricular fibrillation, 32-33, 32i, 286, 299
Ventricular tachycardia, 31-32, 31i

Verapamil hydrochloride, 251t, 272, 276, 280
Virchow's triad, 75
Vitamin K_1, 249t
Vitamin K_3, 249t
Voiding cystourethrography, 216
Vomiting, 89

WXYZ
Warfarin sodium, 77, 249t
Water deprivation test, 101
Water intoxication, 290, 301
Water loading test, 101

i refers to an illustration; t refers to a table.